# Climacteric Medicine

*– where do we go?*

# Climacteric Medicine

## – *where do we go?*

Edited by

**Hermann P. G. Schneider**
President of The International Menopause Society,
and Department of Obstetrics and Gynecology,
University of Münster, Germany

and

**Frederick Naftolin**
Department of Obstetrics and Gynecology,
Yale University School of Medicine, New Haven, USA

Published under the auspices of the
International Menopause Society

Taylor & Francis
Taylor & Francis Group
LONDON AND NEW YORK
A PARTHENON BOOK

First published in the United Kingdom in 2005
by Taylor & Francis,
an imprint of the Taylor & Francis Group,
2 Park Square, Milton Park
Abingdon, Oxon OX14 4RN, UK

Tel.: +44 (0) 1235 828600
Fax.: +44 (0) 1235 829000
Website: www.tandf.co.uk



British Library Cataloguing in Publication Data

Data available on application

Library of Congress Cataloging-in-Publication Data

Data available on application

ISBN 1-84214-261-5

Distributed in North and South America by

Taylor & Francis
2000 NW Corporate Blvd
Boca Raton, FL 33431, USA

*Within Continental USA*
Tel.: 800 272 7737; Fax.: 800 374 3401
*Outside Continental USA*
Tel.: 561 994 0555; Fax.: 561 361 6018
E-mail: orders@crcpress.com

Distributed in the rest of the world by
Thomson Publishing Services
Cheriton House
North Way
Andover, Hampshire SP10 5BE, UK
Tel.: +44 (0) 1264 332424
E-mail: salesorder.tandf@thomsonpublishingservices.co.uk

Composition by AMA DataSet Limited, Preston, Lancashire, UK
Printed and bound by CPI Bath, UK

# Contents

**Section IV Rationale for and availability of therapeutic hormones**



**Section V Current randomized controlled trials and epidemiology**



**Section VI Urgent needs for future research**

**Section VII Position statements**

# List of principal contributors

**E. M. Alder**
Faculty of Health and Life Sciences
Napier University
74 Canaan Lane
Edinburgh EH9 4TB
UK

**D. F. Archer**
Eastern Virginia Medical School
Jones Institute for Reproductive Medicine
601 Colley Avenue
Norfolk
Virginia 23507
USA

**M. H. Birkhäuser**
Division of Gynaecology, Endocrinology and Reproductive Medicine
University of Berne
Inselspital
Effingerstrasse 102
3010 Berne
Switzerland

**H. G. Burger**
Prince Henry's Institute of Medical Research
Level 3, Block E
Monash Medical Centre
PO Box 5152
Clayton
Victoria 3168
Australia

**L. Dennerstein**
Office for Gender and Health
The University of Melbourne
Charles Connibere Building
Royal Melbourne Hospital
Parkville
Victoria 3050
Australia

**A. R. Genazzani**
Department of Obstetrics and Gynecology
Ospedale Sta Chiara
Via Roma 35
56100 Pisa
Italy

**F. A. Helmond**
Organon International
56 Livingston Avenue
Roseland
New Jersey 07068
USA

**D. M. Herrington**
Department of Internal Medicine/Cardiology
Wake Forest University School of Medicine
Winston-Salem
North Carolina 27157
USA

**H. Kuhl**
Universitätsfrauenklinik
J. W. Goethe University
Theodor-Stern-Kai 7
60590 Frankfurt
Germany

**E. Lang**
Novo Nordisk Region Europe A/S
Andreasstrasse 15
8050 Zurich
Switzerland

**K. K. Limpaphayom**
Menopause Clinic
Faculty of Medicine
Chulalongkorn University
Rama IV Road
Bangkok 1-330
Thailand

**R. A. Lobo**
Department of Obstetrics and Gynecology
Columbia University College of Physicians & Surgeons
622 West 168th Street
New York
New York 10032
USA

**F. Naftolin**
Department of Obstetrics, Gynecology and Reproductive Sciences
Yale University School of Medicine
333 Cedar Street, 331 FMB
New Haven
Connecticut 06520
USA

**M. Neves-e-Castro**
Av. Antonio Augusta de Aguiar
24-2 dto
1050-016 Lisbon
Portugal

**M. Notelovitz**
4279 NW 61 Lane
Boca Raton
Florida 33496
USA

**M. Oettel**
Beethovenstrasse 30
07743 Jena
Germany

**S. Palacios**
Institute Palacios of Women's Health
Antonio Acuna 9
28009 Madrid
Spain

**J. H. Pickar**
Clinical Research and Development
Wyeth-Ayerst Research
145 King of Prussia Road
PO Box 42528
Radnor
Pennsylvania 19087
USA

**J. V. Pinkerton**
Midlife Health Center
University of Virginia at Northridge
2955 Ivy Rd, Suite 104
Charlottesville
Virginia 22903
USA

**V. W. Pinn**
Office of Research on Women's Health
Bldg. 1, Room 201
National Institutes of Health
Department of Health and Human Services
Bethesda
Maryland 20892
USA

**V. V. Ragavan**
Care of Women's Health
Novartis Pharmaceuticals
One Health Plaza
East Hanover
New Jersey 7936
USA

**G. Samsioe**
Department of Obstetrics and Gynecology
Lund University Hospital
22185 Lund
Sweden

**H. P. G. Schneider**
Department of Obstetrics and Gynecology
University of Münster
Von-Esmarch-Strasse 56
ZMBE
48149 Münster
Germany

**R. Schürmann**
Schering AG
SBU Gynecology & Andrology
Sellerstrasse 31
13342 Berlin
Germany

**S. Shapiro**
Mailman School of Public Health, Room 1613
Columbia University
722 West 168th Street
New York
New York 10032
USA

**S. Sherman**
Geriatrics and Clinical Gerontology Program
National Institute on Aging, NIH
Gateway Building, Suite 3C-307
7201 Wisconsin Avenue
Bethesda
Maryland 20892-9205
USA

**L. Speroff**
Department of Obstetrics and Gynecology
Oregon Health & Science University
3181 SW Sam Jackson Park Road
Portland
Oregon 97201-3098
USA

**A. Strothmann**
Department of Clinical Pharmacology
Charité/Humboldt-University of Berlin
Invalidenstr. 115
10115 Berlin
Germany

# Foreword

If it is true that 'every cloud has a silver lining', these Proceedings of the 4th Workshop of the International Menopause Society, held in Vienna in December 2003, are glowing because of the effects of evidence-based medicine on the fields of Climacteric Medicine and Geriatrics. Recently, a small number of studies and trials have been widely interpreted to indicate that the practice of hormone therapy should be much more circumscribed than was indicated by the great bulk of previous clinical and preclinical data. This has resulted in great turmoil in the lives of women and confusion among professionals upon whom they depend for advice and care. But, the picture for hormone therapy is still being clarified. This Workshop was convened as a milestone event, to review the important issues regarding the menopause, the methods that are being applied to study them, the interpretation of the new data and the necessary research that will allow these fields to move ahead.

As will be seen, the apparent discrepancies between the data and their application that have been given wide play by the lay press and other publications are now being viewed with more circumspection. Overly broad interpretations of inherently narrow randomized controlled trials and the discrepancies between the populations studied and the clinical populations that are in need of study are coming to the fore; even the best data from the randomized controlled trials are only valid regarding the populations studied. Similarly, it is being appreciated that sheer numbers do not make up for limited quality of experimental design or imprecision in observational studies.

The need for research on the climacteric remains paramount. This is more important than might be appreciated at first glance. The domino effect of allowing insufficient information to limit hormone therapy to a thin slice of the perimenopause will foreclose ever learning about the role of hormone therapy in diseases that require 10–30 years to become manifest clinically. These include, in addition to bone mass depletion and fracture, heart and other blood vessel disease and brain dystrophies attending aging and hormone lack.

These Proceedings underline that the stakes are at historical highs; women regularly live half or more of their lives after the menopause. They also make clear that, in this age of preventive medicine, it is premature to dismiss the preventative advantages of hormone therapy without properly designed research.

To this end, we dedicate this book to the billions of women who have played, and will continue to play, a role in this uncharted voyage into longer life. They need and deserve the best efforts of all concerned in order to fill this new post-evolutionary niche in the most suitable way that biomedical science can provide.

Hermann P. G. Schneider, MD, PhD
Münster, Germany

Frederick Naftolin, MD, DPhil
New Haven, USA

# Introduction

*H. P. G. Schneider*

The climacteric is the phase in the aging of women marking the transition from the reproductive phase to the non-reproductive state. The perimenopause as part of the climacteric extends, for a variable period of years, to before and after the menopause. This definition most adequately describes the period with which the International Menopause Society is concerned. On the other hand, the term 'menopause' describes the permanent cessation of menstruation resulting from the loss of ovarian follicular activity. Natural menopause is recognized to have occurred after 12 consecutive months of amenorrhea, for which there is no other obvious pathological or physiological cause. An adequate independent biological marker for the event does not exist. By that token, there is an ongoing debate as to whether 'menopause' is too narrow a label for the activities of the International Menopause Society. The cessation of menses in many women is perceived as having no influence on subsequent physical and mental health. Women tend to express either positive or neutral feelings about menopause, with the exception of those who experience surgical menopause. Thus, the majority of women who feel healthy and happy do not seek contact with physicians. Medical intervention at this point in life should rather be regarded as an opportunity to provide and reinforce a program of preventive health care. These issues would include family planning, cessation of smoking, control of body weight and alcohol consumption, prevention of heart disease and osteoporosis, maintenance of mental well-being (including sexuality), cancer screening and treatment of neurological problems. Leon Speroff has phrased menopause as 'a wonderful signal occurring at the right time of life when preventive health care is especially critical'. This positive attitude would require an understanding of the epidemiology of menopause, an understanding that is based on the recognition of this event as a normal stage in development. Development - a broader concept than simply aging - incorporates biology, psychology, society, and culture.

Fries has described three eras in health and disease. The first era, which extended into the early 1990s, was characterized by acute infectious diseases. The second era, highlighted by cardiovascular disease and cancer, has now moved into a third era marked by problems of frailty such as fading eyesight and hearing, impaired memory and cognitive function, decreased strength and reserve. Much of our medical effort is still directed towards the first era - 'find the disease and cure it'.

During the process of aging, visible and invisible organic alterations occur. Part of this is a change in complete organic systems such as the endocrine system. These processes occur at the cellular level, with accumulation of DNA mutations and alterations in protein metabolism. Hundreds of theories have been brought forward to explain the aging process. Some refer to 'intrinsic' organic alterations and others to more 'extrinsic' processes. Among genetic 'intrinsic' factors, the telomerase hypothesis has gained acceptance, while external environmental impact relates to oxidative processes. Possibly, we should give preference to both environmental and genetic backgrounds as a rationale for what causes aging.

Damage to mitochondrial DNA, as well as accumulation of oxidated and modified proteins, the basis for the formation of lipofuscein, the aging pigment, is based on the action of free radicals and oxidants. Such accumulation of oxidated proteins may be caused by a growing oxidative impact or an insufficient protein metabolism.

Accumulation of oxidative proteins, formation of autofluorescent materials (lipofuscein) and a fall in intercellular protein metabolism could also be documented in *in vitro* models with human fibroblasts. The lipofuscein-dependent fall in proteolytic activity may be interpreted as a vicious circle of a self-stimulating process. The question is whether these concepts offer the potential of interfering with aging. Hormones have also been associated with anti-oxidant activity.

Independent of an age-related incidence and prevalence of chronic disease, multi-morbidity is an important characteristic of the aging population. In a German population study, 96% of participants aged 70 years and over had at least one and 30% had five or more internal, neurological, orthopedic or psychiatric diseases. There is, however, a discrepancy between objective diagnosis and subjective impairment. While, for example, cardiovascular disease and its risk factors were objectively predominant, subjective complaints were mostly related to orthopedic impairment such as arthrosis and osteoporosis.

Chronic disease and older age are associated with functional deficits, which considerably reduce the quality of life. Their detailed assessment and physicotherapeutic care are critical for the improvement of individual well-being. Not all chronic diseases have an age-related incremental prevalence. Hyperlipidemia and arterial disease will decrease with older age, a partial selective advantage of non-affected individuals.

The tremendous arsenal of positive as well as potentially threatening pharmaceutical intervention in the aging population is reflected by the size of the market. In my country, in Germany, there is an annual turnover of pharmaceutical preparations of about 20 billion Euros. Each 60-year-old and over, on average, is on chronic medication with at least three different specifications. While the over-60-year-olds represent 22% of the population, they consume over 54% of all pharmaceutical products; thus, they are over-represented by a factor of 2.4. This growing medicalization, however, does not produce the alleged peak of health-care expenses during the ultimate months of everybody's life, which has triggered the political issue of denying health care to those on the death ward. Rather, if people manage to postpone clinical illness or successfully prevent it, they will survive longer and compensate for age-driven expenditures. The complexity of medicalization in older people results in an absolute death toll of around 20 000 in Germany, picking up 7% of total mortality as causally related to medicinal products. Of all hospital referrals, 20–25% is related to such side-effects, half of which could have been avoided. The German Medical Curriculum provides for 6–10% of its training in pharmacotherapy. This deficitarian program also relates to neighboring European countries.

Such alarming figures more often result in therapeutic nihilism, which is totally unjustified. Pharmaco-scandals, such as that with cerivastatin causing rhabdomyolysis, led to major confusion and uncertainty among physicians. As a consequence, already established statin use was abandoned. The deadly side-effect of cerivastatin is seen in one case in 100 000 treatment-years with a frequency of 1 in 1 000 000. The 4S Study demonstrated, however, that statins in secondary cardiovascular prevention would save 700 lives in 100 000 treatment-years, an extraordinary positive benefit–risk relationship, unsurpassed by any other medical intervention, not even appendectomy. In absolute figures, statins could potentially save up to 100 000 deaths per annum; this does, however, not happen because practical management (indication and contraindication, selection, dosages, route and mode of application, etc.) does not strictly follow official recommendations. In another local German study on cholesterol-reducing medication in patients with pre-existing coronary heart disease, low density lipoprotein cholesterol targeting below 100 mg/dl was only achieved in 4% of participating patients. Guidelines for diabetics have, in similar ways, been ignored with respect to both therapeutic scrutiny and adherence. The general conclusion is that only continuing medical and lay public education will positively affect the situation.

Certainly, we are also dealing with a challenging environment for hormone therapy. Recent publications have impacted negatively and risks outweigh benefits almost by an order of magnitude. Regulatory bodies have become cautious and restrictive. Doctors are distrustful and worried about the medico-legal implications, and patients are worried and reluctant to take hormones. European women perceive hormone therapy positively with respect to well-being and menopausal symptoms and more negatively as related to memory performance, weight issues and bladder weakness or complaints. Their reasons to start hormone therapy at present would be relief from hot flushes and improvement of general well-being, followed by prevention of osteoporosis; their main reasons for discontinuing hormone therapy, on the other hand, are the disappearance of menopausal symptoms, information about increases in diseases such as breast cancer, or individual observation of weight gain. Particularly in Germany, there is still a tendency to continue hormone therapy for longer than 5 years. However, only one-third of the decision-making is left to the doctor.

The publication of findings from the Women's Health Initiative's randomized controlled trial, followed soon after by those reported from the Million Women Study, has raised major issues as to how the evidence from these and other studies should be interpreted. Therefore, a key issue of this International Menopause Society Workshop is consideration of the background data relevant to the evaluation of the effects of hormone replacement therapy. Is it correct to give randomized controlled trials the pride of place because they are assumed to eliminate or reduce the likelihood of confounding and 'double-blinding' in order to eliminate or reduce the likelihood of bias? It appears that the time has come for a paradigm shift, as Samuel Shapiro has depicted it. Long-term studies, because of a loss of blinding effects and drop-out related problems with randomization, tend to take on the characteristics of an observational study. They need to be interpreted as such. Optimally valid causal research in population studies should incorporate the complementary roles of clinical medicine, biology, and statistics.

One major argument against the Women's Health Initiative Study is the fact that only older, potentially prediseased women have been investigated and only very rarely the age groups of the 50–54- or 50–59-year-old women, which are usually the groups entering hormone therapy. Therefore, the risks of pre-diseased women have been wrongly transferred to the younger healthy group of women in the menopausal transition.

The Workshop was organized such that it started with the natural history and progress of the menopause, and aspects of the current practice of the climacteric, and then moved to the issues of quality of life, currently utilized hormone preparations, the problems of the recent larger trials and epidemiology, and finally the Position Statements generated by various Regional Societies, and our vision of the needs for future research in climacteric medicine.

In clinical terms, about 50% of persons who experience a first myocardial infarction or sudden cardiac death do not have a high level of risk, as estimated by standard risk factors (smoking, hypertension, obesity, lack of physical activity, high and low density lipoprotein cholesterol) routinely used in specially developed algorithms. The development of 'non-conventional' risk factors such as lipoprotein(a), C-reactive protein, ferritin or chlamydial infection was the next step. Today, however, we are looking into genetic polymorphisms and their metabolic traits, which open up a new realm of identifying the individual at risk.

A clinical pharmacologist of the German Safety of Medicines Board has associated the recent epidemiological objections to hormone therapy with the thalidomide catastrophe. This really is an indicator of how much the subject of medical and, in particular, hormonal prevention of age-related frailty and disability has been politicized. The efforts of Medical Authorities and Regional as well as Local Medical Societies are taken in order to provide the practicing physician with guidance to adequate clinical management. And yet, many of us are still left with confusion and uncertainties. With this Workshop, the International Menopause Society is attempting to raise a global voice of contemporary clinical judgement and psychological sanity.

The contributions of the Workshop, by tradition, have been collected for publication in these Workshop Proceedings. At the end of the book, the Position Statement formulated by the Executive Committee of the International Menopause Society during the Workshop has been reproduced, following its publication in *Climacteric.*

# Menopause: lack of Darwinian adaptation drives its physiology

1

*F. Naftolin and S. Richman*

## INTRODUCTION

The battle for survival through evolutionary fitness is won by the natural selection of those characteristics that enhance the number of living offspring produced. Since reproduction is the forge of Darwinian evolution, adaptive reproductive responses rapidly impact fitness. Such adaptations became the bases of contemporary reproductive strategies and are deeply woven into the genetic fabric. These matters often focus on the response to sex steroids under various conditions related to reproduction.

The climacteric, when reproduction starts to falter, and the postmenopausal years are by definition beyond Darwinian adaptation[1]. Thus, the expected physiological repertoire of postmenopausal women to decreased ovarian estrogen is forecast by the response to similar changes in the steroid milieu during reproductive life.

**Table 1** Periods when estrogen (and other sex steroids) fall in reproductive females

- Postnatal female infant
- Following the preovulatory surge of estrogen
- Following the demise of the corpus luteum
- During pregnancy (a functional anti-estrogenic effect of placental steroids, especially progesterone)
- Following functional or surgical castration
- During the puerperium

## ESTROGEN WITHDRAWAL DURING THE REPRODUCTIVE PERIOD

Clinical entities during the reproductive era that resemble the picture seen during the climacteric are listed in Table 1. By process of elimination due to immaturity or lack of stability of the hormonal state, *the puerperium is the most likely candidate reproductive prototype for the menopausal transition and beyond*. While none of these analogies are perfect, for example, the puerperium follows a high-estrogen and progesterone state and has considerable metabolic and endocrine overtones. Although castration does not occur in nature, this does not preclude the use of castrated subjects to study the effects of gonadal deficiency states[2] or learning about the menopause from the puerperium.

What follows is designed to describe relevant aspects of the puerperium and to compare them to the physiological adjustments made during the menopause. The results observed in the postpartum mother can be contrasted with those of the climacteric, especially the postmenopausal period. This allows recognition that the employment of previously adaptive responses after reproduction may no longer be appropriate and may result in responses that would be termed maladaptive if they had been arrived at via Darwinian mechanisms. This furnishes insights necessary for anticipation, prevention and possible treatment of disease states that may develop during the climacteric.

## ADAPTIVE RESPONSES TO LOW ESTROGEN DURING PREGNANCY AND THE PUERPERIUM

The success of the Order Mammalia rests on the continuing responsibility of the mother for the child's welfare; the mother is responsible for more than just gestational fitness. This relationship extends through perinatal protection and nurturing until the F2 is capable of producing the F3 generation. Necessary survival skills for the mother during the puerperium include staying alive, protecting the neonate from accidents, predators and the environment, and providing nutrition[3]. Despite the elevated levels of estrogen, pregnancy is a progesterone-dominated state. Maternal gestational support of the developing fetus and preparation for the puerperium are driven by this antiestrogenic environment. Thus, physiologic adaptations during pregnancy include centripetal fat deposition, weight gain (positive metabolic state), relative insulin resistance to facilitate fetal growth, lax smooth muscles, bone resorption[4] and cognitive alteration[5]. At term, as the balance shifts to an estrogen-dominated state, many of the above-described maternal adaptations recede as the onset of labor approaches. There is a period of preparation for delivery, which in ancestral forms included nesting in a safe location, shielded from the elements. This was likely to be in a covered area, down-wind of predators. The breeze carrying their scent was protective but also cooling.

As indicated in Table 2, hormonal changes subsequent to the loss of the placenta have adaptive effects for postnatal protection and nurturing of the newborn[6,7].

These adaptive responses include increased arterial tone that contracts the blood volume and maintains perfusion pressure to the brain. To nourish the infant, the mother mobilizes both fat and calcium for milk production. The former elevates the blood lipid levels and the latter is at the expense of bone mineral density. The infant receives the full focus of the mother's attention[8]. Even during sleep, the mother's vigilance is maintained by altered states of arousal and depth of sleep. Cutaneous vasodilatation when the infant suckles furnishes warmth. These are all adaptive responses that maximize the likelihood of infant survival. The physical needs of the newborn and mother are succeeded by adaptive behavioral patterns for parenting the child and preparing it for eventual independence. The ovarian cycle, with the passage of time, resumes and the important cognitive and physical work of raising the child assumes increasing significance.

This is a very simplified rendition of the effects of estrogen deficiency during the puerperium. There are many supporting hormonal and environmental signals that also contribute to adaptive function. They are not mentioned here since they are not extant during the post-reproductive period and therefore less germane to this discussion.

**Table 2** Puerperal response: things to do to keep the F2 generation alive and to foster an F3 generation

Immediately postpartum: stay alive

- Estrogen-responsive mucocutaneous areas undergo a bland response to stretching (elasticity, no tears/scars)
- Uterine contractions minimize bleeding
- Increased vascular resistance, curtailing blood flow to non-essential vascular beds maintains blood flow to the brain; and avoids syncope or slowed reaction time
- Reduced stage 4 and REM sleep promotes ease of arousal

## LONGER LIFE BRINGS NEW CHALLENGES

In the USA, current female life expectancy is ~85 years (Figure 1). Beginning with the faltering of ovarian follicular development at ~35 years, the average woman will live half or more of her lifespan in the climacteric[9]. This unprecedented post-reproductive longevity is primarily the result of the development of public health measures such as antibiotics, immunizations, sewage and potable water during the preceding two centuries[10]. Thus, the causes of death have shifted from illnesses related to pregnancy and birth, and accidents and infection, to the sequelae of aging plus changes in lifestyle (diet and insufficient caloric expenditure) and maladaptive responses to gonadal decline. While dietary and lifestyle modification can be expected to improve the health of the aging population, there is no antidote for aging, per se, and, in practicality, being post-reproductive eliminates the possibility of Darwinian adaptation. As a result, the increased longevity of post-reproductive women has changed the profile for causes of death in our contemporary society. Figure 1 shows that, by 1991, the chief cause of death was (coronary) vascular disease, followed by cancers[11]. It has become clear that many of these vascular lesions are outcomes of induced or inherent metabolic syndromes that are exposed by longevity. The decrease of sex steroids in the aging woman contributes to these outcomes by accelerating the

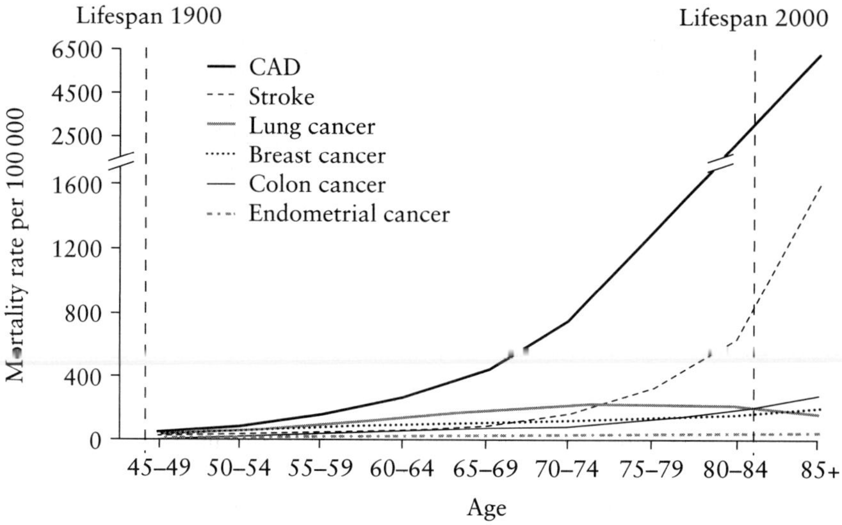


**Figure 1** Leading causes of death in women. Modified from National Center for Health Statistics. *Vital Statistics of the United States, 1992, Vol. II Mortality*. Part A. SEER Cancer Statistics Review 1973–1993. Miller *et al.*, eds. National Cancer Institute, 1997

sequelae of glucose intolerance and immunopathies such as the favoring of Th1 over Th2 responses that may lead to inflammation-driven vascular and dystrophic brain lesions[12,13].

## RESPONSES TO ESTROGEN WITHDRAWAL DURING THE CLIMACTERIC THAT MAY NO LONGER BE ADAPTIVE

While aging, per se, clearly plays a major role in the development and course of these entities; there is also evidence of an active role played by the decline of estrogen[14,15]. These effects, such as bone-wasting and menopausal symptoms, stem largely from the absence of adaptive responses to hormonal decreases during the post-reproductive period. In fact, menopausal responses to estrogen depletion may be viewed as a recapitulation of previously adaptive responses that evolved to insure reproductive success which are detrimental during the climacteric. The combination of aging, smoking, metabolic syndromes, sedentary lifestyle and hormone deficiency will furnish the greatest medical challenges to women in industrial societies in the 21st century. Some of them are listed in Table 3.

**Table 3** Effects of estrogen withdrawal during the climacteric

| | |
|---|---|
| • Cardiovascular | increased arterial resistance |
| • Metabolism | energy conservation |
| • Body fat | increased blood lipids, redistribution |
| • Bone/calcium | increased bone loss |
| • Neurological | hypothalamic autonomic dysfunction |
| | sleep disorders |
| | diminished sex drive |
| | mood disorders |
| | cognitive dysfunction |
| | memory loss |
| • Connective tissue | failure of subcutaneous and other tissues |
| • Breasts | loss of tissue mass |
| • Genitourinary | genital atrophy with scarring/infection |
| | bladder atrophy and incontinence |
| • Immune system | increase of circulating monocytes |
| | increase in specific immune response to foreign antigens (lost immune-sanctuary) |

As can be seen, in the post reproductive period, the same endocrine/metabolic events that supported reproductive function now lead to accelerated atherosclerosis, osteopenia/osteoporosis,

People who develop coronary heart disease grow differently from other people, both *in utero* and during childhood. Slow growth during fetal life and infancy is followed by accelerated weight gain in childhood. Two disorders that predispose to coronary heart disease, type 2 diabetes and hypertension, are preceded by similar paths of growth. Mechanisms underlying this are thought to include the development of insulin resistance *in utero*, reduced numbers of nephrons associated with small body size at birth and altered programming of the micro-architecture and function of the liver. Slow fetal growth might also heighten the body's stress responses and increase vulnerability to poor living conditions in later life.

**Figure 2** The Barker hypothesis of the fetal origins of adult disease. From *Br Med J* 2001;322:949[11], with permission

sleep/mood disorders[16,17], genital/bladder atrophy, and memory loss[18]. The degree and symptomatology depend on cultural expectation, genetic predisposition, body habitus and co-morbidities. The over-nutrition and sedentary lifestyle of modern industrial societies contribute to obesity, insulin resistance, and their sequelae of hypertension, hyperlipidemia, microalbuminuria and fibinolysis - the so-called syndrome X[19]. These all contribute to the effects of age, etc., to increase the rates of illness and death. The genetic blueprint also plays a large role in excursions of morbidity and mortality in affected populations.

## CHANGES IN LIFE HISTORY ARE FORECAST AT BIRTH (THE BARKER HYPOTHESIS)

Recent evidence indicates that the life history of individuals may be impacted by prenatal events (Barker hypothesis). This seems especially evident in the case of cardiovascular disease. The responses of the fetoplacental unit to stresses during pregnancy result in postnatal vascular dysfunction that may set the stage for the effects of the climacteric[20,21]. This is described in Figure 2.

## THE ROLE OF PREVENTION IN THE HEALTH OF AGING WOMEN

Despite the important evolutionary, genetic, developmental imperatives described above, there are many ways that the life history of the average woman can be positively affected by modern medicine. These include traditional medical evaluation plus the use of contemporary tools for assessment of genetic and epigenetic risk[22]. These will lead to rational selection of preventative measures, such as reducing environmental risk (stop smoking), lifestyle modification (diet[23,24] and exercise) and medical interventions (hormones, statins, anti-inflammatory and anti-thrombotic agents[25-28]). These measures have already been utilized and will be more widely employed in the future. We are engaged in the greatest experiment ever; determining whether it is possible to avoid the predictions of the Barker hypothesis. The technical tools are in our hands. We have already surpassed natural selection through the application of modern thought and action in many areas of modern life. It seems only right that these principles should be applied to the health of our aging population.

## CONCLUSION

Comparison of the characteristics of the puerperium with those of the menopausal transition reveals striking similarities. In part, these are secondary to the effects of a hypoestrogenic milleau. Whereas the former state is an adaptive and evolutionarily conserved state, the latter predisposes to cardiovascular morbidity and endocrinopathies, which are worsened by the overfeeding, sedentary lifestyle characteristic of many industrial societies.

## ACKNOWLEDGEMENT

We appreciate the excellent assistance of Ms. Tara Marshall.

# References


1. Lahdenpera M, Lummaa V, Helle S, Tremblay M, Russell AF. Fitness benefits of prolonged post-reproductive lifespan in women. *Nature* 2004;428: 178–81
2. Shadoan MK, Anthony MS, Rankin SE, Clarkson TB, Wagner JD. Effects of tibolone and conjugated equine estrogens with or without medroxyprogesterone acetate on body composition and fasting carbohydrate measures in surgically postmenopausal monkeys. *Metabolism* 2003;52:1085–91
3. Miranda-Paiva C, Ribeiro-Barbosa SR, Cantera NS, *et al.* A role for the periaqueductal grey in opiodergic inhibition of maternal behavior. *Eur J Neurosci* 2003;18:667–74
4. Kalkwarf HJ, Specker BL, Ho M. The effect of calcium supplementation on bone density during lactation and weaning. *J Clin Endocrinol Metab* 1999;84:464–70
5. Dempsey JC, Williams MA, Leisenring WM, Shy K, Luthy DA. Maternal birth weight in relation to plasma lipid concentrations in early pregnancy. *Am J Obstet Gynecol* 2004;190:1359–68
6. Haluska GJ, Wells TR, Hirst JJ, Brenner RM, Sadowsky DW, Novy MJ. Progesterone receptor localization and isoforms in myometrium, decidua, and fetal membranes from rhesus macaques: evidence for functional progesterone withdrawal at parturition. *J Soc Gyn Invest* 2002; 9:125–36
7. Abou-Saleh MT, Ghubash R, Karim L, *et al.* Hormonal aspects of postpartum depression. *Psychoneuroendocrinology* 1998;23:465–75
8. Barbaccia ML, Serra M, Purdy RH, *et al.* Stress and neuroactive steroids. *Int Rev Neurobiol* 2001;46: 243–72
9. Zapantis G, Santoro N. The menopausal transition: characteristics and management. *Best Pract Res Clin Endocrinol Metab* 2003;17:33–52
10. Perls T, Fretts R. The evolution of menopause and human life span. *Ann Hum Biol* 2001;28:237–45
11. Singh R, Hellman S, Heimann R. The natural history of breast carcinoma in the elderly: implications for screening and treatment. *Cancer* 2004; 100:1807–13
12. Satta N, Toti F, Freyssinet JM, *et al.* Hormone replacement therapy and sensitive C-reactive protein concentrations in women with type II diabetes. *Lancet* 1999;354:487–4
13. Mor G, Nilsen J, Horvath T, Bechmann I, *et al.* Estrogen and microglia: a regulatory system that affects the brain. *J Neurobiol* 1999;40:484–96
14. Adamson DL, Webb CM, Collin. Esterified estrogens combined with methyltestosterone improve emotional well-being in postmenopausal women with chest pain and normal coronary angiograms. *Menopause* 2001;8:233–8
15. Ahlborg H, Johnell D, Turner CH, *et al.* Bone loss and bone size after menopause. *N Engl J Med* 2003;349:327–34
16. Slopien R, Meczekalski B. Relationship between climacteric symptoms and serum serotonin levels in postmenopausal women. *Climacteric* 2003;6: 653–7
17. Polo-Kantola P, Erkkola R, Helenius H, *et al.* When does estrogen replacement therapy improve sleep quality? *Am J Obstet Gynecol* 1998;178: 1002–9
18. Tierney MC. Oestradiol concentrations in prediction of cognitive decline in women. *Lancet* 2000; 356;694–5
19. Alebiosu CO, Odusan BO. Metabolic syndrome in subjects with type 2 diabetes mellitus. *J Natl Med Assoc* 2004;96:817–21
20. Eriksson JG, Forsen T, Tuomilehto J, *et al.* Effects of size at birth and childhood growth on the insulin resistance syndrome in elderly individuals. *Diabetologia* 2002;45:342–8
21. Ericksson JG, Forsen T, Tuomilehto J, *et al.* Early growth and coronary heart disease in later life: longitudinal study. *Br Med J* 2001;322:949
22. Xydakis AM, Case CC, Jones PH, *et al.* Adiponectin, inflammation, and the expression of metabolic syndrome in obese individuals: the impact of rapid weight loss through caloric restriction. *J Clin Endocrinol Metab* 2004;89:2697–703
23. Esposito K, Pontillo A, Di Palo C, *et al.* Effect of weight loss and lifestyle changes on vascular inflammatory markers in obese women. *J Am Med Assoc* 2003;289:1799–804
24. Carr MC, Brunzell JD. Abdominal obesity and dyslipidemia in the metabolic syndrome: importance of type 2 diabetes and familial combined hyperlipidemia in coronary artery disease risk. *J Clin Endocrinol Metab* 2004;89:2601–7
25. Loprinzi CL, Michalak JC, Duella SR, *et al.* Megestrol acetate for the prevention of hot flashes. *N Engl J Med* 1994;331:347–52
26. Naftolin F, Silver D. Is progestogen supplementation of ERT really necessary? *Menopause* 2003;9:1–2
27. Schonbeck U, Libby P. Inflammation, immunity, and HMG-CoA reductase inhibitors: statins as anti-inflammatory agents? *Circulation* 2004;109:II18–26
28. Komesaroff PA, Esler MO, Svahir K. Estrogen supplementation attenuates glucocorticoid and catecholamine responses to mental stress in perimenopausal women. *J Clin Endocrinol Metab* 1999; 84:606–10

# A holistic approach to mature women's health and aging

2

*M. Neves-e-Castro*

## INTRODUCTION

The health and aging of middle-aged women are nowadays the subject of many challenging strategies in view of recent important progress in preventive medicine.

Women are cells of a 'social body'. As such, one should study them both in their macrosocial and in their microsocial context, without forgetting that 'everything should be made as simple as possible . . . but not simpler', as said by Albert Einstein.

### Holism

A holistic approach seems to be more realistic and meaningful. Holism is 'the approach to the study of a phenomenon through the analysis of the phenomenon as a complete entity in itself'[1]. It permits one to see 'an individual as a complex system'[2], arising in the body, the psychological life, the ecosocial environment, and the health-care system.

The World Health Organization (WHO) has defined health as a 'state of complete physical, mental, and social well-being and not merely the absence of disease or infirmity'. In itself, this definition is holistic, meaning that the individual is seen as a complex system, as indicated above.

As a matter of fact, 'the *climacteric* is a complex, multifaceted process that responds to the interaction of different *biopsychosocial factors*'[3]. This is, therefore, a very judicious counsel as to how to manage the mature women who come to their doctors seeking advice and help.

### Health

One of the most difficult tasks facing the attending physician is the diagnosis of 'health'. It is far simpler to diagnose a disease. 'It is politically less threatening to view women's health only through the biomedical model but *this denies* the roles social, political and economic circumstances have in shaping and influencing everyone's health'. 'Conflicts over the best approach to women's health arise in large part because *there is no agreed upon, universal definition* of women's health'[4].

Women's health and men's health are different. Heart disease kills 19% more women than men, but 10 years later. Depression is two to three times more common in women than in men. Of those suffering from osteoporosis, 80% are women. Of those with autoimmune disease, 75% are women.

The 2002 WHO World Health Report focused on reducing risks to health in developed countries; the leading risk factors are: 'tobacco, blood pressure, alcohol, cholesterol, overweight, low fruit and vegetable intake, physical inactivity, illicit drugs, unsafe sex, iron deficiency'[5].

### Aging

Aging is another very complex problem. 'It is the most pressing problem of our age'. 'One of the curious features of aging is its *unpredictability* at the individual level.' 'Aging is not a disease; it is a normal part of the life cycle'[6]. There are many theories that try to explain it, including free radicals, metabolic error catastrophe, DNA damage, glycosylation of cross-linkage, finite cell division, immune dysfunction, and neuroendocrine dysregulation.

'The fact that *genes* explain only 25% of individual variability in aging means that 75% *must be accounted for by other factors*, such as life-style variables (nutrition, exercise) and powerful effects of the environment (effects on older age).' 'We can always delay aging but we can never avoid it . . .'[6].

The promotion of health for the elderly is focused on active aging - physically, socially and mentally. Active aging has several determinants: health and social services, behavioral determinants, personal determinants, physical environment, social determinants, and economic determinants[7]. The purpose of all interventions is 'the compression of morbidity'[8] in the last years of one's life.

Following the holistic model based on the WHO definition of health, women's health must be analyzed in its components.

## SOCIAL HEALTH

'In the developed world, the percentage of women over 50 years of age has *tripled* in the last 100 years'[9]. In Japan and Canada, the percentage of population aged 65 and older will increase from 2000 to 2020 by 53.7% and 42.9%, respectively. In Australia, New Zealand, United States and Germany the respective increases will be 39.2%, 33.7%, 32.8% and 31.9%[10]. 'In more developed regions, the proportion of older people already exceeds that of children; by 2050 it will double'[11].

In 1998, the health status of women (45–64 years of age) was such that 57% had one chronic condition and 23% had a disability or limiting illness. After age 65, the percentages were, respectively, 80% and 31%[12]. It is dramatic that the percentage of the population aged 65 and older living alone in 1990 was 41% in Germany, 38% in the United Kingdom and approximately 30% in the United States, New Zealand, France, Canada and Australia. Nevertheless, the number was much lower in Japan (14%), indicating the influence of sociocultural conditions[13].

## MENTAL HEALTH

During the transition from the reproductive to the non-reproductive years, women are usually more perceptive of their mental health. It is, thus, not surprising that emotions and feelings may play an important role in their behaviors and coping and that many of their complaints may be of a psychosomatic nature. Psychosomatics is not a new specialty; it is the true perspective of human medicine.

The woman's perception of her own existence and identity is not only an act of thought, as Descartes put it in his famous 'I think, therefore I am'. Recent research in human models led Damasio (1994)[14] to challenge Descartes and to rephrase his sentence into 'I feel, therefore I am'. This is very important, as exemplified in the effect of a psychosocial treatment on the survival of patients with metastatic breast cancer[15,16]. The survival time from time of randomization and onset of intervention was a mean 36.6 (standard deviation (SD) 37.6) months in the *intervention group*, compared with 18.9 (SD 10.8) months in the *control group*.

Depression also influences components of immune function that may affect cancer surveillance. 'Life stress situations, depression and social isolation have been linked to increased risk of myocardial infarction in women'[17]. Therefore, mental health is an important determinant of physical health.

## PHYSICAL HEALTH

Across all ages, the most frequent causes of death among women are diseases of the circulatory system (accounting for 43% of all deaths), cancer (26%), diseases of the respiratory system (6%), suicide and accidents (5%)[18].

Cardiovascular diseases are the major cause of women's death after age 50. For every 10-year increase in age, their risk for heart disease increases about three times. A family history of premature coronary heart disease (myocardial infarction before age 65 in women) increases the risk for myocardial infarction about two times[17].

The role of female hormones in the primary prevention of cardiovascular diseases has recently been much contested. However, 'It appears that half of the benefits in the prevention of cardiovascular diseases *are not* hormone-related'[19]!

The major concerns about hormonal treatments are related to cardiovascular and breast cancer risks. But . . . will hormones provide benefit or harm? Menopausal hormonal treatments are very good, but treatments without hormones may also be very good for a woman's health[20,21].

And, should one say HRT (hormone replacement therapy) or MHT (menopausal hormonal therapy)[21–24]? This discussion is important because there is a tendency to consider that there is nothing but estrogens to offer to a postmenopausal woman, and that such treatment is obligatory for every woman and for a very long time. This is wrong[22].

In fact, 'there are no really 'safe' biological active drugs. There are only 'safe' physicians'. 'Science . . . is an art of probability. Medicine . . . is an art of uncertainty'[25].

The alarm that was spread all over the world in recent years is the consequence of several well-known clinical trials and of their interpretation in the light of evidence-based medicine. Yet, 'Not everything that can be counted counts; and not everything that counts can be counted' (Albert Einstein).

If one extrapolates the relative risks shown in the trials into NNH (number needed to harm), the reciprocal of relative risk, it becomes apparent that the absolute risks are rather insignificant. 'As with the WHI reports, much emphasis has been given to the relative risks of percentage increases of 30–200%, whereas absolute figures provide a more suitable perspective of the risk. The additional cancers associated with estrogen-only therapy are 1.5 after 5 years and 5 after 10 years, and for combined estrogen–progestin therapy the figures are 6 and 19, respectively per 1000 women by the age of 65 years. Or, put in another way, a doctor would need to give combined estrogen–progestin therapy to 116 women for 5 years or 53 women for 10 years to see one extra case of breast cancer'[26].

In the Heart and Estrogen/progestin Replacement Study (HERS)[27,28], for a relative risk of 26%, the NNH is 833/1 year, whereas, in the WHI trial, for an increase in relative risk of 26%, the NNH is 1250/1 year. Other risks accepted by women and doctors, like obesity[17] – or two alcoholic drinks/day, are indeed far more important than female hormones.

This alarm has caused an enormous drop in hormonal treatments given to postmenopausal women after July 2002[29].

Recent research has emphasized that every medical treatment should be based on evidence. 'It is therefore worrisome if the decline in the use of HRT is followed by an increased use of alternative medicines, with mostly undocumented effects[30]. We have recently critically reviewed all these alarmist trials. The conclusions of these studies suggest that the 'safe woman' (NNH between 600 and 1000) to *initiate* HT is between 50 and 59 years of age, with vasomotor symptoms, less than 10 years after the menopause, being treated with statins, with a good lipid profile, and with a body mass index ≥ 30. This is precisely the profile of the great majority of women who come for consultation after their menopause.

Therefore it seems that what most gynecologists are doing for their predominant population of patients is not unsafe and contributes not only to a good quality of life but to prevention, as well[31].

The interpretation of what should and should not be done to preserve women's health (quality of life, prevention of diseases) is nowadays strongly influenced by the rules of evidence-based medicine and their application to the results of the clinical trials published in the last decade. It is appropriate, therefore, to discuss these problems in the light of their applicability to good clinical practice.

## EVIDENCE-BASED MEDICINE

Since evidence-based medicine is in fashion and considered by most physicians to be the only law to obey, it is pertinent to meditate on some statements and facts. 'Evidence-based medicine and /or medicine-based evidence?'[22]. 'Without clinical expertise, practice risks becoming tyrannized by evidence'. 'Without current best evidence, practice risks becoming rapidly out of date, to the detriment of patients'[32,33]. 'Evidence alone does not make decisions'[34]. 'The new look of evidence-based medicine should be research-enhanced health care'[35]. In fact, evidence-based medicine can be used *to do* . . . and *not to do*.

Here are some astonishing examples of contradictions:

(1) The 'annual physical check-up may be an empty ritual' . . . 'Many tests that are useful, like cholesterol and blood pressure checks, *need not be done every year*, it is said in reports to doctors, policy makers and the public'. There is 'no evidence', it is said, 'that routine pelvic, rectal and testicular exams made any difference in overall survival rates for those with no

symptoms of illness'[35]. Is this a wise economic recommendation?

(2) For estrogen and memory in postmenopausal women: 'New data provide further positive evidence that estrogen treatment might provide positive long-term effects on memory and learning in postmenopausal women.' 'Doctors may be 'throwing the baby out with the bath water' by having their patients stop taking estrogen replacement.' Studies recently published in the *Journal of the American Medical Association* 'have a lot of problems with their methodology'[36]. 'Low physiological levels of estradiol replacement exert dramatic protective effects in the brain. Using an animal model of stroke, we found that estradiol dramatically decreases the degree of brain injury in adult female rats and mice and in the aging female rats'[37].

(3) Coronary heart disease prevention:

(a) A cost-effective prevention strategy would offer aspirin and initial antihypertensive treatment to all patients at greater than 75% 5-year coronary risk[38]. But . . . 'Women who take an aspirin a day – which millions do to prevent heart attack and stroke as well as to treat headaches – may raise their risk of getting deadly pancreatic cancer'[39].

(b) High-fat, no-starch diets do not raise cholesterol. . . .'Patients with atherosclerosis lose weight on a high-fat, no-starch Atkins-style diet, without increasing their blood fat (lipid) levels'[40]. Is this not the opposite of what one recommends?

(c) 'Postmenopausal women who have undergone bilateral salpingo-oophorectomy have a decreased risk of coronary artery disease'[41]. However, 'Hormone replacement therapy is associated with less coronary atherosclerosis in postmenopausal women'[42], although some say that . . . 'Estrogen-only/estrogen-progestin therapy does not appear to increase or decrease atherosclerosis rate'[43].

(d) WHI women have an 81% higher risk of heart attack during the first year of hormone therapy.' But, the same study concludes later[44] that 'women who were less than 10 years postmenopause had an overall hazard ratio of 0.89, while women 20 or more years postmenopause had a hazard ratio of 1.7' and that 'Estrogen-progestin therapy use for 6 years was associated with a 30% decrease in coronary heart disease.'

However, 'Hormone therapy is not risky for heart disease in the first year.' These findings would suggest that the results of early coronary heart disease risk observed in the Women's Health Initiative (trial) might not be applicable to healthy, younger postmenopausal women who seek treatment for menopausal symptoms' and 'healthy women within 5 years of menopause do not experience early harm'[45]. Furthermore, a recent study concludes that HRT given for 13–60 months 'was associated with a small reduction in acute myocardial infarction, but, when used for more than 60 months, there was a substantial risk reduction'[46].

The fact is that 'WHI was very much a study about older women'[47]. Therefore, it is mandatory to meditate, serenely, without passion, on the data that are available in order to merge them, wisely, in each one's experience as contributions for good clinical practice. 'You cannot create experience. You must undergo it' (Albert Camus). 'He who *learns*, but does *not think is lost*. He who *thinks*, but *does not learn* is *dangerous*' (Confucius). 'If we both learn and think . . . *we will neither be lost* . . . *nor dangerous* . . . to our postmenopausal women patients'[48]. It is regrettably true that, after all 'Common sense is not so common' (Voltaire).

Thus, the important questions are: what do we *know* today? And, to know . . . What is it? To know is the selective and critical acquisition of information and its concerted integration in one's mind. Are we being well informed, or well misinformed?

### The information

The information is supplied by clinical trials. 'Researchers from the University of California, at Davis, claim clinical trials are reported with misleading statistics.' 'Most randomized trials of new treatments published in leading medical journals (*Ann Intern Med*, *BMJ*, *JAMA*, *Lancet*) are reported in a potentially misleading way.' '*Most* of the trials report results based on relative risk reduction'! 'Only 18 of the papers reviewed considered absolute risk reduction'! 'Only eight of the 359 trials reported the number needed to treat'[49]!

Concerning clinical trials, how were they performed, what similarities do they have with our clinical practice, and how do we interpret them? 'The popular belief that only randomized, controlled trials produce trustworthy results and that all observational studies are misleading *does a disservice* to patient care, clinical investigation, and the education of health-care professionals'[50]. 'Which clinical studies provide the best evidence?' 'An earlier systematic review also found no consistent difference between randomized controlled trials and observational studies in estimates of the effects of treatment in 22 areas'[51].

'The new studies do not justify a major revision of the hierarchy of evidence, but they do support a flexible approach in which randomized controlled trials and observational studies are complementary'[51].

'. . . the news media generally did a poor job of communicating a basic point about the data from the trial: that there was a considerable difference between the relative and absolute risks of combination hormone therapy'. 'Most articles and broadcast segments tended to focus exclusively on either the small absolute risks or the large relative risks, neglecting the more even-handed picture that presented both'. 'Since the sharply increased relative risks got the most play, news coverage about the trial's findings had an alarming cast'[52].

Based on sound *information*, one must acquire the *knowledge* to find the *truth*.

### The truth?

'The objective of both basic and clinical science is to know the truth.' 'Every epidemiologic study, no matter how good or how large, gives only one view of the truth.' 'It takes many views to come close to seeing the truth'[53].

Which treatments were investigated? Only 'hormone replacement therapy'! Thus, studies based *only* on the use of hormones *do not reflect good clinical practice*! 'We are drawing in information, but starved for knowledge' (John Naisbilt).

Evidence-based medicine, to be clinically useful, must contribute to *know* the *truth*, based on reliable *information*.

## CONCLUSION

Since WHO defined *health* as 'a state of complete physical, mental, and social well-being and not merely the absence of disease of infirmity', one must take into consideration social health, mental health and physical health. Physicians are the health-care providers of *mental* health, *social* health, and *physical* health. As *physicians* and *citizens*, we have *civic* responsibilities, *political* responsibilities, and *medical* responsibilities at both the national and the international level.

### Final reminders

'Menopausal hormone therapy aptly fits the metaphor of the blind men describing the elephant: each touches a part, ear, trunk, tail, body, and draws a different conclusion. We are the blind men. The elephant is the data published in a half-century of medical literature that now includes the report from the Women's Health Initiative.' 'Biased opinions, be they pro or con, dishonor the profession and harm our patients'[32].

It is regrettable that some epidemiologists, with no clinical experience, feel entitled to set the rules for clinical practice as if they were 'hormone legislators'!

It is very true that 'Each time we learn something new, the astonishment comes from the recognition that we were wrong before'. 'In truth, whenever we discover a new fact, it involves the elimination of old ones. *We are always*, as it turns out, fundamentally *in error*' (Lewis Thomas, English Biologist, 1913–1993).

Medical judgment requires: 'The application of accumulated knowledge and understanding acquired not only through our appraisal of the literature but also from our education and experience.' 'The final impact on a patient is never the result of a single, solitary fact or one scientific study'[54].

'Preventing a woman from the benefits of a sound postmenopausal hormone therapy because of the fear of rare side-effects does not seem to be satisfactory medicine'[55].

'And, now that the dust has settled . . .' (about WHI): 'To publish data that may or may not be entirely true or certainly premature is a *disservice to the medical profession and, most important, to our patients.*' The majority of the data that were published are not statistically significant even at the nominal level'[56].

## The message

The message is that we should prescribe postmenopausal hormonal treatments *when clinically indicated*, if not contraindicated. *No answers from ongoing clinical trials are indispensable* to practice today Good Medicine'[31]. Which is the winner – menopause (based) medicine, climacteric (based) medicine, sex (based) medicine, gender (based) medicine, or women's medicine?!

'There is only one medicine'[54]. Therefore, what one must learn is how to practice *good medicine*[20]! Let us not medicalize the Menopause. Instead, let us holistically approach the climacteric and the aging women.

# References


1. Stedman's Medical Dictionary, 1990
2. Ruiz R, Luna CL. La incorporacion de um nuevo modelo en medicina: consequencias teórico-práticas. *Aten Primaria* 1992;10:629–34
3. Dennerstein L. Well-being, symptoms and the menopausal transition. *Maturitas* 1996;23:147–57
4. Curtis M. Guest Editorial: Definition of women's health: a rose by any other name? *Obstet Gynecol Surv* 2003;58:83–5
5. World Health Organization. *The World Health Report, 2002*. Geneva: WHO
6. Kirkwood T. The most pressing problem of our age. *Br Med J* 2003;326:1297–9
7. Kalache A. Gender-specific health care in the 21st century: a focus on developing countries. *Aging Male* 2002;5:129–38
8. Fries JF, Crapo LM. *Vitality and Aging*. San Francisco: W.H.Freeman and Co., 1981
9. Paoletti R, Wenger NK. Review of the International Position paper on Women's Health and Menopause: a comprehensive approach. *Circulation* 2003; 107:1336–9
10. *Percentage of the Population Age 65 and Older, 2000-2020*. United Nations, October 1999
11. *World Population Ageing 1950-2050*. Population Division, DESA. United Nations, 2002:29–32
12. The Commonwealth Fund 1998, Health Status by Age. Survey of Women's Health
13. *Percentage of the Population Age 65 and Older Living Alone, 1970-1990*. OECD, Oct.1999
14. Damasio AR. *Descartes' Error: Emotion, Reason and the Human Brain*. New York: Grosset/Putnam Book, 1994
15. Spiegel, Bloom JR, Kraemer HC, *et al.* Effect of psychosocial treatment on survival of patients with metastic breast cancer. *Lancet* 1989;2:888–91
16. Spiegel D, Giese DJ. Depression and cancer: mechanisms and disease progression. *Biol Psychiatry* 2003; 54:269–82
17. NIH Publication Nº.02-3284. International Position paper on Women's Health and Menopause: a comprehensive approach. Bethesda, MD: National Heart, Lung, and Blood Institute, 2002
18. European Community. Commission Report of 22 May 1997 on the state of women's health
19. Mosca L, Grundy SM, Judelson D, *et al.* Guide to preventive cardiology for women. *Circulation* 1999;99:2480–4
20. Neves-e-Castro M. The *Queen* . . . is naked! *Maturitas* 2001;38:235–7
21. Neves-e-Castro M. Imaginary women. *Maturitas* 2001;40:5–15
22. Neves-e-Castro M. Is there a menopausal medicine? The past, the present and the future. *Maturitas* 2002;43S:75–80

23. Neves-e-Castro M. Where are we now? In Neves-e-Castro M, Wren BG, eds. *Menopause: Hormones and Cancer*. London: Parthenon Publishing, 2002:141–5
24. Sturdee DW, MacLennan A. HT or HRT, that is the question. *Climacteric* 2003;6:1
25. Kaminetzy HA. The men and the children - then the women. *Int J Gynaecol Obstet* 1993;43:245
26. Sturdee DW, MacLennan AH. Is combined estrogen/progestogen hormone therapy worth the risk? *Climacteric* 2003;6:177–9
27. Hulley S, Grady D, Bush T, *et al.* for the HERS Research Group. Randomized trial of estrogen in secondary prevention of coronary heart disease in postmenopausal women: Heart and Estrogen/progestin Replacement Study (HERS) research Group. *J Am Med Assoc* 1998;280:605–13
28. Hulley S, Furberg C, Barrett-Connor E, *et al.* for the HERS Research Group. Non-cardiovascular disease outcomes during 6.8. years of hormone therapy: Heart and Estrogen/progestin Replacement Study follow-up (HERS II). *J Am Med Assoc* 2002; 288:58–66
29. Hersh AL, Stefanick ML, Stafford RS. National use of postmenopausal hormone therapy. annual trends and response to recent evidence. *J Am Med Assoc* 2004;291:47–53
30. Jensen CW, Ottesen B. The aging woman: the role of medical therapy. *Int J Gynecol Obstet* 2003;82: 381–91
31. Neves-e-Castro M. Menopause in crisis post-Women's Health Initiative? A view based on personal clinical experience. *Hum Reprod* 2003;18:1–7
32. Sackett DL. The arrogance of preventive medicine. *Can Med Assoc J* 2002;167:363–4
33. Sackett DL, Rodenberg WM. On the need for evidence-based medicine. *Therapie* 1966;51:212-17
34. Haynes RB, Straus SE. Clinical expertise in the era of evidence based medicine and patient choice. Evidence-based medicine in practice. *ACP Journal Club* 2002;136:A11-2
35. US Federal Agency for Healthcare Research and Quality. *The New York Times*, August 12, 2003
36. Hancur-Bucci CA, Newhouse P, Naylor MR, *et al.* Presented at the *33rd Annual Meeting, Society for Neurosciences*, 2003
37. Wise PM, Bottner M, Dubal DB, *et al.* Presented at *The Endocrine Society's 85th Annual Meeting* 2003;S18-1
38. Marshall T. Coronary heart disease prevention: insights from modeling incremental cost effectiveness. *B Med J* 2003;327:1–5
39. Schernhammer ES, Kang JH, Chan AT, *et al.* A prospective study of aspirin use and the risk of pancreatic cancer in women. *J Natl Cancer Inst* 2004;96:4–5
40. Hays JH, DiSabatino A, Gorman RT, *et al. Mayo Clin Proc 2003*;78:1331-6
41. Johnson BD. Presented at the *14th Annual Meeting of NAMS*, 2003;S-13
42. Akhrass F. Hormone replacement therapy is associated with less coronary atherosclerosis in postmenopausal women. *J Clin Endocrinol Metab* 2003;88:5611–14
43. Hodis HN, Mack WJ, Azen SP, *et al.* Women's Estrogen-Progestin Lipid-lowering Hormone Atherosclerosis Regression Trial Research Group. Hormone therapy and the progression of coronary-artery atherosclerosis in postmenopausal women. *N Engl J Med* 2003;349:535–45
44. Manson JE, Hsia J, Johnson KC, *et al.* Estrogen plus progestin and the risk of coronary heart disease. *N Engl J Med* 2003:349:523–34
45. Lobo R. Presented at the *51st Annual Meeting of ACOG*, 2003
46. Chilvers CE, Knobb RC, Armstrong SJ, *et al.* Postmenopausal hormone replacement therapy and risk of acute myocardial infarction-a case control study of women in the East Midlands, UK. *Eur Heart J* 2003;24:2197–205
47. Stefanick M. *The Wall Street Journal*, Oct. 21, 2003
48. Wenger NK. Hormonal and nonhormonal therapies for the postmenopausal woman: what is the evidence for cardioprotection? *Am J Geriatr Cardiol* 2000;9:204–9
49. Mayor S. Researchers claim clinical trials are reported with misleading statistics. *Br Med J* 2002;324:1353
50. Concato J, Shah N, Horwitz RI. Randomized, controlled trials, observational studies, and the hierarchy of research designs. *N Engl J Med* 2000; 342:1887–92
51. Barton S. Which clinical studies provide the best evidence? *Br Med J* 2000;321:255–6
52. Denzer S. Science, public health, and public awareness: lessons from the Women's Health Initiative. *Ann Intern Med* 2003;138:352–3
53. Bush T. Beyond HERS: some (not so) random thoughts on randomized clinical trials. *Int J Fertil Womens Med* 2001;46:55–9
54. Speroff L. WHI: It's time to be critical! *Am J Obstet Gynecol* 2003;189:620
55. Neves-e-Castro M. When hormone replacement therapy is not possible. In Studd J, ed. *The Management of the Menopause. The Millennium Review*. London: Parthenon Publishing, 2000:91–102
56. Creasman WT, Hoel D, DiSaia PJ. WHI: Now that the dust has settled. *Am J Obstet Gynecol* 2003; 189:621–6

# Natural history of menopause studies and related efforts at the National Institute on Aging, NIH

3

*S. Sherman*

## INTRODUCTION

The significance of menopause in healthy aging and its role in the etiology of the chronic diseases, disorders or conditions of aging (such as osteoporosis, cardiovascular disease, and cognitive decline) are highly controversial. It is well accepted that aging and the decline in ovarian function culminating in menopause constitute a clear challenge to urogenital structures such as the vagina[1] and to the skeletal system by increasing rates of bone turnover and bone loss[2]. However, because of the high variability between populations in the susceptibility to menopause-related symptoms[3] and to the chronic diseases of aging, the 'true' scope of the biological and psychological changes that are attributable to menopause *per se* is unclear.

Established by a US Congressional Act in 1974, the National Institute on Aging (NIA) is one of 27 institutes and centers of the National Institutes of Health. The Institute is at the forefront of a broad national scientific effort to understand the nature of aging and to extend the healthy, active years of life[4]. NIA conducts and supports biomedical, social, and behavioral research, training, health information dissemination and other programs with respect to the aging process(es) and the diseases and other special problems and needs of the aged. The NIA has an extensive research program on menopause, which explores a variety of biological, psychosocial, behavioral, cognitive and demographic domains during the menopause transition and the postmenopausal years. Menopause-related research and activities range from those in basic biology and epidemiological investigations to identify risk factors and predicators of symptoms and changes in susceptibility to chronic diseases, to small- and large-scale intervention studies including randomized controlled trials. Amongst the many NIA-supported studies of aging, three cohort studies of the menopause transition have enrolled 400 or more women and have been in the field for at least 5 years. These are The Massachusetts Women's Health Study, the Study of Women's Health Across the Nation, and the Penn Ovarian Aging Study. Findings from NIA-funded studies underscore the importance of race/ethnicity as a determinant of levels of reproductive hormones (estradiol, testosterone, follicle stimulating hormone (FSH)) and precursors (dehydroepiandrosterone sulfate (DHEAS)). Race/ethnicity is also a prominent predictor of symptom reporting. Because a number of factors (body mass index (BMI), smoking and physical activity) which may be significantly associated with symptom reporting are potentially modifiable, alternative approaches involving lifestyle and behavioral modification may help to reduce the burden of menopause-related symptoms when conventional medical strategies, such as menopausal hormone therapy, are contraindicated or unacceptable.

## STUDIES OF THE NATURAL HISTORY OF MENOPAUSE

### The Massachusetts Women's Health Study

The Massachusetts Women's Health Study (MWHS) began with a large population-based cross-sectional survey using annually compiled Massachusetts census lists to identify a cohort of eligible women who were 45–55 years old as of

January 1, 1982. Eligibility criteria required having menstruated in the preceding 3 months and a uterus and at least one ovary[5]. At the baseline visit, of 2570 predominantly Caucasian women enrolled, all of whom had had a period in the preceding 3 months, 1178 women were premenopausal (reporting the absence of change in cycle regularity), while 1392 were perimenopausal (reportings a change in cycle regularity). The women were followed with six telephone contacts over 5 years.

Major findings from the MWHS include ascertainment of the median age at natural menopause to be 51.3 years, the median age at the inception of the perimenopause to be 47.5 years, and the estimated median duration of the perimenopause to be 3.5 years. Of the factors significantly influencing the timing of the final menstrual period (FMP), age and smoking had the most profound effect, while that of parity had a lesser effect. The median age at the FMP for current smokers was 50.2 years, while for non-smokers it was 52 years. Smokers not only had their FMP at a younger age, but also experienced a shorter duration of the perimenopause. Women who were older at baseline also tended to have shorter perimenopause duration.

Evaluation of symptom reporting in the MWHS showed that 10% of women who were premenopausal reported hot flushes. The proportion of women reporting hot flushes increased as more experienced cycle irregularity and peaked at 50% some 3–9 months before the FMP. Interestingly, women with a shorter duration of perimenopause were less likely to report hot flushes before, during or after their FMP, as evidenced by hot flush reporting by 39% of a shorter-duration subset vs. 50% of the cohort as a whole. Women with a longer perimenopause transition had the highest rate of physician consultations, further suggesting a more onerous symptom experience. Fortunately, only 20% of women were reporting hot flushes 4 years after their FMP, indicting the transitory nature of this symptom for the majority of women undergoing the menopause transition[5].

An important legacy of the MWHS was the identification of a practical algorithm - based on self-reported data - for defining the 'inception of the perimenopause' for application in epidemiological investigations. This algorithm was proposed on the basis of its ability to predict menopause 3 years later and consisted of two items to define the 'inception of perimenopause' - 3–11 months of amenorrhea or increased menstrual irregularity for those without amenorrhea[6]. These definitions/algorithms have been further refined and additional ones for sub-stages of the menopause transition developed for application in other studies such as the Melbourne Women's Midlife Health Project and the Study of Women's Health Across the Nation.

## The Study of Women's Health across the Nation

The Study of Women's Health Across the Nation (SWAN) was a 1993 initiative developed and sponsored by the NIA and its co-sponsors, the National Institute of Nursing Research and the NIH Office of Research on Women's Health[7]. An initiative was required because the current state of knowledge was based in large part on anecdotal reports or studies (primarily clinic-based) of very limited numbers of women. Importantly, the knowledge base on menopause in the early 1990s applied almost exclusively to white women (of Northwest European ancestry) and the minority experience(s) had been neglected. It was appreciated that understanding the impact of race/ethnicity on the menopausal experience and its sequelae was essential in identifying ethnically relevant risk factors for menopause-related symptoms and chronic diseases of aging.

The overarching objective of the initiative which gave rise to SWAN was to implement prospective longitudinal studies of the natural history of menopause and the decline in ovarian function in middle-aged women. The intention was to characterize the biology/endocrinology of the 'perimenopause' in terms of its biological and psychosocial antecedents, short-term consequences and effects on later health and risk factors for age-related disease. A major aim was to distinguish the role of aging from that of menopause in the development of the chronic diseases of old age.

*Features of SWAN*

SWAN is a multi-site, community-based longitudinal cohort study comprised of seven clinical field sites, a coordinating center, central reproductive hormone laboratory, cardiovascular biochemistries laboratory, and a repository for serum, plasma, urine and DNA.

A detailed description of the two-stage recruitment plan of SWAN is provided in reference 8. To briefly summarize, community-based sampling was conducted between 1995 and 1997 in seven locations across the US: Boston, Chicago, Detroit, Los Angeles, Newark, Oakland, CA, and Pittsburgh. The objectives of the first stage were to obtain cross-cultural demographic, health, reproductive and lifestyle data related to the menopause transition in a large, racially diverse group of mid-life women, as well as to identify those eligible for enrollment into the longitudinal cohort. Each site recruited Caucasian women and women from one other site-designated racial/ethnic minority (African American, Chinese, Hispanic, or Japanese), for a total of five different racial/ethnic groups across the seven sites. The cross-sectional interview was conducted with women found to be 40–55 years of age, able to speak English or a designated other language (Spanish, Japanese or Cantonese) and to provide verbal consent, who resided in the appropriate geographic area and self-identified at least partially with one of the site's target racial/ethic groups. At the end of 1997, over 16 000 cross-sectional surveys had been completed in phone interviews with 7771 Caucasian, 4393 African American, 654 Chinese, 845 Japanese, 1942 Hispanic and 542 women of mixed ancestry.

Subsequently, to establish the longitudinal cohort, each clinical site fielded a recruitment effort designed to enroll 450 women, of whom at least 150 would be from the site-designated minority group, with the remainder being Caucasian. To be cohort-eligible, women had to be 42–52 years of age, have an intact uterus and at least one ovary, and have had at least one menstrual period in the past 3 months. Women using medications known to influence ovarian function and/or menstruation (e.g. menopausal hormone therapy, oral contraceptives) were not eligible. Participants in the baseline visit included 934 African American, 1550 Caucasian, 250 Chinese, 286 Hispanic and 281 Japanese women, for a total cohort of 3301. As of February 2004, data collection had been completed for six follow-up visits and is ongoing for a seventh visit.

The definitions of menopausal status used in reports of SWAN findings were based on self-reports of the timing and predictability of the last menstrual period (as indicated earlier). Women were classified as *premenopausal* if they reported a period within the past 3 months and no decrease in menstrual bleeding predictability, *early perimenopausal* if they reported a period within the past 3 months but experienced decreased predictability, *late perimenopausal* if they reported 3–11 months of amenorrhea, *postmenopausal* if they had experienced 12 or more months of amenorrhea (without an obvious cause (e.g. pregnancy, lactation, severe weight loss), or *surgically menopausal* if they had had a hysterectomy or bilateral oophorectomy[9].

*Reproductive hormone levels in the early menopause transition*

It is well established that, with aging and the approach of the menopause transition and ovarian senescence, there is a progressive rise in serum FSH and a decrease in serum estradiol (E2) levels[10]. However, the role of race/ethnicity on changing levels of hormones, hormone precursors (such as DHEAS) and related binding proteins, as women approach and traverse the menopause transition, is poorly understood. SWAN's unique study population is facilitating a much broader understanding of the role of race/ethnicity and other key host factors, such as body mass index on reproductive hormone status and dynamics in mid-life women as they approach and traverse the menopause.

Reports from SWAN have emphasized the powerful effect of BMI on the variation of the hormones and precursors evaluated, with decreases in DHEAS[11], E2, FSH, but increases in testosterone as BMI increases within each racial/ethnic group[12].

Significant racial/ethnic differences in E2, testosterone, and DHEAS, but not FSH, were apparent at the baseline visit[12]. In initial analyses, Chinese and Japanese women had the lowest, and

Hispanic and Caucasian women had the highest E2 levels (Figure 1). Testosterone levels were highest in Caucasian and African American women and lowest in Hispanic women, while DHEAS levels were highest in Chinese and lowest in African American women. After adjustment of the analyses for BMI and other confounders (such as menopausal status, day of the cycle, age, smoking and alcohol use), the differences in E2 levels due to race/ethnicity were no longer significant (Figure 2). However, racial/ethnic differences in FSH now became significant with levels which were highest in Hispanic and African American and lowest in Japanese women. Racial/ethnic differences in DHEAS and testosterone remained significant after adjustment[12].

By design, all the women were either premenopausal (54.3%) or early perimenopausal (45.7%) at the baseline visit. Menopausal status had a significant effect on levels of serum FSH and DHEAS such that (mean ± standard deviation) levels of FSH were lower (19.7 ± 17.5 vs. 29.8 ± 31.9 IU/l) while those of DHEAS were higher (135 ± 80 vs. 128 ± 78 µg/dl) in premenopausal compared to early perimenopausal women. However, after adjustment for host characteristics, the only significant differences remaining between pre- and early perimenopausal women were for FSH (20.5 ± 0.4 vs. 25.5 ± 0.5 IU/l). Neither E2 nor testosterone was significantly associated with menopause status before or after adjustment for confounders[12].

*Symptom reporting*

An increased reporting of symptoms such as hot flushes, night sweats, vaginal dryness, urine leakage and difficulty in sleeping is commonly hailed as one of the hallmarks of the menopause transition[1]. Findings from the SWAN cross-sectional screening survey which collected data from over 16 000 women indicate that large proportions of women,

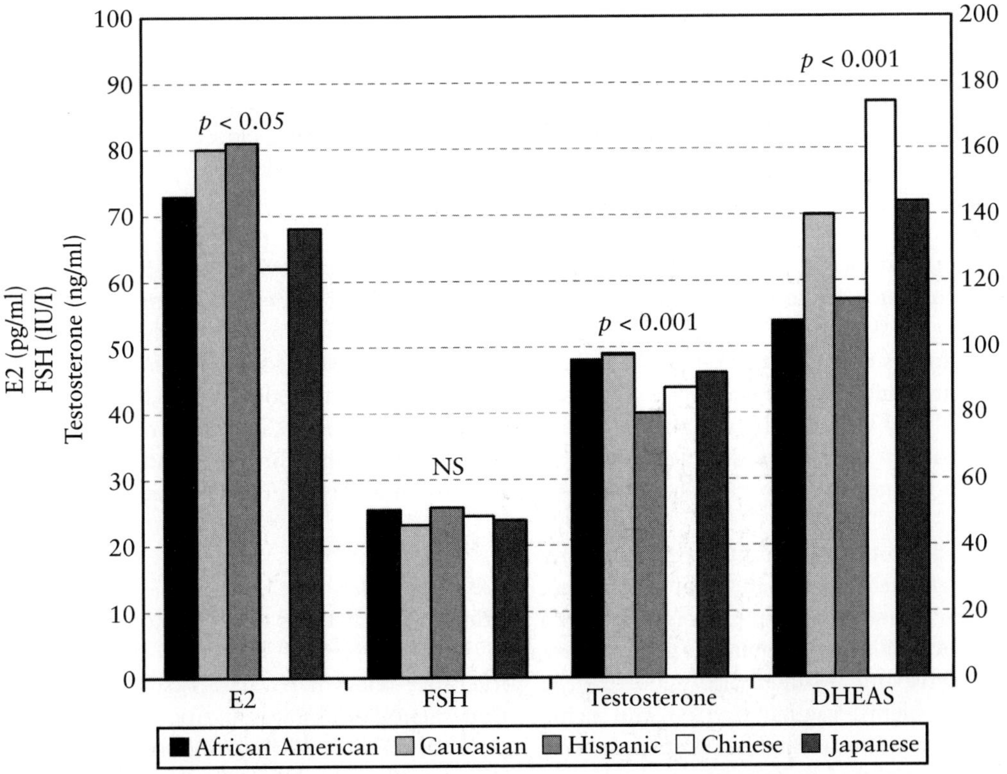


**Figure 1** Unadjusted mean serum hormone concentrations by race/ethnicity. *p* Values are from an ANOVA for racial/ethnic differences. Values are plotted from tables in Randolph JF Jr, Sowers M, Gold EB, *et al. J Clin Endocrinol Metab* 2003;88:1516–22

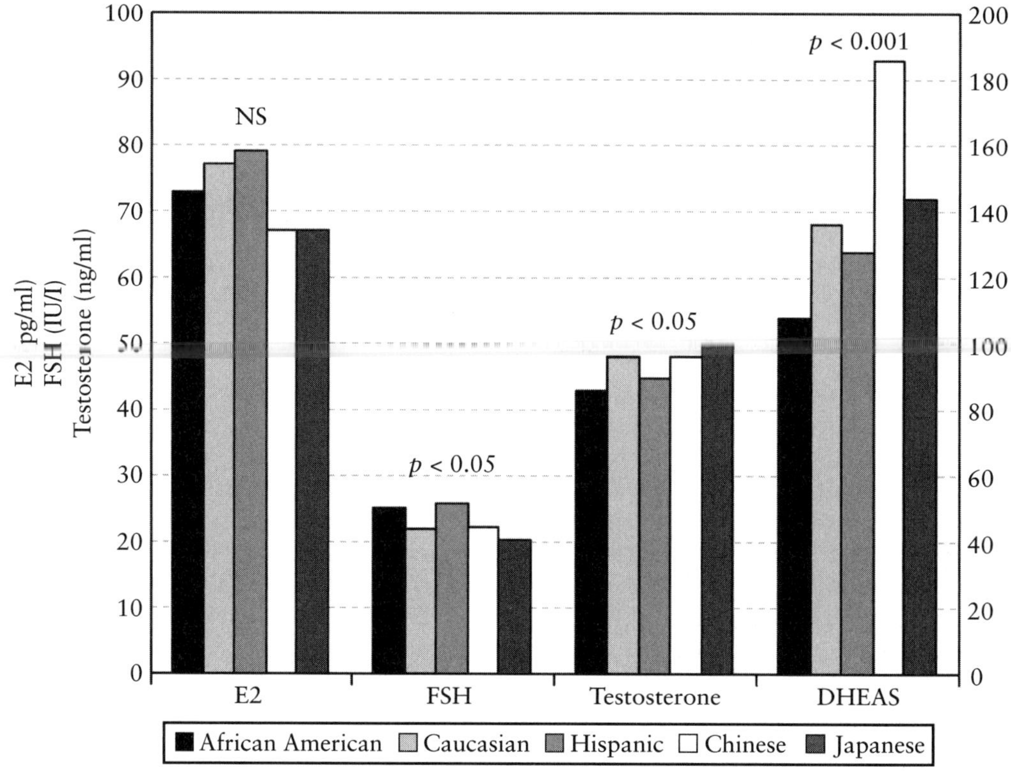


**Figure 2** Adjusted mean serum hormone concentrations by race/ethnicity. Adjusted for menopausal status, day of the cycle, body mass index, age, smoking and alcohol consumption. $p$ Values are from an ANOVA for racial/ethnic differences. Values are plotted from tables in Randolph JF Jr, Sowers M, Gold EB, *et al. J Clin Endocrinol Metab* 2003;88:1516–22

depending on their race/ethnicity, may be affected with symptoms such as hot flushes/night sweats and difficulty in sleeping (Table 1)[9]. The reporting of hot flushes and night sweats (which were combined into one outcome variable as a result of factor analyses) was especially high in African American women (45.6%) and much lower in Japanese and Chinese women (17.6% and 20.5%, respectively).

The second most common symptom, difficulty in sleeping, affected 29% or more of all women, and was reported most often in Caucasian (40.6%) and Hispanic (38.6%) women. A greater proportion of Hispanic women also reported the urogenital problems, vaginal dryness and urine leakage, whereas all four of these complaints were less frequently reported by Japanese and Chinese women. Evaluation of the relationship between menopausal status and symptom reporting showed that the prevalence of hot flushes/night sweat reporting increased from a 'baseline' of 19.4% of premenopausal women to 36.9% of women who had progressed to early perimenopause and then peaked at 56.8% of late perimenopausal women. Symptom reporting was also high in women who had had a spontaneous (48.8%) or a surgical (46.9%) menopause.

*Body mass index*

Multivariate analyses were used to test associations of risk factors with symptoms after adjustment for other relevant covariates (such as age, education, menopausal status, parity, BMI, smoking and physical activity). BMI was significantly associated with hot flushes/night sweats and urine leakage, in that women with a higher BMI (≥ 27 kg/m$^2$) were more likely to report hot flushes (odds

**Table 1** Prevalence of symptom reporting by race/ethnicity and menopausal status. Reproduced with permission from Gold EB, Sternfeld B, Kelsey JL, *et al.* Relation of demographic and lifestyle factors to symptoms in a multiracial/ethnic population of women 40–55 years of age. *Am J Epidemiol* 2000;152:463–73

| | | | *Symptom (%)** | | | |
|---|---|---|---|---|---|---|
| *Characteristics*[†] | *n* | % | *Hot flushes/ night sweats* ($n$ = 3963)[‡] | *Vaginal dryness* ($n$ = 1629) | *Urine leakage* ($n$ = 2135) | *Difficulty in sleeping* ($n$ = 4632) |
| *Race/ethnicity* | | | | | | |
| African American | 3650 | 29.5 | 45.6 | 14.8 | 16.7 | 34.9 |
| Caucasian | 5746 | 46.5 | 31.2 | 11.2 | 18.2 | 40.6 |
| Chinese | 542 | 4.4 | 20.5 | 10.2 | 11.0 | 31.9 |
| Hispanic | 1712 | 13.8 | 35.4 | 20.4 | 19.7 | 38.6 |
| Japanese | 707 | 5.7 | 17.6 | 6.7 | 12.6 | 29.1 |
| *Menopausal status* | | | | | | |
| Premenopausal | 1988 | 16.0 | 19.4 | 7.1 | 12.3 | 30.9 |
| Early perimenopausal | 3547 | 28.6 | 36.9 | 12.9 | 20.6 | 40.6 |
| Late perimenopausal | 611 | 4.9 | 56.8 | 18.2 | 19.6 | 43.9 |
| Postmenopausal | 1753 | 14.2 | 48.8 | 21.2 | 17.7 | 40.4 |
| Surgical | 1988 | 16.0 | 46.9 | 19.4 | 22.1 | 43.5 |

*Crude percentage of women with each symptom (of those reporting) by race ethnicity and menopausal status
[†]Numbers are after exclusions and include those who had missing information for some variables
[‡]$n$ = total number of women reporting 'yes' to a given symptom

ratios ≅ 1.15) and urine leakage (BMI 27–31.9, odds ratio = 1.42 and BMI ≥ 32, odds ratio = 2.18) than women with a lower BMI (19–26.9 kg/m$^2$)[9].

### *Physical activity*

Physical activity was negatively associated with hot flush/night sweats, difficulty in sleeping, vaginal dryness and urine leakage. Women who reported getting much less physical activity than other women their age (the reference group) were more likely to experience these symptoms with odds ratios of 1.64 for vaginal dryness, 1.66 for urine leakage, 1.71 for hot flushes and 2.00 for difficulty in sleeping[9].

### *Smoking*

Previous or current smoking was significantly associated with increased reporting of hot flushes (odds ratios ranged from 1.24 to 1.68, depending on the number of cigarettes smoked). Current smokers were also more likely to report difficulty in sleeping (odds ratios ranged from 1.17 to 1.23). Urine leakage reporting was significantly elevated but only in current smokers of ≥ 20 cigarettes per day (odds ratio = 1.50). There was no clear dose-dependent relationship between number of cigarettes smoked per day and the likelihood of reporting a given symptom[9].

### *Race/ethnicity*

Race ethnicity had a major influence on symptom reporting (Figures 3 and 4). After adjusting for menopause status and demographic and host factors, African American women were significantly more likely to report hot flushes/night sweats and vaginal dryness but less likely to report difficulty in sleeping or urine leakage than Caucasian women (the reference population). Hispanic women were significantly more likely to report vaginal dryness and urine leakage than Caucasian women. Japanese and Chinese women had the lowest odds ratios and thus were least likely to report any of these four symptoms.

### *Menopausal status*

Menopausal status had the most profound associations with symptom reporting compared to other host and demographic predictors (Figure 5 and 6). This was especially true for hot flushes/night

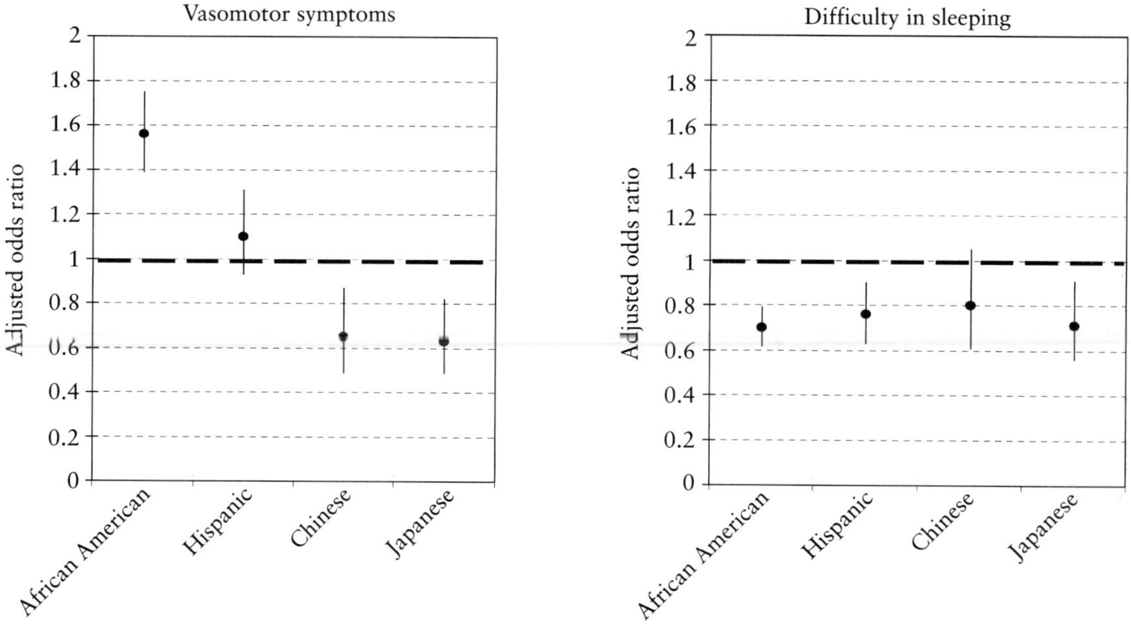


**Figure 3** Racial/ethnic differences in vasomotor symptoms and difficulty in sleeping. Prevalence odds ratios for vasomotor symptoms and difficulty in sleeping by race/ethnicity after adjustment for host factors including age, education, menstrual status, body mass index, smoking, physical activity. Referent category is Caucasian women, depicted as a horizontal dashed line with odds ratio = 1. Odds ratios are plotted from Table 3 in Gold EB, Sternfeld B, Kelsey JL, *et al. Am J Epidemiol* 2000;152:463–73

sweats, where odds ratios ranged from 2 in the early perimenopause to 4.3 in the late perimenopause (compared to the premenopause reference of 1). The likelihood of reporting difficulty in sleeping, vaginal dryness and urine leakage as well as vasomotor symptoms was significantly increased in all subgroups of women who were early perimenopausal or more advanced in menopausal status in comparison to premenopausal women. The patterns of increased symptom reporting across the different stages of the menopause transition varied substantially by the particular symptom under consideration. For example, the likelihood of reporting vasomotor symptoms peaked in the late perimenopause and declined thereafter, whereas the likelihood of reporting urine leakage was highest in the early perimenopause, with subsequent declines in late peri- and natural postmenopause. Women with a surgical menopause had odds ratios for urine leakage comparable to those in the early perimenopause.

*Continuing studies in SWAN*

In elucidating the hormone dynamics of the menopause transition in five different ethnic groups, SWAN investigators hope to also identify sensitive/specific early markers of the onset and various stages of the menopause transition. Other study aims are to determine the impact of the menopause transition and the changing hormonal milieu on quality-of-life domains such as symptoms, cognitive function, mood, sleep, sexuality and depression. Changes in bone density, body composition and risk factors for cardiovascular disease will be comprehensively evaluated to understand the contribution of menopause versus aging on the development of the chronic diseases of old age.

## The Pennsylvania Ovarian Aging Study

The Penn Ovarian Aging Study is a prospective population-based longitudinal cohort study of ovarian aging in 218 African American and 218

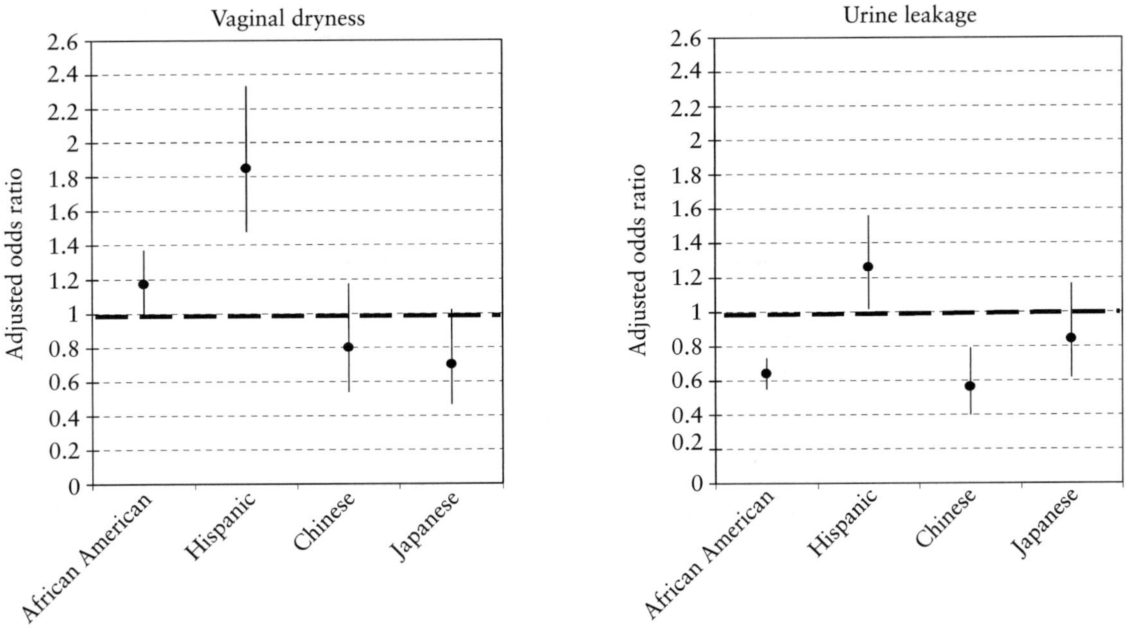


**Figure 4** Racial/ethnic differences in vaginal dryness and urine leakage. Prevalence odds ratios for vaginal dryness and urine leakage by race/ethnicity after adjustment for host factors including age, education, menstrual status, body mass index, smoking, physical activity. Referent category is Caucasian women, depicted as a horizontal dashed line with odds ratio = 1. Odds ratios are plotted from Table 3 in Gold EB, Sternfeld B, Kelsey JL, *et al.* *Am J Epidemiol* 2000;152:463–73

Caucasian women in their late reproductive years[13]. The participants reside in Philadelphia County, were 35 and 47 years at enrollment and will be followed until they are 45–52 years old. Study objectives were to evaluate:

(1) Hormone (FSH, E2, DHEAS, and inhibin) dynamics over the menopause transition;

(2) Menopause-related symptoms and factors influencing their severity;

(3) The associations of alterations in hormone levels with biological and psychological predictors and/or outcomes (e.g. body mass, hot flushes, depression, sleep disturbance); and

(4) Ethnic/racial differences in these associations.

Eligibility criteria required intact ovaries and uterus and menstrual cycles in the range of 22–35 days for the 3 months prior to enrollment.

In analyses of hormone levels measured four times over 9 months in sera from the early follicular phase of the menstrual cycle, Freeman found that mean levels of E2 and FSH (generally > 25 pg/ml and < 10 mIU/ml, respectively) indicated that the cohort had not progressed far, if at all, into the menopause transition. Estradiol levels in this cohort were significantly lower in African American compared to Caucasian women at the initial (37.4 vs. 305 pg/ml) but not subsequent visits[14]. While DHEAS was significantly lower in African American compared to Caucasian women in this cohort (consistent with SWAN findings), there were no differences due to race/ethnicity in either mean FSH or testosterone levels. BMI was a significant predictor of E2 and DHEAS levels but only in the African American group, where increasing BMI was significantly associated with lower E2 and higher DHEAS levels. Similar to the findings in SWAN, increasing BMI was associated with increasing levels of testosterone in both Caucasian and African American women.

Hot flushes were reported by nearly one-third of the women – a surprisingly high prevalence for women who were 35–47 years old (mean age 41

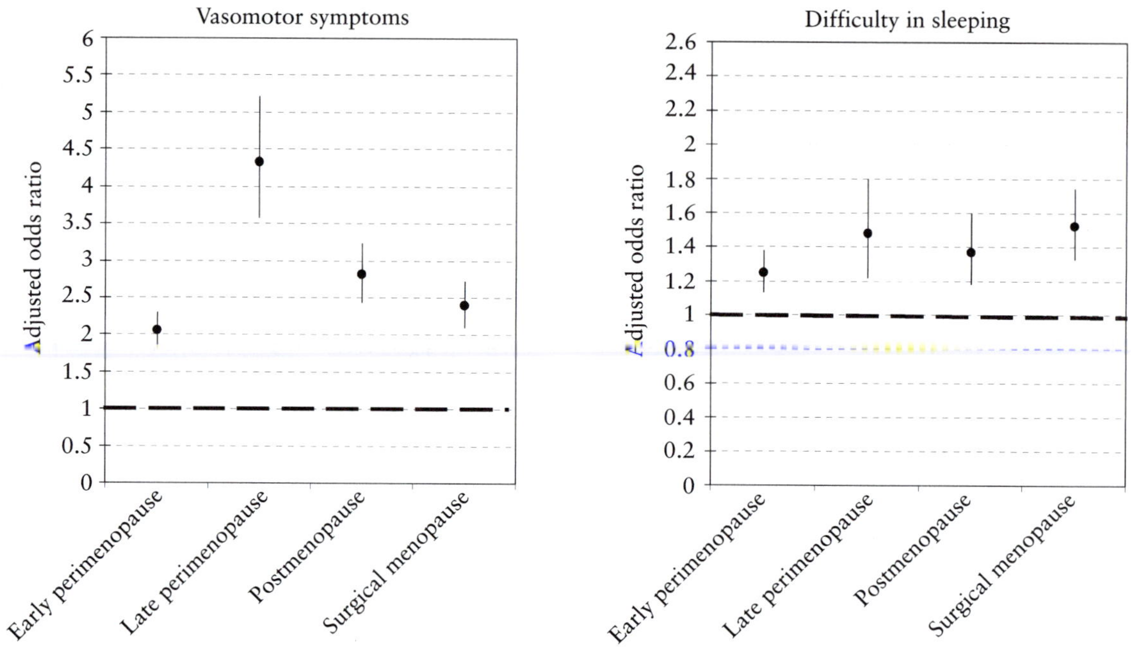


**Figure 5** Differences in vasomotor symptoms and difficulty in sleeping by menopause status. Prevalence odds ratios for vasomotor symptoms and difficulty in sleeping by menopause status after adjustment for host factors including age, education, race/ethnicity, body mass index, smoking, physical activity. Referent category is premenopause, depicted as a horizontal dashed line with odds ratio = 1. Odds ratios are plotted from Table 3 in Gold EB, Sternfeld B, Kelsey JL, *et al. Am J Epidemiol* 2000;152:463–73

years) and still premenopausal with regular periods. Furthermore, there were significant differences due to race/ethnicity ($p = 0.01$), with 38% of African American vs 25% of Caucasian women reporting this symptom. A number of host factors were significantly associated with, and hence predictive of, hot flushes: higher FSH levels (odds ratio = 3.19), anxiety (odds ratio = 1.06), baseline menopausal symptoms (odds ratio = 4.91), alcohol use (odds ratio = 1.09), BMI (odds ratio = 1.04) and parity (odds ratio = 1.20). After adjustment for these factors, the racial/ethnic differences in hot flush reporting were no longer significant. Because a number of factors, such as anxiety, BMI and alcohol consumption are potentially modifiable, these findings may be useful in developing strategies to reduce the burden of hot flushes as women approach reproductive senescence[15].

## CONCLUSION

The findings from SWAN and the Penn Ovarian Aging study underscore the importance of race/ethnicity as a determinant of levels of reproductive hormones (estradiol, testosterone, FSH) and precursors (DHEAS). Race/ethnicity is also a prominent predictor of symptom reporting in women as they enter the menopause transition and progress to their final menstrual period and beyond. SWAN analyses are demonstrating how the prevalence of a given symptom varies additionally by stage of the menopause transition and other demographic and host factors, such as age, BMI, smoking and physical activity. Because a number of factors (BMI, smoking and physical activity), which are significantly associated with symptom reporting, are potentially modifiable, when conventional medical strategies, such as

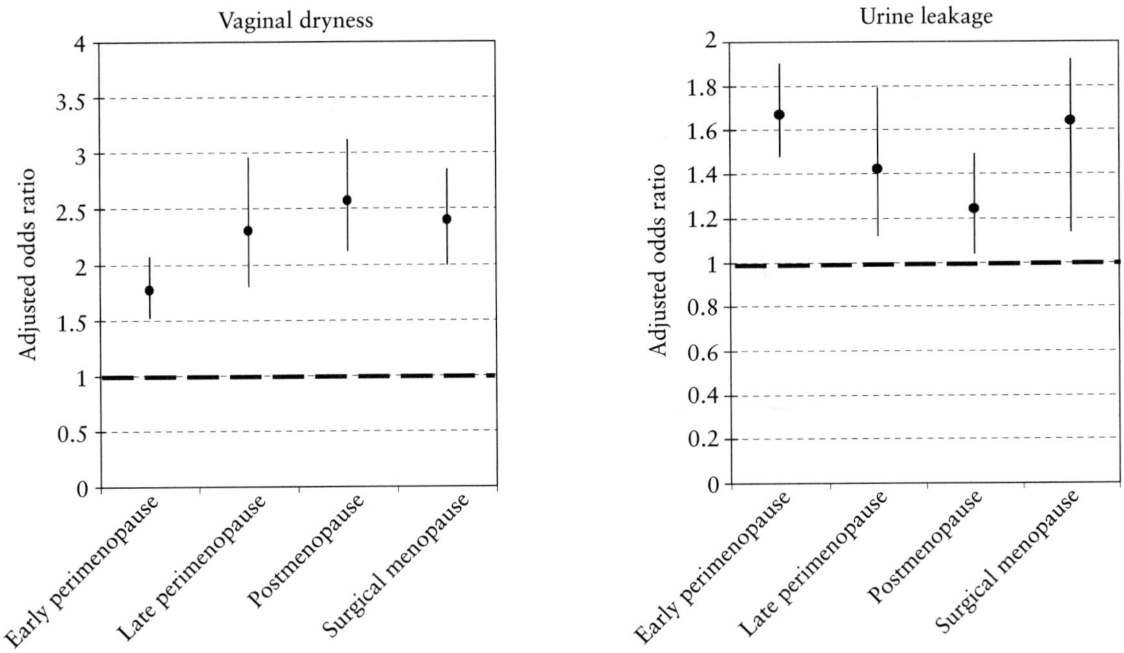


**Figure 6** Differences in vaginal dryness and urine leakage by menopause status. Prevalence odds ratios for vaginal dryness and urine leakage by menopause status after adjustment for host factors including age, education, race/ethnicity, body mass index, smoking, physical activity. Referent category is premenopause, depicted as a horizontal dashed line with odds ratio = 1. Odds ratios are plotted from Table 3 in Gold EB, Sternfeld B, Kelsey JL, *et al. Am J Epidemiol* 2000;152:463–73

menopausal hormone therapy are contraindicated or unacceptable, alternative approaches involving lifestyle and behavioral modification may help to reduce the burden of menopause-related symptoms. These and other scientific advances from NIA-supported studies on menopause will help to pave the way in formulating strategies which are more effective in ameliorating menopause-related symptomatology and preventing or delaying deleterious changes associated with the development of age-related conditions and diseases.

## References


1. Greendale GA, Lee NP, Arriola ER.The menopause. *Lancet* 1999;353:571–80
2. Riggs BL, Khosla S, Melton LJ 3rd. A unitary model for involutional osteoporosis: estrogen deficiency causes both type I and type II osteoporosis in postmenopausal women and contributes to bone loss in aging men. *J Bone Miner Res* 1998;13:763–73
3. Lock M. Menopause in cultural context. *Exp Gerontol* 1994;29:307–17
4. http://www.nia.nih.gov/about/history.htm
5. McKinlay SM, Brambilla DJ, Posner JG. The normal menopause transition. *Am J Hum Biol* 1992;4:37–46
6. Brambilla DJ, McKinlay SM, Johannes CB. Defining the perimenopause for application in epidemiologic investigations. *Am J Epidemiol* 1994;140:1091–5

7. Menopause And Health In Aging Women, RFA AG-94-002, NIH GUIDE, September 3, 1993;22 (32) http://grants2.nih.gov/grants/guide/rfa-files/RFA-AG-94-002.html
8. Sowers MF, Crawford S, Sternfeld B, *et al.* SWAN: a multi-center, multi-ethnic, community-based cohort study of women and the menopausal transition. In Lobo R, Marcus R, Kelsey J, eds. *Menopause.* New York: Academic Press, 2000:175–88
9. Gold EB, Sternfeld B, Kelsey JL, *et al.* Relation of demographic and lifestyle factors to symptoms in a multi-racial/ethnic population of women 40–55 years of age. *Am J Epidemiol* 2000;152:463–73
10. Burger HG, Dudley EC, Hopper JL, *et al.* Prospectively measured levels of serum follicle-stimulating hormone, estradiol, and the dimeric inhibins during the menopausal transition in a population-based cohort of women. *J Clin Endocrinol Metab* 1999;84:4025–30
11. Lasley BL, Santoro N, Randolf J, *et al.* The relationship of circulating dehydroepiandrosterone, testosterone, and estradiol to stages of the menopausal transition and ethnicity. *J Clin Endocrinol Metab* 2002;87:3760–7
12. Randolph JF Jr, Sowers M, Gold EB, *et al.* Reproductive hormones in the early menopausal transition: relationship to ethnicity, body size, and menopausal status. *J Clin Endocrinol Metab* 2003; 88:1516–22
13. Freeman EW, Grisso JA, Berlin J, *et al.* Symptom reports from a cohort of African American and white women in the late reproductive years. *Menopause* 2001;8:33–42
14. Manson JM, Sammel MD, Freeman EW, Grisso JA. Racial differences in sex hormone levels in women approaching the transition to menopause. *Fertil Steril* 2001;75:297–304
15. Freeman EW, Sammel MD, Grisso JA, *et al.* Hot flashes in the late reproductive years: risk factors for Africa American and Caucasian women. *J Women's Health Gend Based Med* 2001; 10:67–76

# Major findings of the Melbourne Women's Midlife Health Project

4

*L. Dennerstein, J. R. Guthrie, J. R. Taffe, P. Lehert and H. G. Burger*

## INTRODUCTION

The Melbourne Women's Midlife Health Project (MWMHP) commenced in 1991 in order to provide documentation about women's experience of the menopausal transition and the relative role of endocrine, psychosocial and lifestyle factors. The study was designed to provide information on risk factors for longer-term health outcomes, such as those of osteoporosis and cardiovascular disease.

In order to reduce the methodological problems of earlier studies related to the use of convenience samples or recall bias, a population sample was chosen and a prospective design. The Melbourne research team was allowed access to a questionnaire used in North American population studies[1,2]. Important differences in the Melbourne study were the use of a validated well-being questionnaire[3], an inquiry about sexual functioning, and annual physical measures and blood collection. The Melbourne Project was established at the outset as collaboration between scientists from a range of disciplines and, over the years, 16 co-investigators have contributed to the project. The questions asked and the methods employed (qualitative and quantitative) reflect the integration of a broad range of approaches (public health, biomedical, psychological, sociological), together with the views expressed by women themselves.

## METHODS

The study was approved by the Human Research Ethics Committee of the University of Melbourne and the procedures followed were in accordance with the ethical standards of the National Health & Medical Research Council. All subjects provided written informed consent for their participation in the study.

The MWMHP was a population-based observational study that included both cross-sectional and longitudinal phases. The first stage was the cross-sectional study of 2001 Australian-born women aged 45–55 years who completed a 20–25-min telephone interview. The second stage was a 9-year follow-up of 438 of these women who at the time of their initial telephone interview had menstruated in the last 3 months (had an intact uterus and at least one ovary) and were not taking hormone therapy (HT) or the oral contraceptive pill. The women in the longitudinal study were interviewed and had physical measurements and blood taken annually in their own homes for 8 years of follow-up. In the 9th year of follow-up, only women who were still menstruating and who had never taken HT were interviewed ($n = 51$).

### Sample derivation

In 1991, a random sample of households in Melbourne was generated from a database of the telephone numbers from the Melbourne telephone directory. The response rate among those women eligible and available for the study was 70.6% ($n = 2001$). The number of subjects eligible for analysis was 1897.

From the cross-sectional cohort, 779 women met the eligibility criteria for the longitudinal study. Interviews were completed for 438 of these women, giving a response rate of 56%.

### Measures and analyses

Fasting morning blood samples were collected annually. Blood was taken between the 4th and 8th days of the menstrual cycle in cycling women. For those not cycling, blood was taken after 3 months or more of amenorrhea. Estradiol was measured using the double antibody radioimmunoassay (RIA) kit purchased from Diagnostic Products Corporation (DPC), Los Angeles, USA. Serum testosterone was measured by double antibody RIA, following sample extraction and polyethylene glycol-enhanced separation of bound from free ligand, using $^{125}$I iodinated testosterone as tracer. Sex hormone binding globulin (SHBG) and dehydroepiandrosterone sulfate (DHEAS) were measured by an automated chemiluminescent enzyme immunoassay (Diagnostic Products) using the Immulite Automated Analyser. Free testosterone index (FTI) was calculated as the ratio of measured testosterone to measured SHBG × 100. Total cholesterol and high density lipoprotein cholesterol (HDL-C) and triglycerides were measured according to standard enzymatic methods on routine automated chemistry systems. Low density lipoprotein cholesterol (LDL-C) was calculated using the Friedwald formula adapted for Systeme International (SI) units. Plasma glucose was measured using the hexokinase method and performed on Dimension clinical chemistry systems (Dade International Inc. Newark, USA). Insulin was measured by RIA using Linco Human Insulin Specific kits (Linco, Missouri, USA).

The following physical measures were recorded annually: body height, body weight, body mass index (BMI) (calculated as weight (kg)/height ($m^2$)), waist and hip circumference, four skin-fold thicknesses - triceps, biceps, subscapular and supra-iliac (measured using Harpenden skin-fold callipers), systolic and diastolic blood pressures. Bone mineral density and total body composition were measured at 2-yearly intervals by dual-energy X-ray absorptiometry, using a Hologic QDR-1000W densitometer.

The core questionnaire included variables relating to education, employment, marital status, parity, well-being[3], interpersonal stress, lifestyle factors, general somatic problems, menopausal symptoms, attitudes to aging and menopause, health behaviors, health status (self-rated health, chronic conditions, other health problems), family medical history, prescription and non-prescription medication use, health-care use, medical procedures, reproductive and menstrual histories, and problematic premenstrual complaints. Menstrual diaries and supplementary questionnaires for information on sexuality, hassles, physical activity, diet, experience of physical and sexual abuse are documented in detail in the specific references. Menstrual status was used to determine menopausal status as follows: premenopause was used to refer to those women who reported no change in menstrual frequency; early menopause transition (EMT) was used to refer to women when they reported changes in menstrual frequency; late menopausal transition (LMP) was used once they reported at least 3 months but less than 12 months amenorrhea; and postmenopause was used when there were 12 or more months of amenorrhea. Women were separately categorized if they used oral contraceptives, hormone therapy or had undergone induced or surgical menopause. The above definitions are similar to those developed by the Stages of Reproductive Aging Conference[4].

Data were analyzed both cross-sectionally and longitudinally. Cross-sectional analyses of the baseline sample of 1897 women enabled the description of the following variables according to menopausal status and the estimate of associations with other factors: well-being[5], self-rated health[6], symptoms[7,8], sexuality[9]. Cross-sectional analysis can only indicate whether associations exist and are unable to determine the direction of causality. Also, cross-sectional analyses cannot control for premenopausal characteristics or separate the effects of aging from those of menopause. The strength of the MWMHP lies in the prospective arm of the study, the results of which are detailed here.

The prospective phase of the MWMHP involved the repeated collection of data or measures from the same individuals followed over time. A number of statistical approaches were utilized and are described in detail in the specific papers. Some analyses involved examining the effect of reaching the final menstrual period and, in this case, analysis of covariance was used after dividing the data into premenopausal/EMT, and LMT/postmenopausal series and adjusting for the premenopausal values. Another technique was repeated-measurement multivariate analysis of variance using a number of contrasts to estimate various effects. Random effect time series regression models were also used and this allowed the separate estimation of the effect of differences between, and the effect of changes within, women with regard to the outcome variable. Structural equation modeling was used for examination in detail of a range of factors that may influence the studied end-point, the presence of feedback and of latent or non-measurable variables. The MWMHP investigators have published discussion papers on the various statistical techniques available for analysis of change in longitudinal studies of the menopause[10], methodological issues related to menstrual diary data[11], the derivation, evaluation, validity and reliability of a short scale to assess female sexual functioning[12-15], and measurement of physical activity in mid-life women[16].

## RESULTS

Comparing the 438 participants with the 341 non-participants[17], more of the study participants reported that they:

(1) Had better health than most in comparison with women of the same age (48.5% vs. 38.1%; $p < 0.005$);

(2) Were in paid employment (71.4% vs. 63.0%; $p < 0.05$);

(3) Had more than 12 years of education (34.3% vs. 24.3%; $p < 0.005$);

(4) Had had a Papanicolaou smear (58.3% vs. 50.0%; $p < 0.05$);

(5) Exercised at least once a week (68.0% vs. 58.1%; $p < 0.005$); and

(6) Had undergone dilatation and curettage (46.5% vs. 38.4%; $p < 0.05$).

Participants did not differ in age, body mass index (BMI), marital status, parity, symptoms, well-being, interpersonal stress, number of surgical procedures, proportion of current smokers, recent alcohol consumption, house-hold composition, proportion who had breast checks in the last year, proportion who had a tubal ligation, use of medications, treatment for chronic conditions, and suffering from premenstrual complaints. Table 1 shows the proportion reaching natural or surgical menopause by year of follow-up[18].

Ten (5%) of the 224 women who had experienced the natural menopause transition reported an unexplained 'menstrual cycle' bleed more than 12 months after their last menstrual period[19].

### Hormonal changes

Figures 1 and 2 show the changes in levels of estradiol, follicle stimulating hormone (FSH), testosterone and FTI, in relation to final menstrual period. Most of the changes in FSH and estradiol were observed during the 18 months on either side of the final menstrual period. Between 2 and 5 years after the final menstrual period, mean estradiol levels reached the sensitivity level for the assay (20 pmol/l)[20].

Mean SHBG levels decreased during the menopausal transition, the time of maximum change being estimated at 2 years before the final menstrual period. SHBG was negatively associated with BMI ($p < 0.0001$) and positively associated with estradiol levels ($p < 0.0001$). Mean levels of testosterone did not vary across the menopausal transition and were also not related to age in this

**Table 1** Longitudinal study phase. $n = 438$ at baseline

| *Follow-up year* | *Women reaching natural menopause* | *Women having surgical menopause* | *Women receiving HT prior to FMP* | *Women who had not reached FMP* | *Women who dropped out* |
|---|---|---|---|---|---|
| Year 3 | 13% | 2% | 18% | 60% | 7% |
| Year 6 | 36% | 7% | 25% | 22% | 10% |
| Year 9 | 51% | 8% | 21% | 8% | 12% |

HT, hormone therapy; FMP, final menstrual period

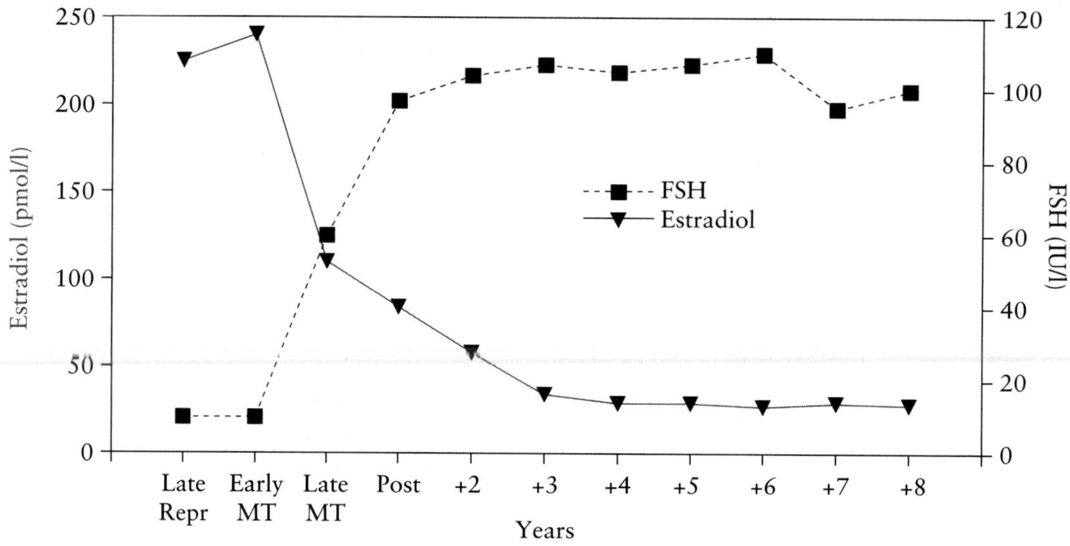


**Figure 1** Hormone changes and reproductive aging. MT, menopausal transition

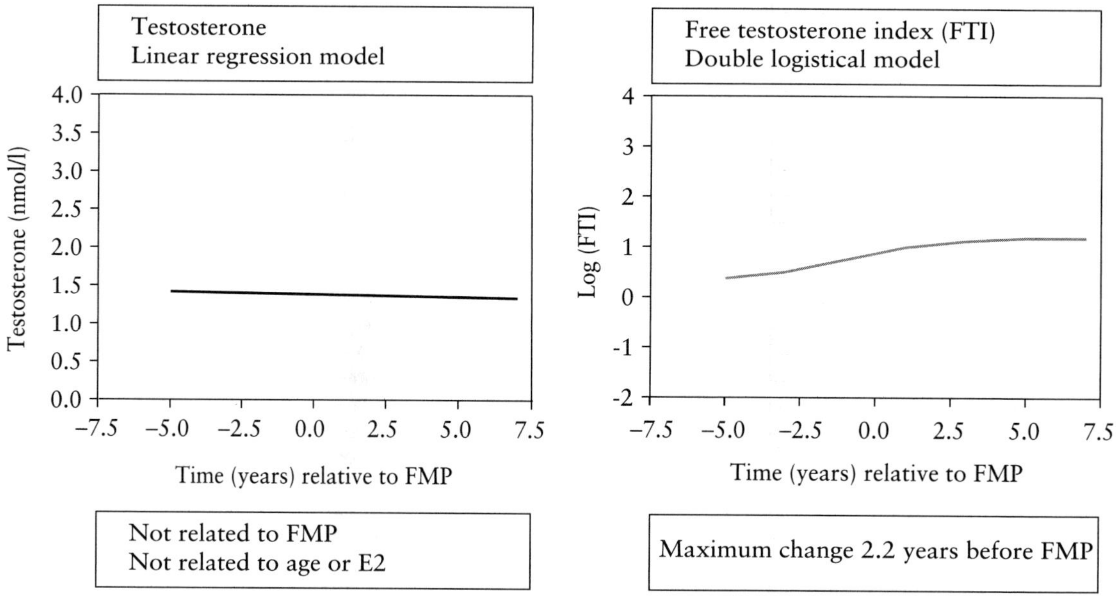


**Figure 2** Testosterone models. FMP, final menstrual period; E2, estradiol

cohort. Mean levels of FTI increased with time relative to the final menstrual period by 80% over a 6-year period, from 1.5 at 4 years before the final menstrual period to 2.7 at 2 years after the final menstrual period. The time of maximum change was estimated to be 2.2 years before the final menstrual period. FTI was also positively associated with BMI, with an average increase of 4% for each unit increase in BMI ($p < 0.001$). Mean levels of DHEAS were not related to the final menstrual period, but decreased with increasing age and BMI (both $p < 0.05$)[21].

## Changes in health outcomes

*Symptoms*

We used summary statistics to compare the rate of bothersome symptom-reporting before and after late menopausal transition, as this is the phase of maximum endocrine change. The symptoms that are specifically related to the hormonal changes of the menopausal transition are vasomotor symptoms, insomnia, vaginal dryness, and breast tenderness (see Figure 3). The reporting of vasomotor symptoms and vaginal dryness increased as women progressed from early to late menopausal transition, whereas breast soreness/tenderness decreased during this period. Insomnia also increased during the transition and was found to reflect bothersome hot flushes and psychosocial factors[22].

The frequency of reporting bothersome hot flushes commences to rise about 2 years before the final menstrual period and reaches a maximum about 2 years after the final menstrual period[23]. There is a gradual decrease in frequency, reaching premenopausal levels after a further 6 years (see Figure 4). Approximately 75% of our cohort reported suffering bothersome hot flushes at some time during the transition. From a list of 22 general somatic and menopausal symptoms, women reported an annual mean of four to five bothersome symptoms.

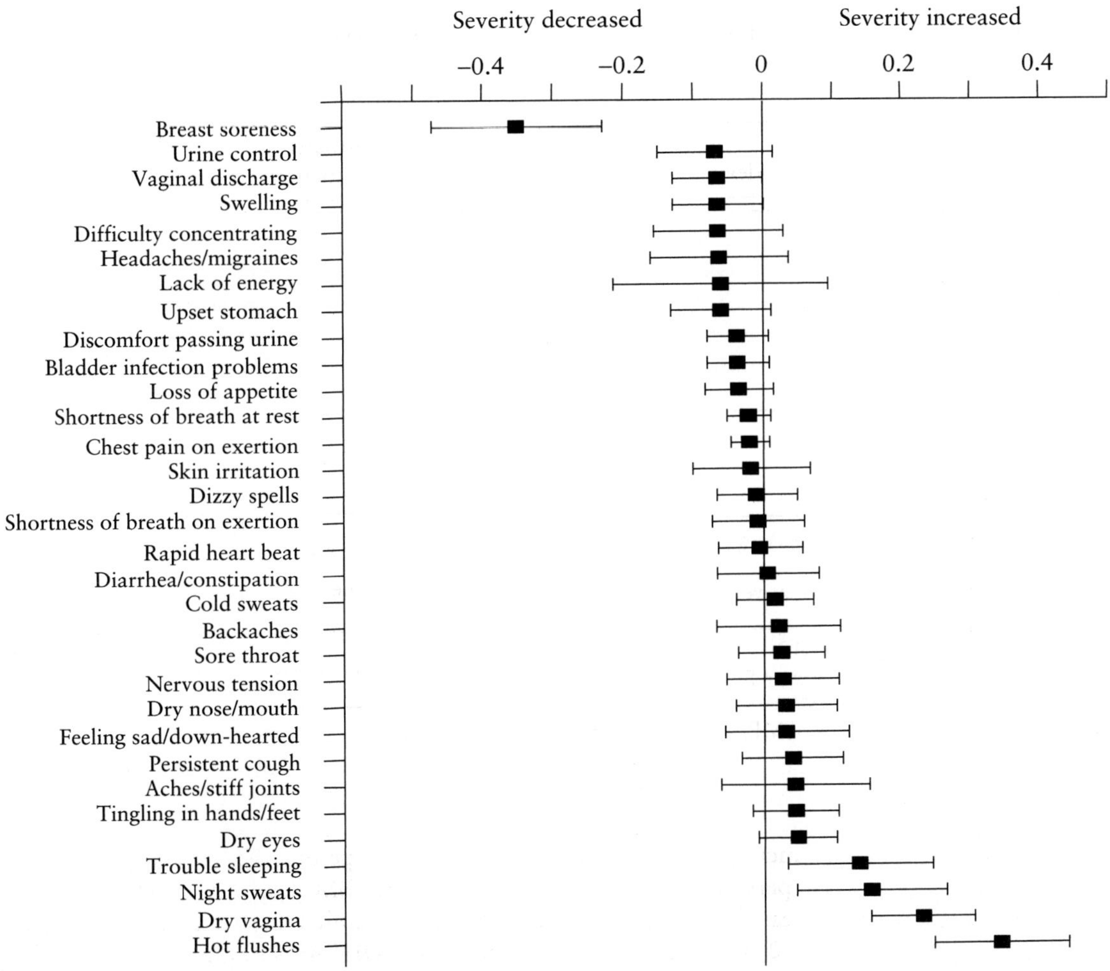


**Figure 3** Mean (± 95% confidence interval) change in symptom scores: pre- and early perimenopause versus late peri- and postmenopause

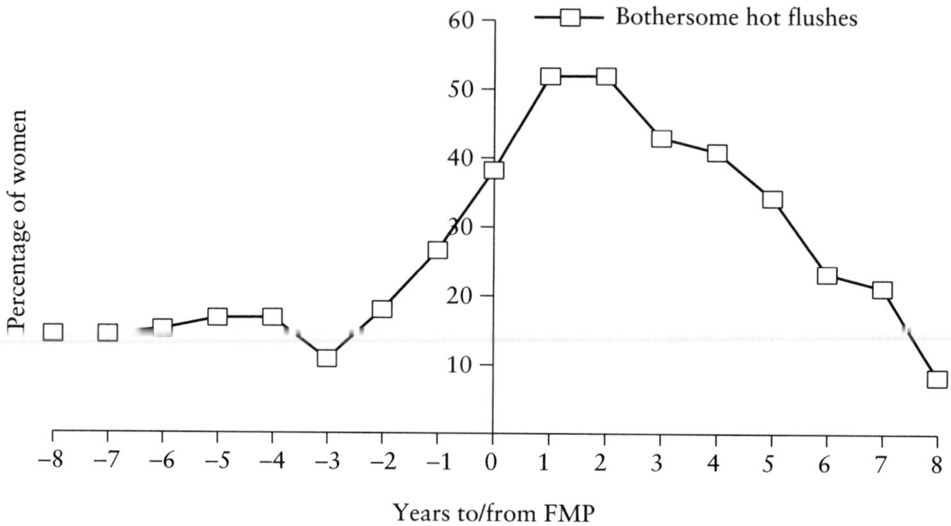


**Figure 4** Hot flushes and final menstrual period (FMP). Adapted with permission from reference 23

After 3 years of follow-up, data were analyzed to evaluate whether a history of menstrually related problems (premenstrual complaints) was a significant predictive marker of a more symptomatic menopausal transition experience. Significant relationships were found between a prior history of both physical and psychological premenstrual complaints and a more symptomatic transition, characterized by dysphoria, skeletal, digestive and respiratory symptoms[24].

*Depression*

Depression was assessed using the negative mood subscale of a validated measure of psychological well-being, the Affectometer 2[3]. Longitudinal analysis of 6 follow-up years using repeated measures multivariate analysis of covariance found that negative mood scores decreased significantly over time and were not directly related to the natural menopausal transition, hormone levels, age or education[25]. The magnitude of negative mood was significantly predicted by baseline reporting of premenstrual complaints, negative attitudes to aging and menopause, and parity of one. During follow-up, the magnitude of negative mood was significantly adversely affected by prior experience of negative mood, experience of bothersome symptoms, poor self-rated health, negative feelings for partner, no partner, current smoking, low exercise, daily hassles, and high stress. Negative mood was reduced by decreasing symptoms, improving health, positive feelings for partner, gaining a partner, and reducing stress. The menopausal transition had an indirect effect in amplifying the effect of stressors such as reducing paid work, poor health and daily hassles[25].

In a separate analysis, we examined the effect on mood of children leaving or re-entering the home. For the majority of women, the departure of the last child from the household leads to positive changes in women's mood state and a reduced number of daily hassles. Return of offspring may have an adverse effect on sexual relating of parents[26].

*Sexuality*

Women's sexuality during the menopausal transition was investigated using the Personal Experiences Questionnaire[12], which was derived from the McCoy Female Sexuality Questionnaire[27]. The questionnaire was shortened using an optimization technique which retained six sexual function domains: feelings for partner, sexual responsivity, frequency of sexual activities, libido, partner problems, dyspareunia/vaginal dryness. A total sex score was obtained by summing the scores for sexual responsivity, sexual frequency and libido.

A total score of 7 or less indicated sexual dysfunction[14].

From early to late menopausal transition, the percentage of women with scores indicating sexual dysfunction increased from 42% to 88%[28]. There was a significant decline in libido, sexual responsivity, frequency of sex activities and women's feelings towards their partner, and a significant increase in vaginal dryness/dyspareunia and partner problems associated with the menopausal transition[29]. In the early menopausal transition, women with low total sex scores had lower estradiol levels but similar androgen levels to those with higher scores[28]. Decreasing total SPEQ scores and sexual domain scores of libido and sexual responsivity correlated with decreasing estradiol levels, but not with androgen levels[28].

Further modeling of sexual functioning found that libido could be classified with responsivity and this new domain was called sexual response[15]. We found that the sexual behavior of a mid-life woman was predominantly determined by her previous behavior, change in partner status and feelings towards her partner. These factors explain more than 50% of the variability on both sexual frequency and response[15]. Using structural equation modeling, estradiol was found to have an additional effect on sexual response and dyspareunia.

## Body composition

*Bone mineral density*

Changes in bone mineral density (BMD), weight, amount and distribution of body fat during the menopausal transition were described and variables associated with these changes determined.

In our cohort, a change in menopausal status from premenopausal/EMT to late menopausal transition was associated with an annual change in BMD of −0.9% at the lumbar spine and −0.7% at the femoral neck. The change to postmenopausal status was associated with a change of −2.5% at the lumbar spine and −1.7% at the femoral neck. All these changes were significantly greater than those in women who remained premenopausal or in the EMT[30]. The Australian-born cohort had multiple risk factors for osteoporosis, but only anthropometric values (BMI, waist, hip, trunk skin-fold measures) were associated with BMD at baseline. Significant changes during the menopausal transition in anthropometric variables and calcium intake were in the direction that could decrease the risk of osteoporosis but were not found to have an effect on bone loss[30,31].

Estradiol was the only endogenous hormone to have a significant effect on BMD during the menopausal transition. An estradiol level of about 240 pmol/l was required for the preservation of BMD during the transition[32].

*Weight*

Suprailiac skin-fold measurements, waist circumference and waist/hip ratio all increased during the menopausal transition. Continuous hormone therapy users showed no gain in mean weight, suprailiac skin-fold or waist measurements over the follow-up period[33]. By the 8th year of follow-up, 58% of the cohort had a BMI of 25 or greater and were classified as being overweight.

*Central abdominal fat*

A sample of the cohort ($n = 102$) had their whole body composition measured using dual-energy X-ray absorptiometry (DXA) in the 6th year of follow-up. Women in the early menopausal transition had significantly lower percentage body fat than women in the later stages of the menopausal transition. The percentage fat in the central abdominal area was estimated from the DXA scans, and multiple regression analysis found it was positively associated with current weight, increase in weight since baseline, baseline FTI and with the increase in free testosterone since baseline[34].

*Cardiovascular health*

Analysis of risk of coronary heart disease (CHD) incorporated a scoring scheme (PROCAM) to estimate the global risk of CHD, and data from 8 years of follow-up were used. This analysis found that higher than average BMI and free testosterone, lower than average estradiol and an increase in BMI and a decrease in estradiol levels during the study period were associated with an increase in CHD risk[35].

## DISCUSSION AND CONCLUSIONS

The MWMHP has enabled description of the underlying hormonal changes of the natural menopausal transition and documented changes in a number of health parameters and in a wide range of determinants including psychosocial, lifestyle and biological factors. We have contributed to the development of rigorous methods and novel analytic techniques for cohort studies of the menopause. The limitations of the project are the lack of ethnic diversity, a possible healthy participant bias, and that the proportion of the sample with adequate exercise or calcium levels to protect against osteoporosis was small.

The longitudinal cohort of the MWMHP is now in the 12th year of follow-up. Areas of investigation include: further cognitive function testing, HT and brain function, prevalence and determinants of osteoarthritis, role of inflammatory markers in bone mineral density, cardiovascular disease and brain function, and determinants of breast density.

In conclusion, this longitudinal study, with adequate measures of health outcomes and data on a range of hormonal, psychosocial and lifestyle variables, has provided important information on changes during the menopausal transition. The project has identified the changes in hormone levels during the natural menopausal transition, those health changes significantly associated with declining estradiol and the risk factors for a range of health outcomes.


## ACKNOWLEDGEMENTS

We would like to thank all the study participants who gave so generously of their time in order to make this project a success. We would like to thank the following co-investigators and researchers who were involved in this study: Adele Green, John Hopper, Peter Ebeling, John Wark, Mark Wahlqvist, Madeleine Ball, Carol Morse, Alastair MacLennan, Anthony Smith, Julia Shelley, Maggi Ryan, David Purdie, Emma Dudley, Corry Garamszegi, Heather Amiconi, Margaret Bolton and Joan Rudder. We would also like to thank Mr Nick Balazs and the staff of the Department of Biochemistry at the Monash Medical Centre for the hormone and lipid assays. The authors would like to thank Margaret Clark and Nicola Blaxill for help with the manuscript.

*Source of funding*: Between 1991 and 2000 research from the Victoria Health Promotion Foundation, the Public Health Research and Development Committee of the Australian National Health and Medical, the University of Melbourne, Australian Dairy Corporation, Percy Baxter Trust, H & L Hecht Trust, Estate of the late Daniel Scott, Ian Potter Foundation, Smorgan Family Trust, Leigh & Marjorie Bronwen Murray Trust, Helen M Schutt Trust, the Australasian Menopause Society, the ANZ Trustees, Eli Lilly Ltd and Pharmacia. Organon Australia Pty Ltd provided a grant to Prince Henry's Medical Research Institute for the blood measurements. The project has a current grant (2002–03) from Wyeth America Pty Ltd.


# References


1. Kaufert P. Women and their health in the middle years: A Manitoba project. *Soc Sci Med* 1984;18: 279–81
2. McKinlay S, Brambilla D, Posner J. The normal menopause transition. *Am J Hum Biol* 1992;4: 37–46
3. Kammann R, Flett R. Affectometer 2: a scale to measure current level of general happiness. *Aust J Psychol* 1983;35:259–65
4. Soules MR, Sherman S, Parrott E, *et al.* Executive summary: Stages of Reproductive Aging Workshop (Straw) [comment]. *Fertil Steril* 2001;76:874–78
5. Dennerstein L, Smith AM, Morse C. Psychological well-being, mid-life and the menopause [comment]. *Maturitas* 1994;20:1–11
6. Smith AM, Shelley JM, Dennerstein L. Self-rated health: biological continuum or social discontinuity? *Soc Sci Med* 1994;39:77–83

7. Dennerstein L, Smith AM, Morse C, *et al.* Menopausal symptoms in Australian women. *Med J Aust* 1993;159:232-6
8. Guthrie JR, Dennerstein L, Hopper JL, Burger HG. Hot flushes, menstrual status, and hormone levels in a population-based sample of midlife women. *Obstet Gynecol* 1996;88:437-42
9. Dennerstein L, Smith AM, Morse CA, Burger HG. Sexuality and the menopause. *J Psychosomat Obstet Gynecol* 1994;15:59-66
10. Lehert P, Dennerstein L. Statistical techniques for the analysis of change in longitudinal studies of the menopause. *Acta Obstet Gynecol Scand* 2002;81: 581-7
11. Taffe J, Dennerstein L. Menstrual diary data and menopausal transition: methodologic issues. *Acta Obstet Gynecol Scand* 2002;81:588-94
12. Dennerstein L, Dudley EC, Hopper JL, Burger H. Sexuality, hormones and the menopausal transition. *Maturitas* 1997;26:83-93
13. Dennerstein L, Lehert P, Dudley E. Short scale to measure female sexuality: adapted from Mccoy female sexuality questionnaire. *J Sex Marital Ther* 2001;27:339-51
14. Dennerstein L, Anderson-Hunt M, Dudley E. Evaluation of a short scale to assess female sexual functioning. *J Sex Marital Ther* 2002;28:389-97
15. Dennerstein L, Lehert P. Modelling mid-aged women's sexual functioning: a prospective population-based study. *J Sex Marital Ther* 2004; 30:173-83
16. Guthrie JR, Smith AM, Dennerstein L, Morse C. Physical activity and the menopause experience: a cross-sectional study. *Maturitas* 1994;20:71-80
17. Burger HG, Dudley EC, Hopper JL, *et al.* The endocrinology of the menopausal transition: a cross-sectional study of a population-based sample [comment]. *J Clin Endocrinol Metab* 1995;80: 3537-45
18. Guthrie JR, Dennerstein L. Studying the menopausal transition: methodological considerations. *Climacteric* 2003;6:354-6
19. Guthrie J, Dennerstein L, Burger H. How reliably does 12-month amenorrhea define final menstrual period? Data from a longitudinal study. *Climacteric* 2002;5:92
20. Burger HG, Dudley EC, Hopper JL, *et al.* Prospectively measured levels of serum follicle-stimulating hormone, estradiol, and the dimeric inhibins during the menopausal transition in a population-based cohort of women. *J Clin Endocrinol Metab* 1999;84:4025-30
21. Burger HG, Dudley EC, Cui J, Dennerstein L, Hopper JL. A prospective longitudinal study of serum testosterone, dehydroepiandrosterone sulfate, and sex hormone-binding globulin levels through the menopause transition. *J Clin Endocrinol Metab* 2000;85:2832-8
22. Dennerstein L, Dudley EC, Hopper JL, Guthrie JR, Burger HG. A prospective population-based study of menopausal symptoms. *Obstet Gynecol* 2000;96:351-8
23. Guthrie JR, Dennerstein L, Taffe JR, Donnelly V. Health care-seeking for menopausal problems. *Climacteric* 2003;6:112-17
24. Morse CA, Dudley E, Guthrie J, Dennerstein L. Relationships between premenstrual complaints and perimenopausal experiences. *J Psychosomat Obstet Gynecol* 1998;19:182-91
25. Dennerstein L, Lehert P, Burger H, Dudley E. Mood and the menopausal transition. *J Nerv Mental Dis* 1999;187:685-91
26. Dennerstein L, Dudley E, Guthrie J. Empty nest or revolving door? A prospective study of women's quality of life in midlife during the phase of children leaving and re-entering the home. *Psychol Med* 2002;32:545-50
27. McCoy NL, Matyas JR. Oral contraceptives and sexuality in university women. *Arch Sexl Behav* 1996;25:73-90
28. Dennerstein L, Randolph J, Taffe J, Dudley E, Burger H. Hormones, mood, sexuality, and the menopausal transition. *Fertil Steril* 2002;77: S42-8
29. Dennerstein L, Dudley E, Burger H. Are changes in sexual functioning during midlife due to aging or menopause? *Fertil Steril* 2001;76:456-60
30. Guthrie JR, Dennerstein L, Wark JD. Risk factors for osteoporosis: a review. *Medscape Womens Health* 2000;5:E1
31. Guthrie JR, Ebeling PR, Dennerstein L, Wark JD. Risk factors for osteoporosis: prevalence, change, and association with bone density. *Medscape Womens Health* 2000;5:E2
32. Guthrie J, Lehert P, Dennerstein L, Burger H, Ebeling P, Wark J. The relative effect of endogenous estradiol and androgens on menopausal bone loss: a longitudinal study. *Osteoporos Int* 2004;online March 24, 2004
33. Guthrie JR, Dennerstein L, Dudley EC. Weight gain and the menopause: a 5-year prospective study. *Climacteric* 1999;2:205-11
34. Guthrie JR, Dennerstein L, Taffe JR, *et al.* Central abdominal fat and endogenous hormones during the menopausal transition. *Fertil Steril* 2003;79: 1335-40
35. Guthrie J, Taffe J, Lehert P, Burger H, Dennerstein L. The association between menopausal changes and the risk of a coronary event: a longitudinal study. *Menopause* 2004;11:315-22

# The Women's Health in the Lund Area (WHILA) study

5

*J. Lidfeldt, C. Nerbrand and G. Samsioe*

## GENERAL BACKGROUND

Several projects have described the health status and risk factor profiles of a variety of diseases in middle-aged men. In contrast, middle-aged women as a group have not been studied so well in Europe. There is considerable uncertainty about the significance of individual risk factors and the possible interactions with lifestyle and other ambient factors, for the risk of middle-aged women developing cardiovascular disease, diabetes, osteoporosis and urinary incontinence, and, further, to what extent the hormonal change affects the course.

### Diabetes and metabolic risk factors

Those men and women who have disturbances in glucose and lipid metabolism run an increased risk of developing cardiovascular disease and diabetes[1]. As a risk factor for cardiovascular disease, diabetes is a 30–40% greater risk in women than in men. Estrogen deficiency and changes in free testosterone and sex hormone binding globulin (SHBG) may be involved, but the possible interactions with other risk factors have not been considered sufficiently. Studies on men with impaired glucose tolerance (IGT) have shown that lifestyle interventions can reduce the risk for diabetes turnover and related cardiovascular complications[2–4], while corresponding data on women are scarce.

Treated and untreated hypertensives of both sexes have higher glucose, insulin, and C-peptide values and are more often obese compared to normotensive persons[5,6]. Not many analyses of 24-h blood pressure levels in women have taken into consideration their hormonal status[7].

Hyperlipidemia, particularly elevated triglycerides, is a risk for myocardial infarction in women[8]. Sex hormones influence the lipid metabolism through complicated mechanisms. *Per-oral* estrogens increase both levels of high density lipoprotein (HDL) cholesterol and triglycerides, meaning that the normally inverted relation between HDL cholesterol and triglycerides is distorted. However, transdermal estrogens seem to lower triglyceride levels, with only minor effect on HDL cholesterol. Progestogens show an opposite effect compared to oral estrogens[9,10]. Androgenoid obesity is an independent risk factor for diabetes and cardiovascular disease[11,12].

### Osteoporosis

The prevalence of osteoporosis increases after the menopausal period, leading to a higher rate of bone fractures[13,14]. There is an increased risk of osteoporosis with early menopause, low body weight, cigarette consumption, premenopausal low physical activity, and strong heredity for osteoporosis and/or low bone density for age[15]. Peri- and postmenopausal osteoporosis is mainly caused by a reduction in estrogen. Reduced risk of osteoporosis has been described in type 2 diabetic patients[16]. However, the mechanisms of the individual factors and to what extent the hormonal status influences bone density in persons with diabetes are not yet fully understood.

### Urinary incontinence

Nearly one-third of postmenopausal women complain of incontinence. This is often a hidden problem, as women hesitate to seek medical attention. However, several new methods for diagnosis as well as treatment are now available, rendering further characterization of this problem an obvious way of reducing health problems in women.

## Sociodemographic and psychosocial factors

Few studies have been made of middle-aged women as regards to personality type, psychosocial support, or social network. It is conceivable that these factors are associated with the women's symptomatology, but the degree of co-variation with biomedical changes, like obesity, hypertension and diabetes[17-19], and osteoporosis, needs to be clarified.

## Main objectives

The general objective of the Women's Health in the Lund Area (WHILA) Study is to analyze the health profile of women aged 50–59 years in a geographically defined area, in relation to biomedical metabolic factors, bone density, quality of life, life style, and different subjective symptoms. The quantitative significance of hormone deficiency in relation to these factors is also studied.

The general hypothesis is that there are interrelations between biological metabolic processes and sociodemographic and psychosocial conditions, and that detection of risk factors at an early stage and intervention in high-risk individuals can delay or prevent the development of cardiovascular disease, diabetes, osteoporosis and urinary incontinence.

The specific objectives are:

(1) *Diabetes*: to investigate the occurrence of IGT and diabetes, to identify risk factors for diabetes in women with IGT, to examine physical and dietary habits among women with IGT, to examine the effect of lifestyle intervention among women with IGT, and to examine the incidence of cardiovascular disease among women at high risk.

(2) *Osteoporosis*: to investigate the occurrence of low bone density, to examine physical and dietary habits among women with osteopenia, to identify and analyze risk factors for progression of low bone density to fractures, and to examine the effect of lifestyle intervention among women with osteopenia.

(3) *Urinary incontinence*: to investigate the occurrence of urinary incontinence, to identify risk factors for urinary incontinence, to examine the quality of life among women with urinary incontinence, and to evaluate the effect of pelvic floor exercise.

(4) *Climacteric symptoms*: to outline factors of importance for the use of hormone therapy, including positive effects as well as side-effects of different HRT regimens.

## Interdisciplinary research

The work is carried out at the Department of Community Medicine, Malmö/Lund, Lund University, with clinical examinations located at the St. Lars Hospital and two primary health-care centers in Lund.

## Study population

The Women's Health in the Lund Area (WHILA) Study invited all women ($n = 10\,766$) living in the Lund area of Southern Sweden by December 1, 1995, and who were born between December 2, 1935 and December 1, 1945 to a screening procedure, which took place from December 1, 1995 until February 3, 2000. The follow-up study ended in 2002. A population registry comprising all inhabitants identified the study population.

Women were told to fill out the questionnaire at home and then bring it to the screening center in conjunction with the health screening process. Of the 10 766 women, 6917 had complete data sets. Non-responders in the cohort were examined via data from official registries.

## Participants vs. non-participants

More non-participants than participants died during the period 1995–98 (2.6% vs. 0.2%; $p < 0.001$), as well as during the following 2 years, 1999–2000 (1.5% vs. 0.3%; $p < 0.001$). The main cause of death in 1995–98 was cancer (non-participants, $n = 64/99$; participants, $n = 10/12$). In the non-participating group, 14 of the 99 deaths were caused by cardiovascular diseases, in contrast to none in the participating group. The cause of death after 1998 has not been analyzed.

During 1998, more participants visited their general practitioner one or more times (53% vs. 44%; $p < 0.001$), as well as consultants at outpatient clinics (49% vs. 43%; $p < 0.001$), while fewer visited a psychiatrist (2.8% vs. 4.4%; $p < 0.001$) or psychotherapist/psychologist (1.7% vs. 2.3%; $p = 0.019$).

During 1998, fewer participants were hospitalized (8.2% vs. 9.8%; $p = 0.005$), both concerning the somatic ward (7.8% vs. 8.9%; $p = 0.049$) and the psychiatric ward (0.4% vs. 0.9%; $p = 0.002$), and, among these women, the participants stayed for shorter periods (9.3 ± 28.1 days vs. 17.4 ± 37.8 days; $p < 0.001$).

The distribution of all types of diagnoses according to the International Classification of Diagnoses (ICD) was analyzed among participating and non-participating women hospitalized during 1998. The analysis showed a difference in women diagnosed with breast or ovarian cancer (0.6% vs. 1.2%, $p = 0.006$), but no difference was seen in total numbers of malignancies. Furthermore, there were differences in diagnoses concerning unstable angina pectoris/myocardial infarction (0.5% vs. 1.0%, $p = 0.005$), chronic obstructive lung diseases (0.2% vs. 0.6%, $p = 0.026$), gastrointestinal diseases (1.0% vs. 1.4%, $p = 0.044$), and in severe alcohol dependence (0.1% vs. 0.4%, $p = 0.012$), but no differences were seen in other types of psychiatric diagnoses.

The postal residences were analyzed between participants and non-participants. There were no differences in the rate of women living in the central city of Lund compared to those living in the suburbs. Among the latter group, five of a total of 21 suburbs showed differences in the distribution between the participants and non-participants ($p = 0.009$ to $< 0.001$), indicating a higher drop-out rate in areas known to have lower socioeconomic status. In total, in these five suburbs, there were 2489 (24.0%) drop-outs from the total invited population.

Of the non-participating group, 408 (10.6%) women had moved from the area recently, prior to when the mail invitation was handed out, but had already been included as part of the study population.

## HEALTH SCREENING PROGRAM

The health screening program included laboratory examinations and a basic questionnaire that was mailed along with the invitation, and collected in conjunction with the first examination (primary screening) (Figure 1).

Women with features of the metabolic syndrome (positive screening) underwent a baseline oral glucose tolerance test (OGTT) 1–4 weeks later. Women with IGT were subsequently invited to participate in a 2.5-year follow-up study. A random sample of subjects without any positive screening variables was also studied.

Informed consent was obtained from participating subjects and approval was obtained from the ethics committee at Lund University as well as from the data registry inspection in Stockholm, Sweden.

## METHODS

### Questionnaires

The basic (generic) questionnaire included 104 questions concerning medical history, drug treatment, family history of diabetes and cardiovascular disease (parents or siblings with events before the age of 60 years), perimenopausal status, smoking and alcohol habits, education, household, working status, physical activity, general dietary habits, physical, social, and mental well-being (quality of life) and subjective physical and mental symptoms. This questionnaire was a composite of several pre-existing and validated questionnaires[20]. To further validate this particular questionnaire, it was mailed twice to 100 women around 55 years old, with a 2-month interval between mailings.

All women who passed the baseline OGTT answered a validated food questionnaire, which described in detail the consumption of fat, fibers, fruits/vegetables and sweets/carbohydrates[21]. Women who were re-examined in the longitudinal follow-up study completed the two questionnaires once again.

All women who answered 'yes' to the question whether they had used hormone therapy received a special hormonal questionnaire comprising five sections, with 39 additional questions on hormone

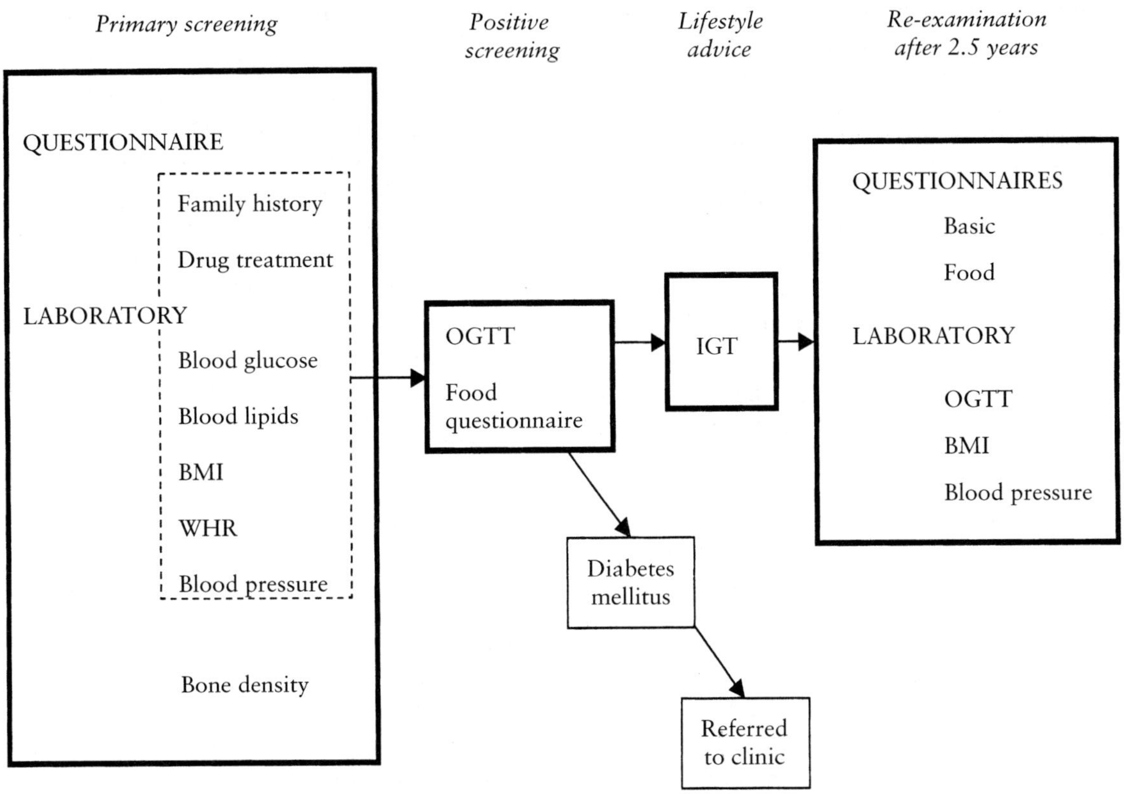


**Figure 1** Screening procedure for women with positive profile and re-examination of women with impaired glucose tolerance (IGT). BMI, body mass index; WHR, waist/hip circumference ratio; OGTT, oral glucose tolerance test

replacement therapy (HRT) use and factors of potential interest for HRT use such as HRT prescriptions, purpose of HRT use, reasons for discontinuation, as well as perceived positive and negative effects of HRT. This questionnaire also contained queries on mood changes such as premenstrual syndrome, postpartum depression and mood changes related to use of hormonal contraception during their reproductive period.

Those women, who on the visual analog scale of problems with urinary continence had marked 2 or higher on a bothersomeness scale from 0 to 10, were given a specific incontinence questionnaire, with an additional 16 questions pertaining to this problem, among which nocturia was also addressed. Numbers of voids per day and night were registered, but it was also possible to address the question of different nocturnal episodes per night as well as different void volumes. Nocturia was defined as at least two nocturnal void episodes at least five nights per week, with a bother index of 2 or more on a visual analog scale from 0 to 10. The frequency and severity of nocturia could then be statistically assessed by regression analysis or the $\chi^2$ test and perceived contributing variables could be assessed.

After completing the specific urologic questionnaire at the screening center, women were interviewed once more on their continence problems. In a subset of women ($n = 400$), the questionnaire was mailed again 2–4 months after the initial one. Of the 369 women returning this second identical questionnaire, responses to questions were identical in 92.1% of cases to the initial urologic questionnaire, as it appeared after corrections by the interview.

A total of 1500 women with self-reported incontinence causing a social and/or hygienic problem, along with 1500 women without incontinence, were selected by computerized randomization from the original WHILA cohort to also receive the Bristol Female Lower Urinary Tract Symptoms questionnaire (BFLUTS)[22].

A specially trained nurse-midwife collected the questionnaires at the time of the examinations and personally interviewed each woman, and potential problems were addressed. At the interview, 19% of the subjects made some corrections in their written answers caused by mistakes or misunderstandings when filling out the forms. The questionnaires were answered before the laboratory results were presented.

## Primary screening

The *physical examination* at the primary screening included measurements of body weight, height, and minimal waist and maximal hip circumference (WHR). Body mass index (BMI) was calculated in kg/m$^2$. To create an estimate, named BMI increase, of how many women had increased their BMI by ≥ 25% during the past 25 years, the actual BMI was compared with self-reported body weight and height at 25 years of age.

*Blood pressure* was recorded twice in the right arm, after 15 and 20 min rest in the seated position, with a mercury sphygmomanometer and a cuff size adjusted to the arm width. Korotkoff phase V was taken as the diastolic blood pressure. The average of the recordings, measured to the nearest 2 mmHg, was the blood pressure used for statistical calculations.

Random blood glucose as well as non-fasting serum levels of triglycerides, total cholesterol, HDL cholesterol and low density lipoprotein (LDL) cholesterol were measured with a Cholestech LDX-instrument (Cholestech Corporation, Hayward, CA, USA) on capillary whole blood. The reason for using non-fasting samples was so that the primary screening could be performed at any time during the day. All measurements were carried out in the same laboratory and by the same examiners. The cut-off values and prevalence figures for the metabolic variables for a positive screening, regarded as features of the metabolic syndrome, are shown in Table 1.

In addition, serum aliquots were stored for future analyses, of which those for estradiol, testosterone, SHBG, androstendione and cortisol are now completed. In a subsample of women with features of the metabolic syndrome, fasting insulin and leptin values were determined. Thyroid stimulating hormone (TSH) was examined in women with the metabolic syndrome and women with low wrist bone density (osteopenia or osteoporosis), and an electrocardiogram was performed.

## Baseline diagnostic OGTT

Women with one or more of the total of eight factors for positive primary screening were defined

**Table 1** Number and percentage of women with screening variables at or above the cut-off level (alone or in combination)

| *Screening variables* | *Cut-off level* | *Positive screening outcome* *n* | *%* |
|---|---|---|---|
| Random capillary blood glucose | ≥ 8.0 mmol/l | 547 | 7.9 |
| Non-fasting serum triglycerides | ≥ 2.3 mmol/l | 1274 | 18.4 |
| Body mass index | ≥ 30 kg/m$^2$ | 944 | 13.6 |
| Waist/hip ratio | ≥ 0.90 | 383 | 5.5 |
| Systolic blood pressure | ≥ 160 mmHg | | |
| *and/or* | | | |
| Diastolic blood pressure | ≥ 95 mmHg | 1254 | 18.1 |
| Family history of diabetes mellitus | | 690 | 10.0 |
| Drug treatment of hypertension | | 1001 | 14.0 |
| Drug treatment of hyperlipidemia | | 123 | 1.8 |

to have features of the metabolic syndrome. A 75-g OGTT in the fasted state and a clinical examination were performed by a physician 1–4 weeks after the primary screening. Venous whole blood samples were collected and a HemoCue instrument (HemoCue AB, Ängelholm, Sweden) was used for glucose analyses. The coefficient of variation was 2.8%. The diagnoses of impaired fasting glucose (IFG), IGT and diabetes were set according to the WHO 1998 guidelines.

The validity of the OGTT used in the study was analyzed by testing the intraindividual variation in 640 women passing two OGTTs with a 14-day interval, with IGT or diabetes at the first measurement. The 95% limits of agreement of the random test–retest differences, expressed in percentage as $100 \times (2SD_{dif}$/median level of individual average score), were 17.9% for fasting glucose and 38.1% for 2-h glucose. If the diagnostic categories in the present study were compared between the first OGTT and a mean of the first and second OGTTs, the comparison showed that 16.1% of women with IGT in the first OGTT were normal according to the mean of both OGTTs.

A computerized randomly selected sample (10%) of women without any features of the metabolic syndrome (negative primary screening) was also offered a baseline OGTT.

## Definitions of obesity and hypertension

Obesity was defined as a BMI ≥ 30 kg/m², according to the recommendations from WHO.

Hypertension was defined as (1) a systolic blood pressure ≥ 160 and/or a diastolic blood pressure ≥ 95 mmHg at the clinical examination or (2) use of antihypertensive drug treatment. The definition of hypertension was based on the WHO recommendations from 1993.

## Bone mineral density measurement

Wrist bone mineral density (BMD) was measured by dual-energy X-ray absorptiometry (DEXA) using an Osteometer DTX 200 (Medi-Tech A/S, Rodovre, Denmark) and expressed as standard deviations (SD) from young healthy women (*t* score) and as age-matched values (*Z* score). One technician performed all measurements. A phantom was used for daily calibration of the instrument. The WHO standard was used to define patients with osteopenia (–1.0 to –2.5 SD) and osteoporosis (< –2.5 SD).

## Perimenopausal status

Women were divided by perimenopausal status into three groups: premenopausal (PM) women, and postmenopausal women with hormone therapy (PMT) or without hormone therapy (PM0). Menopause was defined as a bleed-free interval of at least 12 months.

## Alcohol and smoking habits

Alcohol intake was defined as the weekly consumption of wine, beer and spirits converted into grams of alcohol and divided into four categories: no consumption, ≤ 83 g/week, 84–167 g/week, and ≥ 168 g/week. Twelve grams alcohol was equivalent to one drink.

Smoking was categorized by the lifetime consumption of pack-years. One pack-year corresponded to a consumption of 20 cigarettes per day for 1 year. Subjects were divided into three categories: never smokers (< 1 pack-year), past smokers and current smokers (≥ 1 pack-year for both). Past smokers were those who had stopped smoking at least 1 month prior to the study.

## Leisure time exercise

The subjects reported the duration, frequency and intensity of their leisure time exercise activity performed per week during the last year, corresponding to: hardly any activity, < 30 min/week, 30–60 min/week, > 60–120 min/week and > 120 min/week of jogging and equivalent activities.

## Physical activity at work

Physical activity at work during the last year was categorized into low, moderate and high physical intensity at work. Low referred to sedentary (white collar) work, moderate to mostly walking but not heavy lifting, and high to work with a high degree of walking and lifting. Those without work during the last year were asked to categorize their work at home.

## Dietary habits

The general diet consumption was based on four questions with three sublevels, from an unhealthy to healthy pattern regarding fat, fibers, fruits/vegetables and sweets/carbohydrates. Women with a healthy intake of fat had a low total consumption of fat, especially animal fat, but relatively more vegetable oil, low-fat milk and meat, often fish, seldom sausages, bakeries and whipped cream. A healthy intake of fibers meant high total consumption of fibers, often through fiber-rich bread and whole grain cereals. A healthy intake of fruits/vegetables meant a high total, daily consumption of both fruits and vegetables. A healthy pattern regarding sweets meant hardly ever using extra sugar, eating sweets, cookies or other bakeries. All subjects answered the four basic questions on diet and 40% of these women also completed the validated detailed food questionnaire[21], which ensured that the basic questions discriminated between unhealthy and healthy diet. Women defined as having healthy dietary habits were those indicating a healthy pattern on at least three out of the four basic questions, and with none of the four questions indicating an unhealthy pattern.

## Sociodemographic factors

A household included women living alone or living with a partner or children. Education was categorized into three types: comprehensive school (in total for 9 years), upper secondary school (in total for 12 years), and university degree, according to the highest level of education stated by the respondent. Working status referred to the subjects' relation to the labor market: full-time, part-time, and subjects being unemployed, long-term sick-listed or with disability pension.

## Subjective health

The Göteborg quality-of-life (GQL) instrument measured subjective health[20]. The instrument refers to the WHO definition of health, and divides the subjects' perception of symptoms into physical, social, and mental well-being. Altogether, 19 topics on quality of life were estimated on a seven-step score from 'very bad' (1) to 'excellent, could not be better' (7). Also, 19 physical and ten mental symptoms were listed, to be answered with a 'yes' or 'no', whether the woman had been troubled by any of the symptoms during the last 3 months, or not. Social well-being included all the original GQL variables of family, housing, work, and economy, but also five additional variables: partner, leisure time, sexual satisfaction, appreciation at home, and appreciation outside the home. Physical well-being included the GQL variables of health, fitness, memory, and appetite, but excluded hearing and vision, and included one other variable, bodily perception. Mental well-being included the entire GQL variables of mood, energy, endurance, self-esteem and sleep. The symptoms were assessed as in the original, except that the symptom 'overweight' was excluded. Physical symptoms included eye problems, impaired hearing, headache, dizziness, coughing, breathlessness, chest pain, loss of weight, sweating, feeling cold, pain in the legs, back ache, joint pain, abdominal pain, constipation, diarrhea, loss of appetite, nausea, and difficulty in passing urine. Mental symptoms included restlessness, difficulty in relaxing, nervousness, impaired concentration, sleeping disturbance, irritability, exhaustion, general fatigue, depression, and crying easily.

## Exclusion criteria

Women with known diabetes mellitus, stroke or myocardial infarction within the preceding year, as well as women with a severe, usually malignant, concurrent disease, were excluded from baseline OGTT. The rationale for excluding stroke and myocardial infarction in the following screening process was to avoid the influence of subjects with potentially acute metabolically deteriorated profiles. Women with a previously unknown disease, that required other examinations or treatments, were referred to health-care centers or specialist clinics, but were not excluded from the analyses.

## Follow-up study: exclusion

Women with normal OGTT or isolated IFG were not studied further, but, in the case of obesity, high blood pressure or hyperlipidemia, they were given verbal and written preventive advice and recommended to contact their physician. All women with diabetes, and also those in the subsample without any features of the metabolic syndrome and who had IGT at the OGTT, were informed and given lifestyle advice, and referred to their physician at the primary health-care center.

## Control group at follow-up: women with normal glucose tolerance

A random sample (10%) of women without features of the metabolic syndrome attended baseline OGTT, and those who had normal glucose tolerance served as the control group at the follow-up study. They were not given any specific advice. The OGTT was repeated at follow-up but no information was given at baseline that they would be invited to a re-examination.

## Lifestyle intervention group: women with impaired glucose tolerance

Among women with features of the metabolic syndrome, those who had IGT received initial lifestyle advice and were invited to the 2.5-year follow-up study, ending with a new OGTT.

Individual advice was given for 1 hour by a physician on how to achieve a healthier lifestyle concerning physical exercise, dietary habits, and smoking and alcohol consumption. The subjects' individual answers given in the questionnaire and the results of the physical examination formed the bases for the advice given.

Overall, the recommendations aimed at motivating an increase of leisure time exercise to at least 1 hour or more of moderately intense activities like jogging, cycling or swimming per week. Furthermore, the dietary advice included verbal and written descriptions on reduced total intake of fat and a higher relative proportion of unsaturated fat, increased consumption of fibers and vegetables, and reduced intake of different components of sugar. Smoking women were advised to make a complete stop. A reduction in alcohol consumption was recommended, especially in women with high consumption. However, none was urged to become an abstainer.

The dietary prescription included: fruits ≥ 3 times daily, vegetables ≥ once daily, minimum 25 g fibers daily, 25–30 energy% fat, a higher relative part of unsaturated fat, maximum 10 energy% saturated fat, minimum 1000 mg calcium contents in diet daily. Physical activity recommendations were aimed to increasing energy consumption by 500–1000 kcal/week.

## Intervention for urinary incontinence

Women with urinary incontinence estimated at ≥ 2 on the 0–10 scale were randomized into either one group given information at one occasion, or to a group followed at repeated occasions at their nearby health center. The latter group was given verbal, written and practical information on pelvic floor exercise, under surveillance of a midwife and physiotherapist. A subgroup analysis is conducted in collaboration with the Department of Gynecology and the Department of Urology. Final analyses of the results were performed after 2 years.

## Some initial results of WHILA

All 10 766 women, aged 50–59 years, living in the Lund area were invited, out of whom 6917 attended the baseline study (Figure 2). The study started on December 1, 1995 and the primary screening ended February 3, 2000. The follow-up study ended in 2002.

Among the 6917 women, 7% were PM (mean age 52.7 years), 41% PMT (mean age 55.1 years) and 52% were PM0 (mean age 55.6 years).

In our cohort, the most common HRT preparation was Kliogest, i.e. a continuous combined oral regimen consisting of 2 mg estradiol + 1 mg norethisterone acetate.

Almost 52% had positive primary screening variables, and passed also the baseline OGTT examination; 13.6% were obese (BMI ≥ 30 kg/m$^2$) and 37% had increased in BMI ≥ 25% over the last 25 years. Among hypertensive women, 49% had a corresponding increase in BMI. Blood pressure

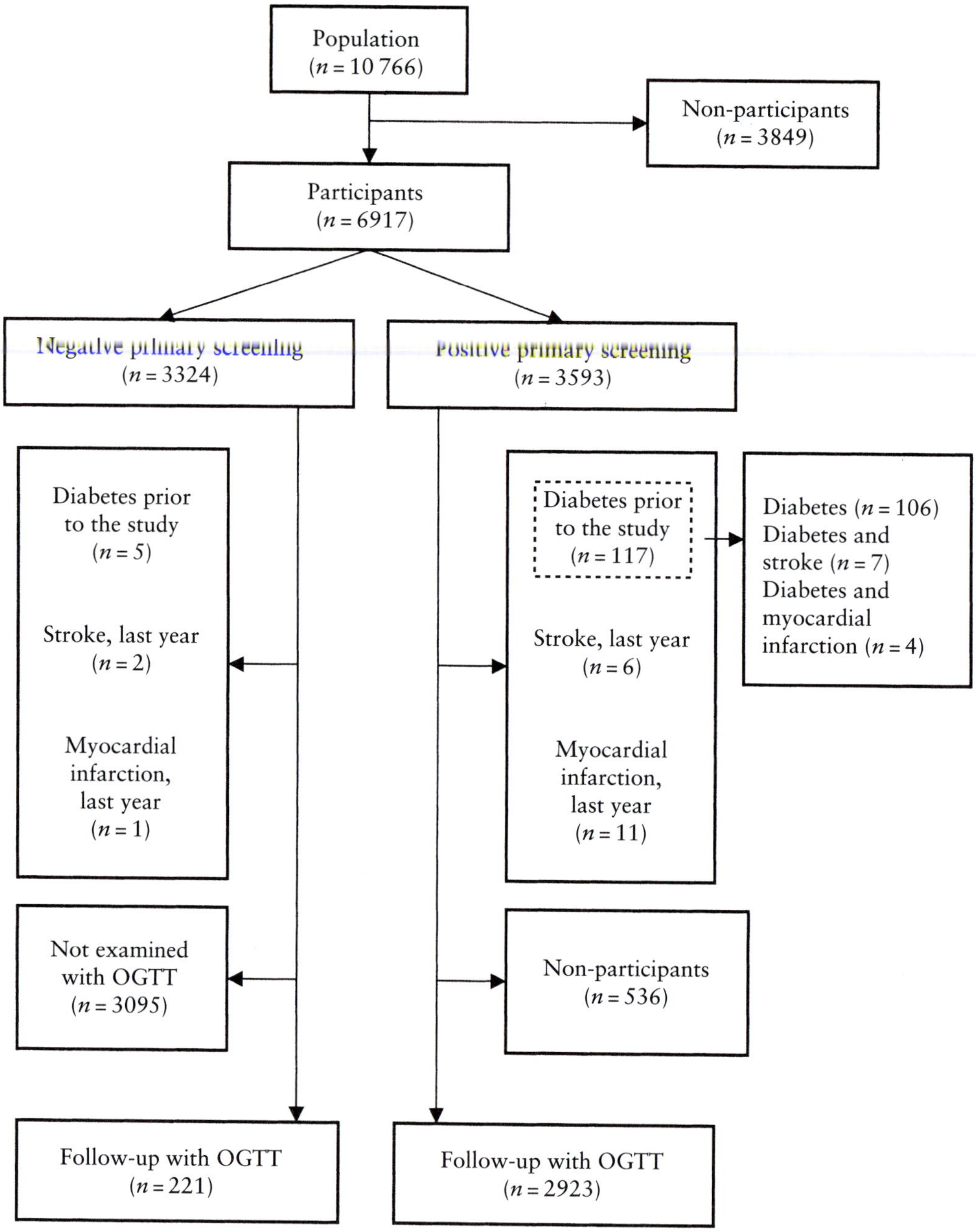


**Figure 2** Study population. OGTT, oral glucose tolerance test

was 160/95 mmHg or higher in 18.1% of the subjects.

Hypertension was more common among those with features of the metabolic syndrome. Hypertension was also more common among women with low education and among those consuming > 84 g alcohol per week (12 g alcohol = 1 glass of wine).

Altogether, 16% were current regular smokers and another 19% past smokers, and 75% of the participants consumed alcohol. Only 34% had healthy dietary and physical activity habits. An unhealthy lifestyle was positively associated with metabolic risk factors, and smoking and alcohol consumption. The results indicate that leisure-time physical activity had higher impact than diet.

*Diabetes and metabolic risk factors*
Features of the metabolic syndrome were found among 3593 women or 51% of the population, and 14% had impaired glucose tolerance and 6.4% diabetes. The general conclusion of the study was that there was a high prevalence of risk markers for diabetes in this population of women, and that many cases of previously unknown IGT and diabetes were found. Biological factors interrelated with sociodemographic and psychosocial disparities, like low level of education, living single and low subjective physical well-being. Low or moderate, but not high, alcohol consumption seemed beneficial on the metabolic profile. The results on smoking were contradictory to previous reports concerning the effect on features of the metabolic syndrome. Smoking showed an independent decreased risk for hypertension and was not associated with the development of diabetes. Menopausal status showed no relation to occurrence of hypertension.

In the longitudinal study, a single baseline occasion of extensive lifestyle advice from a physician seemed enough to significantly reduce the risk for new cases of diabetes. Among these women with IGT at baseline, 38% had normal glucose tolerance at follow-up, while 11.9% had developed diabetes. These results are similar to those that have been found in other more costly intervention studies. According to the results, screening of women at high risk for diabetes should be performed. A model for this procedure has been presented, as well as a description of preventive measures that can be performed in primary health-care settings.

*Osteoporosis*
The osteoporosis and osteopenia prevalences in this study were 7% and 43%, respectively. A positive correlation was found between bone density and impaired metabolic factors such as high body weight, blood pressure and serum lipids. However, women who smoked had low bone density. Hormone replacement therapy seemed to delay the age-dependent bone loss.

*Urinary incontinence*
Urinary incontinence was reported among 32% of the participants at the baseline examination, but this figure was even higher when the latest internationally accepted definition from 2002 was used. Women with low body weight and family history of diabetes more often had incontinence problems, and the most common type was urgency incontinence. Involuntary urinary leakage more than once weekly was considered by the majority of subjects to reduce quality of life. Successful treatment according to urodynamic test results was shown with individually modified programs for pelvic floor exercise.

Since 1999, several papers have been published on various aspects. In general, these data are cross-sectional. The specific WHILA papers published to date are listed below.

## Significance: importance of this work to women's health

This study is unique in examining a total population of women aged 50–59 years, with a broad perspective of focus. Some epidemiological data on middle-aged women's health and related risk factors are still missing. In this population, both women in pre- and postmenopause, with and without hormone replacement therapy, are included. The prevalence of diabetes, cardiovascular diseases and osteoporosis increases substantially in postmenopausal women. At the same time, numerous symptoms set in, influencing quality of life. The study will evaluate this period in women's life and contribute with new understandings of the biological and sociodemographic and psychosocial conditions present during this age period.

## Further study procedures

Further analyses are needed in order to understand better the underlying causes for the increasing numbers of people suffering from diabetes. Previous reports from the WHILA study have indicated that not only biological but also social and psychosocial status is of importance for the risk of developing diabetes. There is reason to believe that more causal relations exist between different social and mental stressor mechanisms and the development of diabetes, and that these relationships need yet to be identified. Individually modified programs that consider most aspects of daily life are warranted, in order to succeed better with preventive measures at an individual level. Such programs could more carefully adjust verbal and written information to differences in, for example, educational level, household, housing, and working conditions as well as other social and psychosocial circumstances. Much of the shortcomings in primary and secondary prevention experienced so far could be explained by that too simplified a model has been used for people at risk, independent of other background factors.

In order to understand better differences in risk factor profiles, measurements of serum levels of insulin, leptin, cortisol, estradiol, testosterone, androstenedione and SHBG have been performed on blood samples collected from participants at the baseline examination, and will be analyzed further.

Analyses of alcohol consumption and use of psychotropic drugs will continue, and also regarding work load and long-term sick leave.

Previous obstetric journals among women with IGT or diabetes will be studied. Risk factor analyses will be performed concerning the interrelations between biomedical factors, drug treatment, social factors, lifestyle and the influence on bone tissue density and the risk of bone fractures.

DXA densitometry used for measuring wrist bone density will be compared with a method used on a subgroup given a vertebral and hip bone densitometry.

Serum cadmium will be compared between groups regarding the differences in smoking and dietary habits and the influence on bone density and kidney-related diseases. The risk markers protein HC (human complex forming protein), NAG (*N*-acetyl-β-D-glucosaminidase urine), and cysteine C will also be studied.

The influence of differences in serum levels of sex hormones, cortisol and insulin for the development of urinary incontinence will be analyzed. Special studies will be performed on women with nycturia and women who have undergone hysterectomy. Further studies will also be performed concerning aspects of quality of life among women with urinary incontinence.

### Follow-up of total cohort

A follow-up of the initial responders ($n = 6917$) using the same technique is planned for 2005, to yield an average follow-up time of 9 years. The same questionnaires will be used, with the addition of queries about health issues, between the first and second time. In addition to the laboratory tests, whole blood will be collected for analyses of genetic markers.

## References


1. Nilsson P, Lindholm LH, Schersten BF. Life style changes improve insulin resistance in hyperinsulinaemic subjects: a one-year intervention study of hypertensives and normotensives in Dalby. *J Hypertens* 1992;10:1071–8
2. Xiao-Ren P, Guang-Wei L,Ying-Hua H. Effects of diet and exercise in preventing NIDDM in people with impaired glucose tolerance, the Da Qing IGT and Diabetes Study. *Diabetes Care* 1997;20:537–44
3. Hu FB, Sigal RJ, Rich-Edwards JW. Walking compared with vigorous physical activity and risk of type 2 diabetes in women. *J Am Med Assoc* 1999; 282:1433–9
4. Tuomilehto J, Lindström J, Eriksson JG. Prevention of type 2 diabetes mellitus by changes in lifestyle among subjects with impaired glucose tolerance. *N Engl J Med* 2001;344:1343–50

5. Nilsson P, Lindholm L, Schersten B. Hyperinsulinaemia and other metabolic disturbances in well-controlled hypertensive men and women; an epidemiological study of the Dalby population. *J Hypertens* 1990;8:953–9
6. Engstöm I, Lindholm LH. Blood pressure in middle-aged women: a comparison between office-, self, and ambulatory recordings. *Blood Pressure* 1992; 6:375–9
7. Fontbonne A, Eschwege E, Cambien F. Hypertriglyceridaemia as a risk factor of coronary heart disease mortality in subjects with impaired glucose tolerance or diabetes: results from the 11-year follow-up of the Paris Prospective Study. *Diabetologia* 1989;32:300–4
8. Stevenson JC, Crook D, Godsland IF. Effects of age and menopause on lipid metabolism in healthy women. *Atherosclerosis* 1993;98:83–90
9. Crook D, Cust MP Gangar KF, Stevenson JC, Whitehead M. Comparison of transdermal and oral estrogen/progestin hormone replacement therapy: effects on serum lipids and lipoproteins. *Am J Obstet Gynecol* 1992;166:950–5
10. Modan M, Karasik A, Halkin H. Effect of past and concurrent body mass index on prevalence of glucose intolerance and Type 2 (non-insulin dependent) diabetes and on insulin response. *Diabetologia* 1986;29:82–9
11. Mokdad AH, Ford ES, Bowman BA. Diabetes trends in the U.S.: 1990–1998. *Diabetes Care* 2000; 23:1278–83
12. World Congress on Osteoporosis, Amsterdam 1996: Consensus Development Statement. *Osteoporosis Int* 1997;7:1–6
13. Lindsay R, Cosman F, Nieves J. Estrogen: effects and actions in osteoporosis. *Osteoporosis Int* 1993; 1:150–2
14. WHO. *Assessment of fracture risk and its application to screening to postmenopausal osteoporosis.* WHO Technical Report Series 843. Geneva: World Health Organization, 1994
15. Barrett-Connor E, Kritz-Silverstein D. Does hyperinsulinemia preserve bone? *Diabetes Care* 1996; 19:1388–92
16. Bouillon R. Diabetic bone disease. *Calcif Tissue Int* 1991;49:155–60
17. Marmot MG, Smith GD, Stansfeld S, *et al.* Health inequalities among British civil servants: the Whitehall II study. *Lancet* 1991;337:1387–93
18. Suadicani P, Hein HO, Gyntelberg F, *et al.* Socioeconomic status and ischemic heart disease mortality in middle-aged men: importance of the duration of follow-up. The Copenhagen Male Study. *Int J Epidemiol* 2001; 30:248–55
19. Rosvall M, Ostergren PO, Hedblad B, *et al.* Occupational status, educational level, and the prevalence of carotid atherosclerosis in a general population sample of middle-aged Swedish men and women: results from the Malmo Diet and Cancer Study. *Am J Epidemiol* 2000; 152:334–46
20. Tibblin G, Tibblin B, Peciva S, *et al.* 'The Göteborg quality of life instrument' - an assessment of well-being and symptoms among men born 1913 and 1923.Methods and validity. *Scand J Prim H Care* 1990;1:33–8
21. Asp NG, Isaksson Å, Johansson U. Dietary habits among adults in Olofström - a baseline study. *Scand J Nutr* 1992;36:106–14
22. Jackson S, Donovan J, Brooks S, Eckford L, Swithinbank L, Abrahams P. The Bristol Female Lower Urinary Tract Symptoms questionnaire; development and psychometric testing. *Br J Urol* 1996;77:805–12

## WHILA publications

Samsioe G, Heraib F, Lidfeldt J, *et al.* Urogenital symptoms in women aged 50–59 years. A preliminary report from the Women's Health in Lund Area (WHILA) Study Group. *Gynecol Endocrinol* 1999;13: 113–17

Li C, Samsioe G, Lidfeldt J, Nerbrand C, Agardh C-D. Important factors for use of hormone replacement therapy: a population-based study of Swedish women. The Women's Health in Lund Area (WHILA) Study. *Menopause* 2000;7:273–81

Svartvik L, Lidfeldt J, Nerbrand C, Samsioe G, Scherstén B, Nilsson PM. Dyslipidemia and impaired well-being in middle-aged women reporting low sense of coherence. The Women's Health in the Lund Area (WHILA) Study. *Scand J Prim Health Care* 2000;18:177–82

Li C, Samsioe G, Lidfeldt J, Nerbrand C, Agardh C-D, Scherstén B. Effects of norethisterone acetate addition to estradiol in long term HRT. A population based study of Swedish women. The Women's Health in Lund Area (WHILA) Study. *Maturitas* 2000;36:139–52

Samsioe G, Lidfeldt J, Nerbrand C, Enström-Granath I, Agardh C-D, Scherstén B. Blood pressure in middle aged women. Results from the Women's Health In the Lund Area (WHILA) project. *J Menopause* 2000;7:3–5

Lidfeldt J, Nerbrand C, Samsioe, G, Scherstén B, Agardh C-D. A screening procedure detecting high-yield candidates for OGTT. The Women's Health In the Lund Area (WHILA) study: a population based study of middle-aged Swedish women. *Eur J Epidemiol* 2001;17:943–51

Lidfeldt J, Holmdahl L, Samsioe G, *et al.* The influence of hormonal status and features of the metabolic syndrome on bone density: a population based study of Swedish women aged 50 to 59 years. The Women's Health in the Lund Area (WHILA) Study. *Metabolism* 2002;51:267–70

Li C, Wilawan K, Samsioe G, Lidfeldt J, Agardh CD, Nerbrand C. Health profile of middle aged women. The

Women's Health in Lund Area study. *Hum Reprod* 2002;17:1379-85

Gunnarsson M, Teleman P, Mattiasson A, Lidfeldt J, Nerbrand C, Samsioe G. Effects of pelvic floor exercises in middle aged women with a history of naïve urinary incontinence - a population based study. *Eur Urol* 2002;41:556-61

Enström I, Lidfeldt J, Lindholm LH, Nerbrand C, Pennert K, Samsioe G. Does blood pressure differ between users and non-users of hormone replacement therapy? The Women's Health In the Lund Area (WHILA) study. *Blood Press* 2002;11:240-3

Lidfeldt J, Nyberg P, Nerbrand C, *et al.* Biological factors are more important than socio-demographic and psychosocial conditions in relation to hypertension in middle-aged women. The Women's Health In the Lund Area (WHILA) Study. *Blood Press* 2002;11:270-8

Teleman P, Gunnarsson M, Lidfeldt J, Nerbrand C, Samsioe G, Mattiasson A. Urodynamic characterisation of women with naïve urinary incontinence: a population based study in subjecively incontinent and healthy 53-63 years old women. *Eur Urol* 2002:42;583-9

Lidfeldt J, Nyberg P, Nerbrand C, Samsioe G, Scherstén B, Agardh C-D. Socio-demographic and psychosocial factors are associated with features of the metabolic syndrome. The Women's Health In the Lund Area (WHILA) Study. *Diabetes Obes Metab* 2003; 5:106-12

Jernström H, Bendahl P-O, Lidfeldt J, Nerbrand C, Agardh C-D, Samsioe G. A prospective study of different types of hormone replacement therapy use and the risk of subsequent breast cancer. The Women's Health in the Lund Area (WHILA) study. *Cancer Causes Control* 2003;14:673-80

Håkansson C, Svartvik L, Lidfeldt J, *et al.* Self-rated health in middle aged women: associations with sense of coherence and socioeconomic and health-related factors. *Scand J Occupational Therapy* 2003;10:99-106

Teleman P, Gunnarsson M, Lidfeldt J, Nerbrand C, Samsioe G, Mattiasson A. Urethral pressure changes in response to squeeze: a population based study in healthy and incontinent 53- to 63-year-old women. *Am J Obstet Gynecol* 2003;189:1100-5

Cederfjäll J, Lidfeldt J, Nerbrand C, Samsioe G, Öjehagen A. Alcohol consumption among middle-aged women: a population based study of Swedish women. The Women's Health In the Lund Area (WHILA) Study. *Eur Addict Res* 2004;10:15-21

Li C, Samsioe G, Borgfeldt C, Lidfeldt J, Agardh CD, Nerbrand C. Menopause related symptoms. What are background factors? A population-based study of Swedish women. The Women's Health in Lund Area (WHILA) study. *Am J Obstet Gynecol* 2003;189:1646-53

Håkansson C, Lidfeldt J, Nerbrand C, Samsioe G, Nilsson P, Eklund M. Wellbeing and occupational roles among middle-aged women. The Women's Health in Lund Area (WHILA) Study. *Work* 2004;in press

Nerbrand C, Lidfeldt J, Nyberg P, Schersten B, Samsioe G. Serum lipids and lipoproteins in relation to endogenous and exogenous female sex steroids and age. The Women's Health in Lund Area (WHILA) study. *Maturitas* 2004;48:161-9

Khatibi A, Samsioe G, Li C, Lidfeldt J, Agardh C-D, Nerbrand C. Does hormone replacement therapy increase allergic reactions and upper gastrointestinal problems? Results from a population based study of Swedish women. The Women's Health in Lund Area (WHILA) study. *Maturitas* 2004;in press

Teleman P, Lidfeldt J, Nerbrand C, Samsioe G, Mattiasson A. Overactive bladder - prevalence, risk factors and relation to stress incontinence in middle-aged women. *Br J Obstet Gynaecol* 2004;in press

# Adequately assessed quality of life 6

*E. M. Alder*

## INTRODUCTION

There are many different ways of assessing quality of life in general, and many health professionals may need measures of quality of life (QoL). Some approaches to measuring quality of life have been developed for disease-specific conditions (which could include menopause, although it is not a disease) and some are generic. Quality of life may be seen positively in terms of life satisfaction and feelings of well-being, and goals and expectations that have been achieved. It can also reflect loss, and be seen as reflecting symptom severity, level of impairment or handicap. Quality of life can be described in terms of subjective well-being (does your health interfere with your social life?) or functional status (can you dress unaided?). Quality of life in the menopause can be measured in terms of symptoms, *or* personal experience *or* functional ability, *or* a combination of all three. This paper will discuss the meaning of quality of life, discuss assessment problems and then relate these to assessment in the climacteric.

## WHAT IS QUALITY OF LIFE?

There is no universally accepted definition of quality of life and it is constantly being redefined. The World Health Organization (WHO) defined health as 'complete physical, mental and emotional well-being'[1]. Hunt and McKenna in 1992 pointed out that there was no agreed definition, no theoretical base, inappropriate use of measures, lack of recognition of the social basis of definitions and measurement, and confusion between the quality of life and quality of care[2].

In 1993, WHO defined quality of life as 'individuals' perceptions of their position of life in the context of the culture and value systems in which they live and in relation to their goals, standards and concerns'[3]. The definition includes six domains: physical health, psychological state, levels of independence, social relationships, environmental features, and spiritual concerns. It would probably now be agreed that quality of life is a multidimensional concept and includes both positive and negative aspects of life.

A biopsychosocial approach can be helpful in understanding how life is affected by a number of different parameters. In 2001, WHO developed a conceptual model which advocates that the outcome of a health program or technology (in this case, we might suggest hormone replacement therapy (HRT) or some other management of menopausal symptoms) should be assessed in three domains, namely, impairments, abilities and participation, all affecting quality of life (the WHO International Classification of Functioning, Disability and Health, ICF)[4]. Figure 1 shows how activities are influenced by health condition, environmental factors and personal factors. The interaction between body functions and structures (menopausal status) and participation (tasks and involvement in life situations of mid-aged women) with activities reflects their quality life. Any change in any of these domains will affect their quality of life. Using this model, a reduction in menopausal symptoms would affect activities but so also would a change in personal factors. The ICF model states that these domains should be assessed independently and that researchers should look for associations between these domains if and where they exist. Such an assessment will not only reveal how the therapy has removed or reduced impairments of body structures and systems, but also the impact of therapy that may reduce functional deficits and improve participation in life's activities. Participation in life's activities obviously varies between individuals, and individual expectations and goals are important to quality of life.

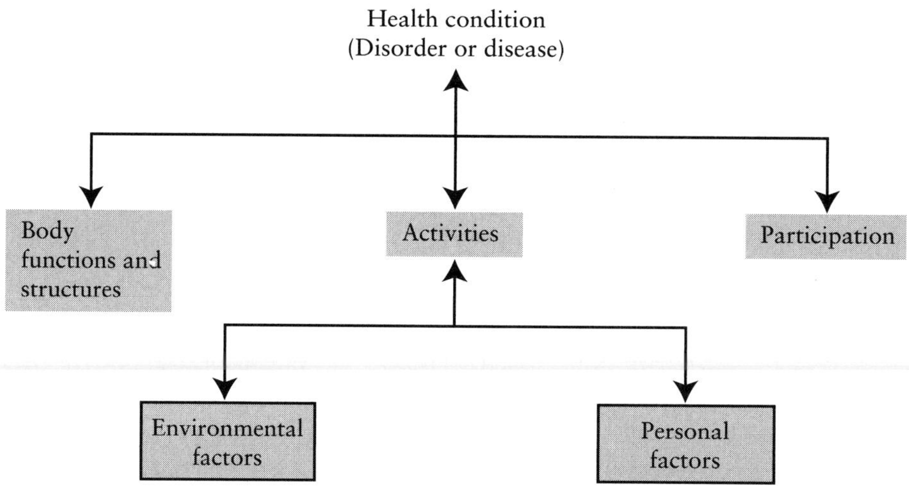


**Figure 1** World Health Organization International Classification of Functioning, Disability and Health, 2001

## WHAT IS AN ADEQUATE ASSESSMENT?

For an assessment to be adequate is an essential minimum, but it may not be enough to do justice to an important aspect of health care. Perhaps we need a more than adequate assessment, but it can be argued that, in the past, assessments of quality of life in the menopause have been inadequate. Garratt and colleagues[5] reviewed quality-of-life measures across specialties. They identified nearly 4000 English language reports between 1990 and 1999. Most (1819) reported the development and evaluation of specific measures, 865 reported generic measures, 690 dimension-specific measures, 409 utility measures and 632 individualized measures. Among the generic measures, the SF-36[6], the Nottingham Health Profile[7] and the Sickness Impact Profile[8] were most often reported, and have been translated into several languages and across numerous patient populations. Garratt and colleagues point out that most development work has taken place in cancer, rheumatology and musculoskeletal medicine, and there has been less development and evaluation in gynecology, in spite of the psychosocial distress reported in gynecology clinics[5]. They admit that the selection of measures can be daunting. Evaluation of measures within primary research involves comparative evaluation of reliability, validity and responsiveness, but they criticise the quality of reviews and suggest that researchers should review the literature carefully before constructing a new measure.

Two examples illustrate inadequate assessment. The agendas of the medical profession and their women patients may not be the same. A review[9] of making decisions about hormone replacement therapy illustrates the confusion of current medical advice and the impact of the result of the Heart and Estrogen/progestin Replacement Study (HERS)[10] and the Women's Health Initiative (WHI) study[11]. The review includes benefits and risks of the effects of relief of menopausal symptoms and quotes only one study on the effect of estrogen on quality of life, in which quality of life is measured by a utility model. Benefits and risks of osteoporosis, cardiovascular disease, thromboembolic disease, colorectal, breast, endometrial and ovarian cancer are reviewed. They conclude, that for symptomatic perimenopausal women, sequential hormone replacement therapy for 1–2 years is likely to improve quality of life with minimal risk, but it is not clear what is meant by quality of life other than reduction of menopausal symptoms.

Many mid-aged women expect that HRT will alleviate their menopausal symptoms and improve their quality of life. The results of the study reported by Hays and colleagues[12] challenge this expectation. In the large WHI study, women with an intact uterus were randomly assigned to estrogen plus progestin. After an increased risk of adverse events was found, the trial was stopped after 5 years. The participants were also assessed at baseline and at 1 year on a number of quality-of-life measures. The results clearly showed that HRT had no benefit in any quality-of-life measures. In women with moderate to severe vasomotor symptoms at baseline, there was a small benefit in sleep disturbance but no benefit in the other quality-of-life measures, and Grady[13] concludes that there is no role for hormone therapy in the treatment of women without menopausal symptoms. The study used a checklist of menopausal symptoms but no standardized validated measure with accepted psychometric properties. The response categories were summed to give an overall score, although previous research has used factor analysis, which shows that symptoms are not independent or of equal weight.

The rationale for the choice of the other quality-of-life measures is not clear. The measure of sexual functioning was a single item and gave no measure of arousal, responsiveness or libido. The Modified Mini Mental state examination is not a sensitive measure of cognitive improvement in healthy, relatively intelligent adults. There was no measure of social functioning, or of self-esteem. One inherent problem with longitudinal studies is that assessment techniques may be out of date by the time of follow-up and it is difficult to interpret the results of this study on healthy women.

## HOW CAN QUALITY OF LIFE BE MEASURED IN THE CLIMACTERIC?

The assessment of quality of life depends on the question asked. The reduction of vasomotor symptoms might be expected to enhance self-esteem, and improve psychological health and social relations, if this was a problem for the individual woman. However, if vasomotor symptoms were not a problem or if her psychological health was affected more by other factors, then a significant reduction in symptoms may not improve her quality of life. Although a woman may consult because of reported vasomotor symptoms, there may be an underlying depression. HRT may relieve the symptoms and relieve the depression or there may be other factors affecting the depression, which need further investigation. Sometimes, sexual desire, function and general well-being are used as proxy for quality of life and then HRT is likely to show a benefit in symptomatic women[14,15].

Assessments of quality of life can be categorized into a particular aspect of health, e.g. depression; disease- or population-specific measures, e.g. asthma; generic measures, e.g. SF-36; individualized measures; and utility measures used by health economists. For a specific aspect of health, e.g. depression, a specific psychological scale can be used, e.g. Beck's depression inventory (BDI) or the Hospital Anxiety and Depression scale (HADS).

Disease- or population-specific scales can be used in specific conditions or social contexts. Schneider[16] reviews their development in menopause research. The Greene Climacteric Scale[17] and the Women's Health Questionnaire[18] have been developed in the UK from clinic populations, based on factor analysis, and have good psychometric properties. In Germany, the Menopause Rating Scale (MRS)[19] provides three subscales and makes good many deficiencies of the Kupperman index. It has good psychometric properties with high levels of reliability[20]; the highest correlations were in physical role functioning, bodily pain, vitality and emotional role functioning. Jacobs and colleagues[21] developed a condition-specific questionnaire to assess quality of life in menopausal women. They analyzed a 48-item questionnaire from over 1000 women aged between 40 and 63 years, recruited from two English Health authority lists and a national women's magazine. Items were quality of life derived from interviews and focus groups. Women reported their own menopausal status. Factor analysis revealed seven factors: sleep, energy, cognition, symptoms' impact, feelings, social interaction and appetite, which were combined to give a total Menopausal Quality-of-Life score (MQOL). Mean scores showed an inverted U-shaped pattern across the stages of the menopause, with lowest scores in the middle of the menopausal transition. The MQOL was highly correlated with a global quality-of-life scale (QOL)[22]. However, the subscales of social interaction and symptom impact showed a steady decline across the menopausal transition. If the end of the menopausal transition coincides with an increasing level of quality of life, this may confound studies of the effect of HRT over time.

Generic measures include The Nottingham Health Profile[7], a simple scale that can be used in community studies. It gives a very functional assessment. The SF-36 was developed the USA with subsequent validation in the UK[23,24]. The SF-36 provides eight subscales covering physical and social functioning, role limitations, pain, energy/vitality and general and mental health. This is the measure most widely used and is probably the scale of first choice.

The Patient Generated Index of Quality of Life takes an individual approach[25]. It asks people to generate their own list of five areas relating to quality of life and to allocate a value to reflect their relative importance to them. This allows individuals to generate their own priorities. It would allow mobility to be considered more important than pain. It is probably particularly useful in assessing change in areas of health that are more individually determined than societal.

Standardized measures of health-related quality of life are almost necessarily culturally value-laden. The WHOQOL used focus groups of health professionals, patients and people in the community in different countries to generate items for the WHOQOL[26]. They were allocated into the six domains and then analyzed nationally[27]. This enabled country-specific items to be added to the core items, making a culture-specific measure.

Scales used to measure symptoms or to measure other domains of quality of life must have certain psychometric properties of validity, reliability and acceptability. These are described in standard psychological texts and more specialized textbooks[23,28,29] and some of the issues relevant to studies of HRT are discussed in Alder[30].

## CONCLUSION

A good measure of menopausal symptoms would appear appropriate to menopausal women, would correlate positively with other scales, include relevant items such as libido, and would distinguish between premenopausal and perimenopausal women. There would be a high correlation with scores on other measures of menopausal symptoms. However, quality of life means more than the presence or the severity of menopausal symptoms.

Hyndland[31] points out that quality-of-life scales are not like thermometers where the reading is independent of the patient. The best scale is always best for a particular purpose, where purpose is defined in terms of disease, population, and treatment.

He also suggests that the most successful scales are those that have the most successful promoters and that quality-of-life researchers always recommend their own scales. If a scale is required to measure change, then those items that are sensitive to change should be selected. This will help in the evaluation of the effectiveness of treatment, but will not tell us about the person's quality of life and does not take into account other aspects of life that may be important to the patient. Here, we have a conflict between a sensitive scale that can measure change and one that is salient to the patient's experience.

Hunt[32] suggests that studies of quality of life in women give different results because there is no agreed definition of quality of life; they use different measures, measures are not condition-specific, populations differ and menopausal status is not consistently defined. The problems and issues in measuring quality of life in studies in the menopause and hormone replacement therapy are not unique, and we need to improve our measurements of quality of life in studies in the menopause.

# References


1. *Constitution of the WHO*. Geneva: World Health Organization, 1946
2. Hunt S, McKenna S. Do we need measures other than QALYs? In Hopkins A, ed. *Measures of the Quality of Life and The Uses to Which Such Measures May be Put*. London: Royal College of Physicians, 1992
3. WHO Division of Mental Health. WHO-QOL study protocol: The development of the World Health Organization quality of life assessment instrument (MNG/PSF/93). Geneva: WHO, 1993
4. The WHO international classification of function (ICF). Geneva: WHO, 2001
5. Garratt A, Schmidt L, Mackintosh A, Fitzpatrick R. Quality of life measurement: bibliographic study of patient assessed outcome measures *Br Med J* 2002;324:1417–19
6. Ware JR, Sherbourne CD. The MOS 36-item short-form health survey (SF-36). I. Conceptual framework and item selection. *Med Care* 1992; 30:473–83
7. Hunt S, McEwen J, McKenna S. Measuring health status: a new tool for clinicians and epidemiologists. *J R Coll Gen Pract* 1985;35:185–8
8. Bergner M, Bobbitt RA Carter WB, Gilson BS. The sickness impact profile: development and final revision of a health status measure. *Med Care* 1981;19:787–805
9. Rymer J, Wilson R, Ballard K. Making decisions about hormone replacement therapy. *Br Med J* 2003;326:322–6
10. Hulley S, Grady D, Bush T, *et al.* Randomized trial of estrogen plus progestin for secondary prevention of coronary heart disease in post menopausal women. *J Am Med Assoc* 1998;280:605–13
11. Women's Health Initiative Investigators. Risks and benefits of estrogen plus progesterone in healthy postmenopausal women. *J Am Med Assoc* 2002; 288:321–33
12. Hays J, Ockene JK, Brunner RL, *et al.* Effects of estrogen plus progestin on health-related quality of life. *N Engl J Med* 2003;348:1839–54
13. Grady D. Postmenopausal hormonal - therapy for symptoms only. *N Engl J Med* 2003;348:191–3
14. Gambacciani M, Ciaponi M, Cappagli B, *et al.* Effects of low-dose, continuous combined estradiol and norethisterone acetate on menopausal quality of life in early postmenopausal women. *Maturitas* 2003;44:157–63
15. Freedman M. Quality of life in the menopause: the role of estrogen. *J Women's Health* 2002;11: 703–18
16. Schneider HPG, Behre HM. Contemporary evaluation of climacteric complaints: its impact on quality of life. In Schneider HPG, ed. *Hormone Replacement Therapy and Quality of Life*. London: Parthenon Publishing, 2002
17. Greene JG. *Guide to the Greene Climacteric Scale*. Glasgow, UK: University of Glasgow, 1991
18. Hunter M. The Women's Health Questionnaire: a measure of mid aged women's perceptions of their emotional and physical health. *Psychol Health* 1992;7:45–54
19. Schneider HPG, Heinemann LAJ, Rosemeier H-P, Potthoff P, Behre HM. The Menopause Rating Scale (MRS): reliability of scores of menopausal complaints. *Climacteric* 2000;3:59–64
20. Schneider HPG, Heinemann LAJ, Rosemeier H-P, Potthoff P, Behre HM. Menopause Rating scale (MRS): comparison with Kupperman index and quality-of-life scale SF-36. *Climacteric* 2000;3:50–8
21. Jacobs PA, Hyland ME, Ley A. Self rated menopausal status and quality of life in women aged 40–63 years. *Br J Health Psychol* 2000;5:395–411
22. Hyland ME, Sodegren SC. Development of a new type of global quality of life scale and the comparison of performance and preference for 12 global scales. *Qual Life Res* 1996;5:469–80
23. Jenkinson C, McGee H. *Health Status Measurement*. Oxford: Radcliffe Medical Press, 1998
24. Jenkinson C, Stewart Brown S, Paterson S, Plaice C. Assessment of the SGF-36 version 2 in the United Kingdom. *J Epidemiol Commun Health* 1999;53: 46–50
25. Ruta DA, Garratt AM, Leng M, Russell IT, Macdonald LM. A new approach to the measurement of quality of life: the patient generated index (PGI). *Med Care* 1994;32:1109–26
26. WHOQOL Group. The World Health Organization quality of life assessment (WHOQOL): development and general psychometric properties. *Soc Sci Med* 1998;46:1569–85
27. Skevington SM, Bradshaw J, Saxena S. Selecting national items for the WHOQOL: conceptual and psychometric consideration. *Soc Sci Med* 1999;48:473–87
28. Rust J, Golombok S. *Modern Psychometrics. The Science of Psychological Assessment*. London: Routledge, 1989
29. Bowling A. *Measuring Health*, 2nd edn. Buckingham: Open University Press, 1997
30. Alder EM. How to assess quality of life: problems and methodology. In Schneider HPG, ed. *Hormone Replacement Therapy and Quality of Life*. London: Parthenon Publishing, 2002
31. Hyndland M. Recommendations for quality of life scales are not simple (Letter). *Br Med J* 2002; 325:599
32. Hunt SM. The problem of quality of life. *Qual Life Res* 1997;6:205–12

# Quality of life: the Asian perspective 7

*K. K. Limpaphayom*

## INTRODUCTION

Over two billion people, slightly more than one in three inhabitants of the planet, live in rural Asia, more than double the population of Latin America and America combined. Helping such a huge and growing population to achieve fulfilling lives is a daunting challenge. People need many things to live fulfilling lives. Sustenance and security, freedom and community, wealth and health, self-actualization and and self-esteem: all these contribute to the quality of human life. Across the rural segment of the developing world, a focus on income is associated with a concentration on improving agricultural productivity, with the expectation that rising agricultural output will promote higher rural incomes, automatically leading to improvements in quality of life. This perspective is supported by considerable evidence showing links running from agriculture through income to a broad range of quality-of-life indicators.

Recent thinking and related evidence, however, suggest that there is more to quality of life than income alone. Health, education, political freedom, participation in civil society, and the status of women are all important components of the concept of quality of life. These factors are bound to each other, and to income, in a complex network of two-way relationships. Educated people tend to be healthier. Healthier people are better able to work and thus become wealthier, while rich people have more money to spend on health. The positive feedback between education and income is also well recognized.

Income, meanwhile, is not a wholly reliable measure of quality of life. It is usually measured in averages and does not take into account the distribution of wealth within groups. Nor do income measures value amenities that are not priced in the market, such as environmental quality, physical security, freedom, or unpaid work (mostly undertaken by women). A focus on income has also led many policy-makers to believe that technological change and rising capital stocks are the most natural and effective drivers of income. This has depressed investment in human and social capital, which can affect economic growth and improved living standards.

## QUALITY-OF-LIFE CONCEPT

Quality of life, in simple terms, means 'How good is your life for you?' The answer to this question is a measure of a person's quality of life. Every person's life is different, and thus the way in which each person experiences a quality life is unique. Individuals lead complex lives that have many dimensions. A quality-of-life approach recognizes that there are many different aspects of living that may contribute to quality.

One of the main features of the world population within the next few decades will be the rapid increase in the absolute and relative numbers of older people in both developing and developed countries. Our global population is aging and aging at an unprecedented rate. Fertility decline and urbanization arguably have been the dominant global demographic trends during the second half of the twentieth century, as well as the rapid improvement in life expectancy[1]. The total number of elderly people (defined as 60 years of age and older) world-wide is expected to increase from 605 millions in 2000 to 1.2 billion by the year 2025. The United Nations, in 1999, reported that, for the year 2050, there will be more people aged 60 years and older than children under 14 in many developing countries[2]. Population aging could be compared to the silent revolution that will impact on all aspects of society. The 'older' nations will experience relatively little change compared with many developing nations.

## THE DEMOGRAPHY OF AGING IN ASIA

During the period 2000–2030, studies of the projected increases in the elderly population range from 14% in Bulgaria to 372% in Singapore and other Asian nations (Figure 1).

The most prominent factor in population aging had been the decline in fertility. Asia is one of the regions of the developing world, except for Japan and Singapore, where fertility change has been recent and more rapid, with most regions having achieved major reductions in fertility rates over the last 30 years. The total fertility rate, or births per woman, in China is 1.8, in South Korea 1.7, in Thailand 1.9, and in Singapore 1.2; these are now below the replacement level[3]. When considering aggregate elderly proportions of a regional population, two important factors must be kept in mind. First, the diversity, for example, Bangladesh and Thailand may be close geographically, but these two countries have divergent paths of expected population aging; second, percentages by themselves may not give the sense of population momentum. In Thailand, the child : elderly ratio can be calculated as shown in Table 1[3].

In 1975, the ratio of the number of children to the number of elderly people in Thailand was exceptionally high at 5.0; for the year 2000, it had decreased to 4.3. According to the United Nation projection for Thailand, in the year 2025 the ratio will be lower than the world average; by the middle of the twenty-first century, the ratio in Thailand may not be so different from that in the West. As a result of declining infant and age-specific mortality, the life expectancy at birth of the Thai population has been increasing. Life expectancy at birth in the year 2000 was 71.74 years for women and 67.36 years for men; in the year 2020, it will be 74.11 years for women and 70.07 years for men[4]. The fact that the female elderly live longer than their male counterparts will be the phenomenon of feminization among the aged population in Thailand as well as in the other nations[5]. Also, the fastest growing proportion of the elderly population in many nations are those

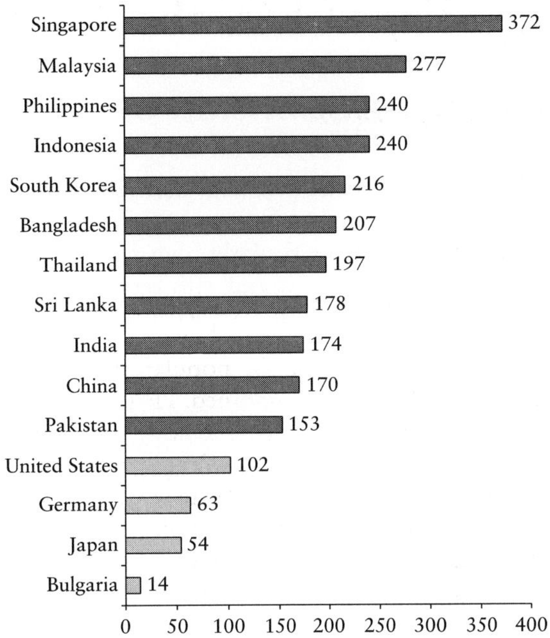


**Figure 1** Percentage increase in the elderly population: 2000–2030

**Table 1** The decreasing ratios of number of children to number of elderly for the World, Europe and Thailand

| *Year* | *World* | *Europe* | *Thailand* |
|---|---|---|---|
| 1950 | 6.6 | 3.2 | 14.2 |
| 1975 | 6.5 | 2.1 | 15.0 |
| 2000 | 4.3 | 1.2 | 4.3 |
| 2025 | 2.3 | 0.7 | 1.6 |
| 2030 | 1.2 | 0.6 | 0.9 |

aged 80 and over, referred to as the oldest old. These rapidly expanding numbers of the oldest old people will represent a social phenomenon. The growth of numbers of the oldest old is silent to public policy because individual needs and social responsibilities change considerably with increased age.

This rapidly aging society of Thailand and other Asian nations is soon likely to face us with the situation of the population consisting of more elderly people than children. There will be debate over health-care costs, social security, and intergenerational equity that has already emerged in Europe and North America[6].

## THE SOCIAL DIMENSION OF AGING IN ASIA

Why is aging a social problem? The last years of life are accompanied by an increase in disabilities and sickness, with particularly high demands on social and health services and with very high costs in relation to the provision of such services. The aging of the world population is likely to result in an increasingly large proportion of the global population living in absolute poverty. The most fundamental difference between developed and developing countries is with respect to the proportion of the population covered by social security and health-care schemes. All countries in Asia are mostly developing and this problem seems to be more obvious. Poverty is associated with feelings of helplessness, lack of control and continuing feelings of uncertainty[7]. These feelings of uncertainty and lack of control are strong predictors of health and well-being. Poverty is a life experience with profound implications for health.

Most elderly Asian couples live with their children or grandchildren. There are growing concerns in developing countries about the extent to which the twin processes of modernization and urbanization will change family structures[8,9]. Data for most of the developing world are insufficient to document changes in the living arrangements of the elderly. In Japan, there is the notion of 'intimacy at a distance', that is, as the financial and to some extent health status of elderly peoples improve, a large proportion of the elderly are able to afford to live alone and choose to do so in independent developments, while at the same time maintaining close familial contact and exchange of support[10,11].

## MAJOR GERIATRIC CONCERNS FOR ELDERLY COUPLES IN ASIA

A number of conditions compromise independence and quality of life in older persons; these are both communicable and non-communicable diseases for the elderly couple in Asia. These conditions result in increased suffering, service utilization and health-related costs. The disease burdens for the top ten leading causes in the world between 1990 and 2020, measured in disability-adjusted life years, are shown in Table 2.

For Thailand in the year 2000, the prioritization of diseases was based on disability data from the National Health examination survey 2, using 'Population attributable risk fraction' as criterion[13].

## ENHANCEMENT OF SOCIETAL ROLES AND INTERPERSONAL SUPPORT AND REDUCTION OF SOCIAL ISOLATION

Social support and continued involvement in useful activities have been shown to foster positive

**Table 2** Change in rank order of disease burden for top ten leading causes in the world: 1990 and 2020 (Source: Murray and Lopez, 1996)[12]

| | *Disease or injury* | |
|---|---|---|
| *Rank* | *1900* | *2020* |
| 1 | Lower respiratory infections | Ischemic heart disease |
| 2 | Diarrheal diseases | Unipolar major depression |
| 3 | Conditions arising during the perinatal period | Road traffic accidents |
| 4 | Unipolar major depression | Cerebrovascular disease |
| 5 | Ischemic heart disease | Chronic obstructive pulmonary disease |
| 6 | Cerebrovascular disease | Lower respiratory infections |
| 7 | Tuberculosis | Tuberculosis |
| 8 | Measles | War |
| 9 | Road traffic accidents | Diarrheal disease |
| 10 | Congenital anomalies | Human immunodeficiency virus |

effects on health and longevity. Being part of an active network also increases the opportunity for productive activities, whether paid or voluntary. For most older men and women, a substantial amount of productive work and contributions can continue throughout life. The identification of valued roles and continued social integration have been associated with health outcomes and self-assessed well-being.

Older people in most Asian countries are regarded as the 'pillar of the family'; they remain independent, active and productive in later life. Older people, both men and women, are now working in paid jobs, doing essential voluntary work, maintaining a household, and supporting grandchildren. Regular physical activity and exercise unquestionably promote dramatic benefits for health and life for people of almost all ages and abilities. Typically, physical activity can provide opportunities for adding years of active independent life. Furthermore, activity can reduce disability and contribute to the quality of life for middle-aged and older individuals[14].

An effective advocacy strategy that helps to promote health policies within each community is greatly needed. University professors, research assistants and graduate students can act as ambassadors. They serve as resources for information and assistance on health and fitness. In order to lead people to sound behavioral modifications, one should avoid phrases such as 'enhance your health and quality of life' and focus on objectives such as 'recover your health and maintain your quality of life'. This is simply because enhancement or improvement seems to be a non-achievable assignment for the majority of older citizens. If health and wellness programs rely on well-trained allied health professionals, then many average citizens may tend to lose their own will-power (strong desire or mental vitality) to achieve an independent, self-motivated way of living. An advocacy strategy that cooperates with or recruits non-qualified but capable health-fitness leaders should be implemented in the new initiatives. Whether one has an exercise leader's licence is not so important for actual leadership. Whether one is competent to help people to modify inadequate health behaviors is much more essential than having a licence. Orientals tend to accept this sort of idea more than Westerners do.

More emphasis should be placed on the combined values of exercise and diet. It is unrealistic for most individuals with chronic illnesses to expect to gain significantly large benefits from physical activities. Most researchers investigating physical activities want their findings from experiments and epidemiological studies to be incorporated into health policies. However, it is more important to help people to gain a real sense of satisfaction from their participation in physical activities. The public may not need any more laboratory data to convince them of the value of exercise. Scientists involved in exercise physiology should be making an all-out effort to inform the public about the potential harm of unhealthy lifestyles. The mass media can be extremely influential in these efforts.

Older adults and family members are sometimes faced with decisions about retirement finances, health and life insurance and medical treatment. In most Asian countries, due to close family links, these problems are encountered somewhat less; the government should prepare health-care delivery systems to support the old and oldest old, and to inform society about the issues of health finances for the family in late life.

## CONCLUSIONS

In the next half century, the proportion of elderly couples in Asia is expected to increase rapidly and to become more diverse. Health-care providers need to consider for these elderly and the oldest old how to live without a disease or disability. Improved diagnosis and treatment of major medical conditions will lead to growth in the of number of people living with one or more chronic conditions, which impact not necessarily on the length of life, but on the quality of life. It is important to understand the special needs of elderly persons so as to improve health status and quality of life for all older people.

# References


1. United Nations. World Population prospects. The 1998 Revision, 1999
2. The World Health Report. *Health systems: Improving Performance*, 2000:156–63
3. United States Census Bureau. International Data Base, 2000
4. Human Resources Planning Division, National Economic and Social Development Board, Population Projections for Thailand 1990-2020. Bangkok, Human Resources Planning Division, National Economic and Social Development Boards, 1995
5. Jitapunkul S, Bunnag S. *Aging in Thailand, 1997*. Bangkok: Thai Society of Gerontology and Geriatric Medicine, 1998
6. Office of Population Censuses and Surveys. *Population Projections 1987-2027*. London: HMSO, 1989: 2, No.16
7. Wallerstein N. Powerlessness, empowerment and health: implications for health promotion programs. *Am J Health Promotion* 1992;6:197–205
8. Anh ST, Cuong BT, Goodkind D, *et al.* Living arrangement patrilineality and sources of support among elderly Vietnamese. *Asia-Pacific Pop J* 1997; 4:69–88
9. Knodel J, Chayovan N. Family support and living arrangements of Thai elderly. *Asia-Pacific Pop J* 1997;4:51–68
10. Kamo Y. A note on elderly living arrangements in Japan and the United States. *Res Aging* 1988; 10:297–305
11. Stehouwer J. The household and family relations of old people. In Ethel Shanas, *et al.*, eds. *Old People in Three Industrial Societies.* New York: Atherton, 1968:177–226
12. Murray CJL, Lopez AD, eds. *The Global Burden of Diseases: a comprehensive assessment of mortality and disability from diseases, injuries, and risk factors in 1990 and projected to 2020.* Cambridge, MA: Harvard School of Public Health, 1996 (Global Burden of Disease and Injury Series, Vol. I)
13. Jitapunkul S. *Elderly Women in Thailand: Current Status*. Bangkok, Thailand: Chulalongkorn University Printing House, 2000:34–5
14. Teoman N, Özcan A, Acar B. The effect of exercise on physical fitness and quality of life in postmenopausal women. *Maturitas* 2004;47:71–7

# Alternatives to hormone therapy in menopausal women

8

*J. V. Pinkerton and R. Santen*

## INTRODUCTION

The recent Women's Health Initiative (WHI) study demonstrated that excess risks outweigh benefits for many women taking combination estrogen and progestogen therapy (EPT)[1]. Discussions with women about menopausal problems should include these findings as well as evidence-based information about hormone therapy and alternatives. Following release of the early results from the WHI in July 2002, many women became fearful or cautious about the use of hormone therapy (HT). Some abruptly stopped HT; others were weaned off by their providers. Concerns about breast cancer represent a major conceptual issue. Two-thirds of breast cancers in women living in western countries occur during the postmenopausal period. Survivors of breast cancer are an important subgroup of women confronting these new data. In premenopausal women who develop breast cancer, chemotherapy frequently induces the abrupt onset of ovarian failure and acute symptoms related to ovarian hormone deficiency. HT is often abruptly discontinued with the diagnosis of breast cancer. Survivors of breast cancer are fearful of the potential adverse effects of HT on their underlying breast cancer and particularly on the possibility of stimulation of undiagnosed tumor micro-metastases and a reduction in duration of survival. They are also concerned about development of contralateral breast cancer. For these reasons, alternatives to the use of hormone therapy for management of menopausal problems provide an important therapeutic strategy[2]. Key targets include vasomotor instability, urogenital atrophy, neurocognitive dysfunction, accelerated bone loss or development of heart disease. In this review, we will first examine the evidence that HT increases the risk of breast cancer and then use an evidence-based approach to compare the efficacy of HT to its alternatives for specific problems related to menopause.

## EVALUATION OF EVIDENCE

Evidence from large, properly controlled, randomized trials allows conclusions to be drawn which generally stand the test of time. Less compelling data lead to conclusions which may be changed when more substantial information becomes available. Evidence from observational studies, case reports, clinical impressions, and case-control or cohort studies may lead to conclusions which are later superseded by more compelling evidence from controlled trials.

### Types of evidence

To provide a standardized means of judging the validity of evidence, we utilize the US Preventative Task Force Criteria[3]:

*Level I* evidence – data from at least one properly randomized, controlled trial

*Level II* evidence – data from well-designed, controlled trials without randomization or from well-designed cohort or case-control analytic studies, preferably from more than one center or research group

*Level III* evidence – based upon the opinion of practicing physicians or upon the opinion of a panel of experts whose charge is to develop a consensus.

According to US Preventative Health Criteria procedures, the quality of individual trials is evaluated as to several fundamental factors including treatment confounders, blinding, statistical power and sample size, population characteristics, 'a priori' specification of hypothesis, data analysis methods, and proportion of persons lost to follow-up. If these quality issues are not appropriately dealt with, evidence from prospective, properly randomized, blinded, controlled studies is considered to be level II rather than level I evidence.

## EVIDENCE LINKING HORMONE THERAPY TO BREAST CANCER

### Clinical trials and breast cancer risk

*Women's Health Initiative (WHI) trial: relative risk*

The prospective, randomized, placebo-controlled WHI[4] study provides level I evidence regarding the effect of HT on breast cancer risk. A total of 16 608 menopausal women between 50 and 79 years of age with an intact uterus were randomized to receive 0.625 mg conjugated equine estrogen (CEE) and 2.5 mg of medroxyprogesterone acetate (MPA) or placebo. Compared with placebo users, those assigned to combination HT experienced a higher incidence of breast cancer. The increase in breast cancer relative risk reached statistical significance, with a relative risk (RR) of 1.24 (95% confidence interval (CI), 1.01–1.45)[4], which translated into a yearly relative risk increase of 5.2% (i.e. 26% increase at 5 years equals 5.2% per year). Based largely on the excess risk of breast cancer breaching preset limits, the WHI EPT arm of the trial was discontinued early after an average follow-up of 5.2 years. The breast cancer data remained significant (RR, 1.24; $p < 0.001$) according to standard statistical analyses after adjudication and complete entry of trial data, but lost significance when adjusted for sequential monitoring (CI, 0.97–1.59)[5].

*WHI estrogen-alone study results*

A separate study in the WHI Hormone Trial compared the use of estrogen alone (ET) with placebo in nearly 8000 women without a uterus[6]. This study was halted 1 year early, in 2004, because early results showed an increase in stroke without finding any reduction in risk of heart disease in women using estrogen alone. Continuing the study to planned conclusion in 2005 was felt not to add new information. Interestingly, there was no increased risk of breast cancer seen with estrogen alone; instead, there was a trend towards a decreased risk of breast cancer.

*Million Women Cohort Study*

The Million Women Study[7] confirmed the findings from the WHI of an increased risk of breast cancer for current users of estrogen and progestin (RR, 2.0; CI, 1.88–2.12), compared to an overall RR of 1.66 (CI, 1.58–1.75) for both ET/EPT. It also confirmed prior observational studies that estrogen therapy alone increases the risk of breast cancer (RR, 1.30; CI, 1.21–1.40). The follow-up was 2.6 years for cancer incidence and 4.1 years for mortality. In current users, the risk of breast cancer became apparent within 1–2 years of starting treatment and increased with duration of HT use. The risk appeared to be linear over time and was less in heavier women. Increased mortality was seen, but of borderline statistical significance. Past use did not increase the risk of incidence or mortality. The risk of breast cancer decreased with time since last use and reached the same level as non-users by year 5. Very little variation was found between specific estrogen and progestin products, their doses, their routes of administration or whether the regimen was continuous or sequential. Notably, for estrogen alone, increased risk was observed with oral, transdermal and parenteral formulations. Vaginal formulations of estrogen did not increase the risk (RR, 0.67; CI, 0.30–1.49). Because this is an observational study, with only a small number of HT prescriptions verified, there are potential confounding factors which could lead to errors. However, the study leads credence to the WHI findings of a small increase in absolute risk of breast cancer with EPT.

Prior observational studies have suggested that ET alone increases the risk of breast cancer (RR, 1.3). Ten years of HT with ET alone is estimated to result in five (CI, 3–7) additional breast cancers per 1000 women, and EPT combination to result in 19 (CI, 15–23) additional cancers per 1000 women. In contrast to the Million Women study which had much larger numbers, the randomized controlled WHI estrogen-only arm found 218 cases of cancer with a HR (hazard ratio) of 0.77 (95% CI, 0.59–1.01), non-significant but suggesting a trend towards a decreased risk of breast cancer in those women on estrogen only[6].

## Definitions of risk: relative, absolute and attributable

Interpretation of data from the WHI and Million Women studies requires understanding of the statistical terms used. Relative risk represents the ratio of breast cancer cases in women receiving HT to those not taking HT. Absolute risk is the number of women who are diagnosed with breast cancer at a specific time point and is usually expressed as number per 1000 per year. Attributable or excess risk refers to the number of women who develop breast cancer because of HT use and is calculated as the difference in absolute risk between HT users and non-users.

To help women make decisions about HT, the WHI and other trial results should be interpreted in terms of absolute and attributable risks and not relative risk[8]. For example, a 26% increase in relative risk does not mean that 26% of women will develop breast cancer. Instead, it indicates a 26% increase in the number of breast cancers diagnosed in a population of women. The attributable (excess) risk is most meaningful for a patient, as it conveys the actual chances that she will develop breast cancer as a result of taking HT. To determine attributable risk of breast cancer in a woman receiving HT, one first calculates the incidence of breast cancer in an age-matched population to determine absolute risk without HT. One then multiplies this by the relative risk imparted by HT. The difference between absolute risk with and without HT represents attributable or excess risk.

Attributable risk of developing breast cancer from HT depends on age. For an average 60-year-old woman, the underlying absolute risk of breast cancer is 16.9 cases per 1000 women per 5 years. Based upon the WHI data, the estrogen plus progestin combination causes a 26% increase in relative risk at 5 years. The absolute risk of breast cancer in women taking HT is then 16.9 multiplied by the relative risk of 1.26 or 21.3 per 1000 over 5 years. The difference in risk (attributable risk or excess risk) is then 4.4 per 1000 women over 5 years. Considered in another way, a woman will have a *1 in 225* chance of getting a breast cancer that she would not otherwise have had if she takes HT for a period of 5 years.

### *WHI estrogen/progestin study: absolute and attributable risks*

Absolute risk in the WHI study was expressed as the number of women per 1000 per year who developed events. These risks were compared in those receiving placebo vs. those taking estrogen/progestin (CEE/MPA)[4]. In the placebo group, 3.0 per 1000 women per year developed breast cancer vs. 3.8 receiving estrogen/progestin. For coronary artery disease events, this was 3.0 per 1000 women per year in comparison with 3.7 per 1000, and for stroke, 2.1 versus 2.9. Data were expressed in the same way when HT caused protective effects. Thus, for colorectal cancer, the absolute rate was 1.6 per 1000 women per year in women taking placebo vs. 1.0 for those receiving CEE/MPA, and for hip fracture 15 vs. 10. Attributable risk (excess risk) was expressed as events per 10 000 woman-years. The updated and adjusted results of the WHI study showed that estrogen/progestin users experienced six excess coronary events[9], seven excess strokes[10], 18 excess venous thromboembolisms[4], eight excess pulmonary embolisms[4], eight excess breast cancers[5], 23 excess cases of dementia[11], six fewer colorectal cancers[4] and five fewer hip fractures[4].

### *WHI estrogen-only study: absolute and attributable risks*

As in the estrogen/progestin study, absolute risk in the WHI study was expressed as the number of women per 1000 per year who developed events and compared against the risk in those receiving placebo[6]. In the placebo group, 3.2/1000 women per year developed stroke vs. 4.4/1000 receiving estrogen therapy. For venous thromboembolic events, there were 1.5/1000 among those on placebo and 2.1/1000 receiving estrogen; for coronary heart events, 5.4/1000 for placebo and only 4.9/1000 on estrogen. Hip fractures were reduced, with 1.7/1000 on placebo and 1.1 on estrogen. For breast cancer, there were 3.3/1000 on placebo and 2.6/1000 on estrogen (not statistically significant). There were slightly more cases of colorectal cancer, with 1.6/1000 on placebo and 1.7/1000 with estrogen (not statistically significant). Overall, there was an increase in stroke and venous thromboembolism, and no significant effect on heart events, breast cancer, or colorectal cancer and a decrease in hip fractures. Attributable risk (excess risk) was expressed as events per 10 000 woman-years. In the WHI estrogen-only study, estrogen users experienced 12 excess strokes, six excess blood clots, five fewer heart events (not statistically significant), seven fewer breast cancers (not statistically significant), one excess colorectal cancer (not statistically significant), six fewer hip fractures, with three more deaths (not statistically significant).

## WHI in comparison with prior observational studies

Observational studies (level II data) published over the past three decades often came to conclusions disparate from those of the WHI. The Collaborative Group meta-analysis[12], involving over 50 000 women with breast cancer provided four reasons for the conflicting conclusions regarding observational studies of HT and breast cancer risk.

(1) The increased risk of breast cancer with HT dissipates within 3–5 years after stopping this medication. Thus, studies comparing 'ever-users' with 'never-users' would be unlikely to demonstrate a risk from HT unless most of the 'ever-users' were still taking estrogens.

(2) The risk of breast cancer from estrogens is linear over time, with a 2.3% increase in relative risk per year of use. Most earlier studies included women taking HT for a relatively short period of time and thus only at a minimally increased risk.

(3) The risk of breast cancer from HT seems to be limited to thin women with a body mass index of less than 25. Studies which included a high proportion of obese women would not be expected to demonstrate an increased risk from HT.

(4) The risk of breast cancer falls for a 4-year period after the menopause; thus, groups of women who have been menopausal for a similar duration are needed to detect an increased risk of breast cancer.

## Addition of a progestin to estrogen

Investigators once believed that progestins might protect the breast from cancer but the opposite conclusion appears likely. Schairer and colleagues[13] examined this issue in a large observational study and reported that estrogen-alone increased the relative risk of breast cancer by 1% per year and estrogen plus a progestin by 8% per year. The Nurses' Health Study[14] confirmed the conclusions of Schairer and colleagues. Women followed for 860 000 patient-years exhibited a 2% increase in relative risk per year with estrogens alone and a 9% increase per year with estrogen plus a progestin. Additional studies by Ross and colleagues[15] and by Magnussen and colleagues[16] also support the conclusion that progestins add to the risk of breast cancer imparted by estrogens. The risk of breast cancer with HT may increase linearly with time, arguing against use of long-term estrogen/progestin therapy to prevent osteoporosis or heart disease. Based upon the Nurses' Health Study, 10 years of use of estrogen plus a progestin would increase the relative risk of breast cancer by 90%. In contrast, 1 year of use to prevent hot flushes would only be associated with only a 9% increased relative risk[14].

## Breast cancer diagnosed in women on HT

The WHI study[5] found that women diagnosed with breast cancer while on combination estrogen/progestin therapy had slightly larger tumors (1.7 cm vs. 1.5 cm) than those on placebo. In addition, local spread to the regional lymph nodes occurred more commonly at the time of diagnosis (25.9%) in the HT group than in those receiving placebo (15.8%). There was no difference in the incidence of distant metastases (1% vs. 1%). This suggests that use of HT might result in the appearance of larger and more aggressive tumors at the time of diagnosis. Since HT can render the reading of mammograms more difficult because of increased breast density, it is possible that HT resulted in delay in diagnosis. These results of the WHI are in contrast to those of observational studies which have shown smaller tumor size and better survival in women diagnosed with breast cancer while on HT. Longer follow-up will be necessary to determine the ultimate outcome of the women diagnosed with breast cancer in the WHI and Million Women studies.

*Summary of use of HT and risk of breast cancer*
Level I evidence indicates that an estrogen/progestin combination (CEE/MPA) increases the relative risk of breast cancer by 5.2% per year. Level II evidence suggests that estrogen alone increases the relative risk of breast cancer by 1% per year. No significant differences were found between specific types or doses or regimens of estrogen or estrogen and progestin therapy and the increased risk of breast cancer in the Million Women study. Final conclusions regarding estrogen alone await development of level I evidence.

### Biologic perspective of estrogen/progestin therapy effects on breast

At the present time, we do not have level I evidence that estrogens alone increase the risk of breast cancer. However, we consider it prudent to err on the conservative side and conclude that the risk is highly plausible. Experimental data in animals and epidemiologic studies in humans strongly suggest that estrogens are promoters in the breast. Administration of estrogen to certain animal species results in an increase in breast cancer. In women, the relative degree of lifetime exposure to estradiol increases the risk of breast cancer. For example, early menarche, late menopause, obesity, a 20 kg weight gain after age 21, increased plasma estradiol levels, increased bone and breast density are all associated with an increased risk of breast cancer. Each of these parameters provides a biologic surrogate reflecting long-term exposure to estradiol. Oophorectomy before the age of 35 reduces the lifetime risk of breast cancer by 75% in women[17,18]. Selective estrogen receptor modulators (SERMs) such as tamoxifen cause a 50% reduction in diagnosed breast cancer when taken over a 4–5-year period[19].

*Use of hormone therapy in breast cancer survivors*
Based upon all available data, what can be concluded about HT use in breast cancer survivors? Only anecdotal observations have suggested that use of HT induces tumor recurrence or more rapid tumor growth in breast cancer survivors[20]. In contrast, highly selected women, given estrogen following a diagnosis of breast cancer, experience no increase in rate of recurrence or diminution of survival[21–23]. A recent randomized trial of placebo versus HT in breast survivors reported a similar rate of disease recurrence and no compromise in survival. This study, however, was small and only a fraction of the women asked to participate agreed to do so[24]. Caution is recommended since data are largely observational and include women highly selected for evidence of cure of their underlying breast cancer. Larger, controlled, prospective trials are needed to resolve the issue of safety in breast cancer survivors. In this group, the use of alternatives to HT is considered a reasonable first approach to managing problems related to menopause.

## BACKGROUND: USE OF ALTERNATIVES TO HT

Major therapeutic goals to be achieved by estrogen alternatives include the relief of vasomotor instability and urogenital atrophy, neurocognitive changes, and the prevention of heart disease and osteoporosis[19]. Estrogen therapy may also reduce Alzheimer's disease, macular degeneration, colon cancer, and mandibular bone loss but data supporting these uses are controversial[18]. This review will examine data regarding the relative risks and benefits of HT vs. non-estrogen alternatives to provide a logical means to approach decision-making and patient education.

## VASOMOTOR INSTABILITY

Vasomotor symptoms are a significant problem in menopausal women and include hot flushes, night sweats, sweating, insomnia or early morning awakening, mood disturbances, muscle aching, and fatigue. The Northern American Menopause Society (NAMS) recently published a comprehensive position statement on the treatment of menopause-associated vasomotor symptoms[25].

## Estrogen

Vasomotor symptoms respond well to hormone therapy which, based on level 1 evidence, is considered the therapeutic standard[25,26]. Treatment of moderate to severe hot flushes, defined as greater than seven hot flushes per day or 50–60 per week, is the primary indication for systemic estrogen therapy. Because of the increased risk of uterine cancer with unopposed estrogen, women with a uterus need progestin to oppose the estrogen effect on the uterus[27].

Evidence is accumulating that lower-dosage[28]. HT may provide similar benefits but potentially with improved safety profile and fewer side-effects. In their position statements, NAMS, The American College of Obstetricians and Gynecologists, and the FDA all recommend that, if HT is used, the lowest effective dose be used for the shortest period of time consistent with treatment goals[26]. Current lower doses of ET and EPT include 0.45 mg and 0.3 mg conjugated estrogens, 0.3 mg esterified estrogens, 0.25–0.5 mg oral 17β-estradiol, and 0.025 mg 17β-estradiol patch. The safety of lower doses of estrogen, use of vaginal/intrauterine progestin therapies and longer-interval intermittent dosing of progestin needs to be determined.

## Placebo

Placebo effect is consistently seen in vasomotor trials, reducing the number and severity of hot flushes from about 25–50%[25]. In order to recommend other alternatives to HT for patients not at high risk for breast cancer, long-term, adequately powered, randomized, placebo-controlled clinical trials are needed for safety and efficacy in patients with moderate to severe vasomotor symptoms with defined hot flush frequency entry criteria.

## Lifestyle modifications

Changes that the women herself can make include lowering air temperature, avoiding hot foods or drinks that raise core temperature, non-perspiration exercise, smoking fewer or no cigarettes, paced respiration, and engaging in relaxing activities such as yoga or massage[25,26]. Evidence of efficacy is primarily anecdotal.

## Non-prescription remedies

When vasomotor symptoms are mild, non-proven therapies may be considered[29,30]. Vitamin E[31] results in statistically significant improvement over placebo but effects are minimal (i.e. one hot flush reduction per person per day).

### *Dietary phytoestrogens/isoflavones*

The popular literature suggests that soy products and phytoestrogens may be effective for treating hot flushes but objective studies[32–35] show conflicting results. Eleven studies examining soy or isoflavone supplementation were recently reviewed. Only three of eight studies lasting longer than 6 weeks demonstrated significant improvement and the longest study to date (24 weeks) was negative[25,29]. A recent randomized, placebo-controlled, double-blind trial of postmenopausal women comparing 59 women who drank a soy beverage compared to 64 with a placebo (rice beverage) found no significant difference between soy and placebo, although both reduced hot flushes[33]. The isoflavone, red clover, has been studied in small, short-duration, randomized, placebo-controlled studies which have shown no benefit for hot flush treatment over placebo. One trial found 80 mg/day effective (Promensil), but the study had a low placebo response of 16%[36–38].

### *Herbal products*

Studies have shown no effect for dong quai[39], ginseng[40], evening primrose oil, and vitamin E plus evening primrose oil[41]. Vitex/Chasteberry, DHEAS, melatonin, and St. John's Wort are often used but lack efficacy, and safety/toxicity data are lacking.

### *Black cohosh*

Studies on black cohosh (*Cimicifuga racemosa*)[42,43] have primarily used the commercial product

Remifemin. Three randomized, placebo-controlled trials compared black cohosh to estrogen. The most recent[43] showed that black cohosh at a dose of 40 mg/day had no significant effect on hot flushes compared with placebo. Although most reports[44] suggest that black cohosh is not estrogenic, caution should be used, particularly in patients with breast cancer or use longer than 6 months.

*Topical progesterone*

Progesterone creams made from wild yam and soybeans contain progesterone precursors (disogenin) but humans lack the enzyme to metabolize disogenin to progesterone. Therefore, USP progesterone must be added for the topical progesterone cream to be pharmacologically active. Although some studies have found efficacy in reduction of hot flushes[45], most studies have found no effect and minimal elevations in serum progesterone levels[45–47]. There is no evidence that these creams, when applied topically, protect against estrogen-induced endometrial hyperplasia[29].

## Prescription therapy: hormonal

Progestins alone effectively decrease hot flushes[48–50]. Megestrol acetate (40 mg daily), as well as oral and intramuscular MPA, appears to be as effective as estrogen, with an approximately 80% level of control of hot flushes. Maximal effect of progestin therapy on hot flush reduction may take 4–6 weeks. Long-term safety of progestins, particularly in patients surviving breast cancer, is not known. Bone loss has been reported with intramuscular long-acting depot MPA. Side-effects include weight gain, increase in appetite, irregular uterine bleeding, exacerbation of diabetes and increase in venous thromboembolic events.

## Prescription therapy: non-hormonal

*Serotonin uptake inhibitors*

The selective serotonin reuptake inhibitor (SSRI) class of drugs decreases hot flushes more effectively than placebo[25], with postulated effects related to effects on central serotonin or norepinephrine concentrations. Onset of action is more rapid (e.g. 1–2 weeks) for hot flush reduction than for relief of depression (e.g. 6 weeks). Most studies have enrolled small numbers with entry criteria of only two to three hot flushes per day. The FDA requires more than seven hot flushes per day or 50 hot flushes per week for entry into trials. Many studies included breast cancer survivors or women at high risk for breast cancer who concomitantly received tamoxifen, raloxifene or other medications. Larger clinical trials are needed in symptomatic menopausal women to determine safety and efficacy.

*Venlafaxine* has been studied in a double-blind, randomized, 4-week trial[51] of 229 women with at least 14 hot flushes per week; 69% of those enrolled were on tamoxifen. Placebo produced a 27% reduction in number of hot flushes ($n = 56$) compared to a 37% decrease with venlafaxine at 37.5 mg ($n = 56$), a 61% reduction with 75 mg ($n = 55$) and a similar reduction of 61% with 150 mg ($n = 54$). Side-effects of dry mouth, decreased appetite, nausea, constipation and sexual dysfunction were significantly higher at doses of 75 and 150 mg. These findings suggest that doses lower than those needed for depression will be effective (level 2 evidence). *Fluoxetine* (20 mg) was studied in a small, randomized, double-blind, cross-over trial[52] in women with breast cancer with at least 14 hot flushes per day and resulted in a decrease in hot flush score (frequency times average intensity) of 50% vs. 36% placebo response. A double-blind, placebo-controlled, 6-week trial[53] used controlled release *paroxetine* in a trial of 165 women with two to three hot flushes per day. This study found that, at doses of 12.5 or 25 mg/day, hot flush composite scores decreased by 62.2% and 64.6% compared to a 37.8% placebo response.

*Gabapentin*

A level 1, randomized, controlled trial[54] of 59 postmenopausal women with seven or more hot flushes per day confirmed Loprinizi's pilot study[55] on the efficacy of gabapentin, 300 mg three times daily. After 12 weeks, hot flush frequency was decreased by 45% and composite hot flush score by 54%. Placebo response was 29% and 31%. Side-effects included dizziness and light-headedness, particularly at initiation of therapy, and peripheral edema; 50% reported at least one adverse event and 13.3% withdrew. Based upon these early findings, gabapentin could be considered for off-label use for treatment of hot flushes, although side-effects may limit use. A starting dose as low as 100 mg/day may be needed, particularly in older women. Larger and longer controlled clinical trials are needed.

### *Antihypertensives and bellergal*

Bellergal (phenobarbitol, ergotamine, levorotatory alkaloids of belladona) and methyldopa provide limited efficacy with significant side-effects. In contrast, clonidine may be somewhat effective. One randomized, placebo-controlled study of 194 breast cancer patients, taking tamoxifen, demonstrated reduction of hot flush frequency by 38% after 8 weeks with orally administered clonidine, compared with a 20% decrease with placebo[56]. Transdermal clonidine[57] also reduced hot flushes significantly ($p < 0.0001$) in a randomized, double-blind study in women with a history of breast cancer on tamoxifen, but was only moderately clinically effective, with a 20% reduction from baseline in hot flush frequency and 10% reduction in severity. Side-effects include dry mouth, constipation, itchiness, drowsiness, fatigue, and hypotension.

## UROGENITAL ATROPHY

Symptoms include frequent urination, urinary urgency or leakage, vaginal dryness, itching or burning in the vagina or vulva, and dyspareunia. Oral estrogens relieve these symptoms and reduce the frequency of urinary tract infections. Vaginal moisturizers[58] and lubricants can be helpful in patients not willing to take estrogens, but do not completely relieve symptoms in the majority. One moisturizer, Replens[59], used three times weekly, was compared to conjugated estrogen cream at a dose of 1.25 mg/day in a randomized 12-week trial with 30 patients. This study showed that Replens reduced vaginal pH to 4.8, compared to estrogen at 4.4, diminished atrophy in 60% of patients, compared to 100% with estrogen, and relieved symptoms, but not to the same extent as estrogen.

Another approach is to use sufficiently low doses of vaginal estrogen to achieve local effects without systemic estrogen absorption. Standard doses of vaginal estrogen have been found to increase plasma estrogen levels. However, very low doses of vaginal estrogen do not increase plasma levels substantially and yet can be effective. Plasma estrone and estradiol levels were measured in women receiving vaginal Premarin[60], with gradual increases in doses from 0.3 to 2.5 g per day. At the highest dose used, systemic levels of estradiol significantly increased up to 60 pg/ml, comparable to those seen with oral Premarin. However, the lowest dose (0.3 g/day) produced complete maturation of vaginal mucosa, with only minimal increases in plasma estrone and estradiol. Using this very low-dose regimen, Handa and colleagues[60] showed no increase in plasma estrone over baseline after 6 months of use. Disadvantages of the vaginal method involve irregular application intervals, bolus absorption and low-absorption capacity of a fat-based vehicle, necessitating use of emollient (which results in stickiness, messiness and compliance issues). Absorption rates vary, based on the severity of the vaginal atrophy.

Estrogen can be delivered locally into the vagina, without significant systemic absorption, with a vaginal estrogen ring device (Estring)[61,62] and with vaginal tablets[63,64]. The vaginal ring provides nearly complete relief of symptoms. Use of this device is associated with a decreased frequency of urinary tract infections in elderly women[62]. In open-label studies (but with blinded review of vaginal cytology), similar efficacy was observed with the vaginal ring device as with conjugated systemic estrogens with respect to vaginal secretions, color, tissue integrity, urethral meatus integrity and patient acceptance. Data reviewed indicate minimal systemic absorption from this device[63,64]. Only 4% of women using the ring had endometrial thickness greater than 5 mm measured by ultrasound, compared with 10% using the vaginal cream. Three percent experienced vaginal withdrawal bleeding from the ring, compared to 21% using vaginal cream. The Estring was associated with an increase in bone density in postmenopausal women, suggesting some degree of systemic absorption.

Very low doses of estradiol given vaginally achieve local vaginal effects without systemic absorption of estradiol[65]. Currently available radioimmunoassays for estradiol may not be sufficiently sensitive to detect minor increments in plasma estradiol with use of Estring or vaginal creams[64]. For example, use of a 25 μg vaginal estradiol tablet, now available, caused no detectable increments in estradiol levels[64]. Our studies using an ultrasensitive estradiol bioassay detected small increases in plasma estrogen after administration of 10 μg into the vagina[65]. Further studies are required to determine the safety of vaginal estradiol in women surviving breast cancer, as these patients could potentially be highly sensitive to even minimal amounts of circulating estradiol. Dessole and colleagues[66] recently showed, in a well-designed study of incontinence using urocytometrics, that vaginal estriol ovules improved urinary incontinence over placebo. Taken together, these data suggest that low-dose local vaginal estrogen allows treatment of genitourinary atrophy with less systemic estrogen exposure. Risk for endometrial cancer is present if vaginal estrogen is unopposed. Safety has not been established in women with prior breast cancer, although the Million Women Study showed no increase in breast cancer risk with local vaginal estrogen.

## NEUROCOGNITIVE DYSFUNCTION

Observational studies suggested that estrogen therapy may have a positive effect on memory and particularly verbal memory and may decrease the incidence and severity of Alzheimer's disease. However, the WHI recently reported an increase in dementia[10] in women who initiated EPT at age ≥ 65 years (hazard ratio (HR), 2.05; CI, 1.21–3.48; $p = 0.01$), with an absolute risk of adverse[10] effect of 23/10 000 women/year. No increase was seen in mild cognitive impairment, considered a precursor to dementia. These studies call into question the beneficial effects of estrogen on memory and Alzheimer's prevention. Accordingly, the alternatives to estrogen require focus on depression and sleep disturbance, symptoms likely to be related to estrogen deprivation. Depression should be identified and treated with antidepressants and mood stabilizers. The SSRI class of drugs should be as effective in women with menopause-associated depression as in endogenous depression not associated with estrogen deficiency. However, this issue has not been studied with carefully controlled studies. More research is needed to identify the frequency and severity of these symptoms and the use of non-estrogenic medications for their treatment. Trazodone or intermittent use (every 3 days) of benzodiazepines and hypnotics has been used for symptoms of sleep disturbance.

**Table 1** 2003 National Osteoporosis Foundation Guidelines for bone mineral density (BMD) testing

- Women 65 and older regardless of risk factors
- Postmenopausal women less than 65 with one or more risk factors (besides Caucasian race) such as:
  - Family history of osteoporosis
  - Personal history of fragility fracture (low trauma) after age 45
  - Current smoking
  - Low body weight of less than 127 lbs
- Postmenopausal women who present with fractures (to confirm the diagnosis and determine disease severity)
- Women considering therapy if BMD would influence their decision
- Women who have been on menopausal hormone therapy for prolonged periods

**Table 2** NOF Recommendations for treatment

- Prior vertebral or hip fracture
- *T* score - 2SD, regardless of other risk factors
- *T* score -1.5 with one or more risk factors

*Additional recommendations*
- Adequate calcium, 1200 mg/day
- Vitamin D, 400–800 IU /day
- Encourage weight-bearing physical activity
- Smoking cessation
- Avoiding excess alcohol

National Osteoporosis Foundation. Physician's Guide to Prevention and Treatment of Osteoporosis, 2003
NIH Consensus Development Panel. Osteoporosis prevention, diagnosis and therapy. *J Am Med Assoc* 2001;285:785–95

## PREVENTION AND TREATMENT OF OSTEOPOROSIS

Osteoporosis is defined[67] as a skeletal disorder characterized by compromised bone strength,

**Table 3** FDA-approved therapy for osteoporosis

| *FDA-approved therapy* | *Prevention* | *Treatment* |
|---|---|---|
| Hormone therapy | yes | no |
| Raloxifene | yes | yes |
| Alendronate | yes | yes |
| Risedronate | yes | yes |
| Calcitonin | no | yes |
| Parathyroid hormone | no | yes |

which predisposes a person to increased risk of fracture. Bone quality is influenced by bone turnover, microarchitecture, damage accumulation and mineralization. Bone mineral density (BMD) is the most useful measure available but gives no information on bone quality. The National Osteoporosis Foundation (NOF) recommendations[68] for when to obtain BMD measurement are given in Table 1 and the WHO classification of bone loss in Table 2. Level I and II studies have established the importance of fractures as independent predictors of subsequent fracture risk. The presence of at least one vertebral fracture at baseline increases the risk of sustaining a vertebral fracture five-fold compared to those without prior vertebral fractures, even with similar BMD[69,70]. The NOF recommends therapy for women who have a *T* score of –2 standard deviations (SD) in the absence of risk factors and –1.5 if other risk factors are present. Younger women with –2 SD are at less risk for fracture than older women. FDA approved medications are available (Table 3) for prevention and/or treatment of osteoporosis. The antiresorptive therapies prevent bone loss while the newer anabolic therapies increase bone formation.

## Exercise

Physical activity throughout life contributes to high peak bone mass. Weight-bearing activities such as walking, exercise against resistance, weight training and high impact exercise can increase BMD, perhaps by 1-2%. Once the exercise program is stopped, the gains in bone density are lost. Fitness may indirectly decrease fractures by improving mobility, muscle strength and reducing the risk of falls.

## Reducing the risk of hip fracture: non-pharmocologic methods

In the Study of Osteoporotic fractures, the independent risk fractures for hip fracture[71] included maternal family history of hip fracture, height at age 25, history of hyperthyroidism, poor depth perception, poor contrast sensitivity, failure to spend more than 4 hours each day on one's feet, inability to rise from a chair without using one's arms, and a history of prior fractures after the age of 50. Risk of falls can be reduced through regular exercise to increase muscle mass and strength, balance exercise programs such as Tai Chi, follow-up and correction of problems with visual acuity and depth perception, avoidance of medications that induce hypotension or sedation, avoidance of slippery floors and loose rugs, putting up handrails, and adequate lighting with night lights. Hip protectors (energy-absorbing external hip padders) reduce hip fractures[72] by 50% compared to controls, if properly and consistently used. Long-term adherence data are lacking.

## Antiresorptive therapy

Antiresorptive agents, including estrogen, the bisphosphonates, calcitonin, and the SERMS, improve bone density and preserve microarchitecture. FDA-approved therapies for prevention and/or treatment of osteoporosis are listed in Table 3 and their use is supported by level I evidence. Adequate calcium intake is considered a physiological requirement.

## Calcium

Low calcium intake provokes secondary hyperparathyroidism and resultant calcium mobilization from the skeleton. In recently menopausal women, calcium supplements alone have proven largely ineffective in preventing the accelerated bone loss that results from estrogen deficiency. In women more than 5 years postmenopausal, however, calcium supplementation slows loss in women with initially low dietary calcium intake[73]. One prospective but not randomized trial suggested that calcium in osteoporotic women decreased the incidence of vertebral fractures[74].

A randomized, controlled, 3-year trial[75] in community-dwelling men and women over the age of 65 showed that 500 mg of calcium plus 700 IU vitamin D decreased bone loss at the spine, femoral neck, total body, and decreased the risk of non-vertebral fractures. In elderly patients, calcium and vitamin D have been shown to reduce hip fracture[76]. Largely on the basis of level II evidence, it is reasonable to suggest daily intake of 1200–1500 mg of elemental calcium and 400 IU of vitamin D daily for postmenopausal women not on hormone therapy. Vitamin D supplementation improves intestinal calcium absorption in women over 65. Treatment with pharmacologic amounts of vitamin D or its metabolites (calcitriol) should probably be restricted to those with limited sunlight exposure or vitamin D intake, malabsorption, multiple anticonvulsants or poor calcium absorption.

## Estrogen therapy

Alternatives to estrogen therapy for osteopenia or osteoporosis should be compared with estrogen to determine relative efficacy. A variety of observational studies have provided evidence that estrogens are beneficial for prevention of osteoporosis and fracture[77-82]. A series of 20 studies[77] revealed a risk reduction of approximately 50%, with a range of zero to 80%. Several studies estimated a lifetime reduction of vertebral and hip fractures and increased overall survival from prevention of these events[78,79]. A prospective cohort study (The Study of Osteoporotic Fractures)[80] among 9704 women 65 and older, found the relative risk for non-spinal fractures for women on estrogen to be 0.66. Current users experienced a reduced hip fracture relative risk of 0.60. For women who started estrogen within 5 years of menopause, the RR was 0.29 for hip fracture and 0.50 for all non-spinal fractures. A recent meta-analysis reported a 27% decrease in rate of total fractures with HT[81]. This reduction was only significant for younger women.

The first randomized trial sufficiently large to present level I evidence was the WHI study[4]. Overall fractures were decreased, with a RR for total fractures of 0.76 (CI, 0.69–0.85), vertebral fractures 0.66 (CI, 0.44–0.98) and for hip 0.66 (0.45–0.98). The WHI study, in contrast to the meta-analysis of Togersen and colleagues, demonstrated a decrease in total fractures as well as hip fractures in a relatively young population (average age 63). This substantiates the efficacy of estrogens for fracture prevention in younger as well as older women. Data from this trial are supported by the PEPI study[82] in which a 2% increase in hip bone mineral density and 4% in the lumbar spine were documented after 3 years of therapy. These data provide the standard against which alternatives to estrogen should be compared. It should be noted, however, that concerns about long-term risk/benefit ratio limit the enthusiasm for long-term use of HT for routine use to prevent osteoporosis or fractures. Once HT is discontinued, bone loss occurs[83,84] similar to that with menopause and the benefits are lost within 5 years of therapy cessation[85].

## Bisphosphonates

Bisphosphonates inhibit osteoclast-mediated bone resorption to the same or to a greater extent than hormone therapy. Both alendronate and risedronate have level I evidence of effectiveness at increasing BMD and reducing fracture rates and are FDA-approved for prevention and treatment of osteoporosis. Etidronate is also effective but has been reported to induce a mineralization defect after long-term use. The oral bioavailability of all bisphosphonates is low, between 1 and 3% of the dose ingested, and is impaired by food, calcium, iron, coffee, tea and orange juice. Because bisphosphonates have an extended duration of action, weekly administration of both alendronate and risedronate is available, which reduces the inconvenience of daily dosing. Similar bone density increases are seen with daily or weekly dosing schedules but fracture data are not available for weekly therapy.

For women with breast cancer, bisphosphonates may be particularly attractive because of reduced risk of fractures from skeletal metastasis and potential for slowing of progression of metastasis[86], with reductions in pathologic fractures, surgery for fracture or impending fracture, radiation, spinal cord compression and hypercalcemia. For patients with radiologic evidence of bone destruction, intravenous pamidronate 90 mg over 2 hours or zoledronic acid 4 mg every 3-4 weeks has been used[87], although not FDA-approved for this indication. Starting patients at high risk for future bone metastasis without evidence of either lytic destruction of bone or osteoporosis is currently not recommended.

### *Alendronate*

*Bone mineral density* A meta-analysis of 11 randomized, placebo-controlled trials of alendronate in postmenopausal women with osteoporosis that lasted at least 1 year[88] revealed increases in the BMD in the lumbar spine, femoral neck and total body in both early postmenopausal women and those with established osteoporosis. The increase in BMD was dose-related, with greater increases seen with 10 mg compared to 5 mg daily use[88]. After 3 years of treatment with a daily dose of 10 mg, the pooled estimate for difference between alendronate and placebo was 7.48% in lumbar spine (CI, 6.12-8.85), 5.6% for femoral neck (CI, 4.80-6.39), 2.08% at the forearm (CI, 1.53-2.63) and 2.73% for total body (CI, 2.27-3.20). These well-designed level I trials show that alendronate is effective at preventing vertebral and non-vertebral fractures when compared to placebo. Ten mg appears to be the most effective dose; 70 mg weekly is considered the equivalent dose with proven similar BMD efficacy, but fracture data are lacking. Long-term use appears safe despite theoretical concerns about oversuppression of resorption (frozen bone). Limited data from long-term extensions[89] of phase 3 studies reported at 10 years confirm continued linear improvements in bone density, estimated at 13.7%. There is evidence of small decreases in hip and forearm BMD during years 8-10. Unlike discontinuation of HT, discontinuation of alendronate after 5 years does not lead to accelerated bone loss.

Data regarding the relative efficacy of the bisphosphonates versus estrogen are available for effects on bone density but not for fracture prevention. Alendronate at low dose (5 mg per day) appears to exert antiresorptive potency similar to that of estrogen. The Early Postmenopausal Intervention Cohort (EPIC)[90,91] study of recently menopausal women included placebo, alendronate (2.5 or 5 mg/day) and open-label estrogen/progestin. Patients receiving placebo plus calcium lost bone. Those receiving either 2.5 or 5 mg of alendronate/day increased bone mass between 1 and 2% over baseline, while the estrogen/progestin group increased BMD by 2%[92].

*Vertebral fracture efficacy* Double-blind, placebo-controlled studies provide compelling level I evidence of the vertebral antifracture efficacy of alendronate. The first[93] study involved 994 postmenopausal women (mean age, 64 years) with osteoporosis who received either placebo for 3 years, alendronate 5 mg/day for 3 years, alendronate 10 mg/day for 3 years, or alendronate 20 mg/day for 2 years and then 5 mg/day for the third year. BMD increased in those receiving alendronate and decreased in the placebo group. Vertebral fractures occurred in 6.2% of patients receiving placebo and 3.2% of patients receiving alendronate; this represented a 48% reduction in numbers of women sustaining fractures ($p < 0.04$). Two or more new vertebral fractures occurred in 4.2% of patients receiving placebo and 0.6% of patients receiving alendronate, a risk reduction of 87%. Patients in the placebo group who sustained new fractures lost 23.3 mm in height. Alendronate-treated patients who sustained one or more fractures lost only 5.9 mm in height, consistent with less severe fractures. Non-vertebral fractures occurred in 60 of 590 women receiving placebo and 73 of 1012 receiving alendronate. The cumulative incidences (placebo vs. alendronate) were 12.6% and 9%, a 29% reduction in risk compared with placebo ($p < 0.05$).

In the Fracture Intervention Trial (FIT)[94-96], 2027 women (mean age, 71 years) with one or more vertebral fractures at baseline and reduced BMD, were randomized to receive either placebo ($n = 1005$) or alendronate ($n = 1022$, 5 mg/day for 2 years, 10 mg/day in year 3). After 3 years, BMD increased significantly by 6.2% above placebo at the spine and by 4.7% above placebo at the total hip region. The rate of new, clinically apparent vertebral fractures decreased by 47%, compared to placebo. Similar decreases were seen in the frequency of hip and wrist fractures, but not for other types of fractures. Of note in a follow-up study of women without prevalent vertebral fractures, only those with osteoporosis (i.e. bone density at the femoral neck of > 2.5 SD below the normal adult mean) responded with a significant reduction of clinically evident fractures[97]. The radiologically detected fractures were reduced by 44% in the total group of women taking alendronate (RR, 0.56; CI, 0.39–0.80), but subgroup analysis demonstrated a significant reduction only in those with a baseline bone density *T* score of > 2.5 SD.

*Hip fracture efficacy* In the FIT trial, alendronate reduced the risk of hip fracture. In postmenopausal women with osteoporosis defined as either a prevalent vertebral fracture and BMD *T*s core of < 1.6 or a BMD *T* score < 2.5 at femoral neck in absence of a prevalent vertebral fracture, treatment with alendronate (5 mg daily for 2 years, then 10 mg daily), the risk of hip fracture was reduced by 53%. This is confirmed in the meta-analysis[88] of 11 placebo-controlled trials, where the summary RR for hip fracture was 0.63 (CI, 0.43–0.92).

### *Risedronate*

*Bone mineral density* A meta-analysis[98] of eight randomized, placebo-controlled trials (level I data) of risedronate in postmenopausal women with osteoporosis revealed increases in BMD of lumbar spine, femoral neck and total body. The increase in BMD was dose-related, with greater increases seen in the 5 mg daily dose compared to the 2.5 mg daily dose. In comparison to placebo, the pooled estimate showed an increase of 4.54% at lumbar spine, 2.75% at the femoral neck and less than 1% at the forearm. This compares with the VERT data, where BMD increased significantly compared with placebo at the lumbar spine (5.4% vs. 1.1%), femoral neck (1.6% vs. –1.2%), femoral trochanter (3.3% vs. –0.7%), and midshaft of the radius (0.2% vs. –1.4%). The overall safety profile of risedronate, including gastrointestinal safety, was similar to that of placebo. Risedronate is available in daily or weekly tablets. BMD improvements and reduction in bone turnover were similar for daily and weekly dosing. Fracture reduction data are not available for weekly dosing.

*Vertebral fracture efficacy* Two large level I studies[99,100] support the efficacy of risedronate in fracture prevention. In each study, postmenopausal women received risedronate or placebo, supplemental calcium and/or vitamin D[70]. Pooled data from five of the eight trials were used in the meta-analysis to give an estimated RR of vertebral fractures of 0.64 (CI, 0.54–0.77). Using only the data from those receiving the 5 mg daily dosing, the RR for vertebral fractures was 0.62 (CI, 0.51–0.76) and 0.68 (CI, 0.53–0.87) for non-vertebral fractures. Amalgamation of the VERT studies[101] showed a 69% decrease between placebo and treatment, with benefits apparent by the end of 12 months and positive trends observed as early as 6 months. The fourth and fifth year extensions of the risedronate data show maintained benefit, with a 59% benefit (CI, 19–79; $p = 0.01$) in years 4 and 5. Mean increase in BMD from baseline in lumbar spine was 9.3% ($p < 0.001$) over 5 years[100,102].

*Hip fracture* Risedronate reduces hip fractures. The Hip Intervention Program (HIP), with hip fracture as the primary end-point[103] studied 5445 osteoporotic women aged 70–79 years (*T* score > –4 SD or > –3 SD plus an additional risk factor) and 3886 women at least 80 years old who had either low BMD or at least one non-skeletal risk factor for hip fracture. Participants were randomized to risedronate (2.5 mg or 5 mg daily) or placebo for 3 years. Overall, there was a 30% reduction in the incidence of hip fracture in women who received risedronate (RR, 0.7; CI, 0.6–0.9; $p = 0.02$). The most pronounced effect was seen in the small group of patients aged 70–79 with initial osteoporotic BMD. In this group, risedronate reduced the risk of hip fracture from 1.9% on risedronate compared to 3.2% on placebo (RR, 0.6; CI, 0.4–0.9; $p = 0.009$). Risedronate significantly reduced the risk of hip fracture among elderly women with confirmed osteoporosis but not among older women selected on the basis of risk factors other than low bone density.

### *Side-effects and toxicity of bisphosphonates*

Reports of gastrointestinal symptoms, including erosive esophagitis, have been reported with bisphosphonates, although no significant differences have been found in controlled studies compared to placebo. In the meta-analyses[88,98] of randomized, placebo-controlled trials, no significant difference was found in discontinuation rates for adverse events between active drug and placebo. However, to minimize the risk of esophagitis and to improve drug absorption, it is recommended that both alendronate and risedronate be taken first thing in the morning, on an empty stomach, with 8 ounces of water, and to remain upright for 30 min. Oral bisphosphonates should not be used in patients with mechanical esophageal problems such as esophageal stricture, dysmotility or achalasia or with severe renal dysfunction. Most upper gastrointestinal symptoms that occur are probably not directly related to the medication; however, bisphosphonates have been associated with esophagitis, gastritis, gastroduodenal perforation, symptomatic ulcers and upper gastrointestinal tract bleeding. If serious upper gastrointestinal symptoms or signs develop, the bisphosphonates should be discontinued and medical therapy instituted. Rechallenge may be appropriate at a later date after resolution.

For patients who cannot tolerate oral bisphosphonates or who have contraindications, intravenous preparations are available but are not currently approved for the treatment of osteoporosis. Zolendronic acid, an intravenous bisphosphonate preparation, has been shown in preliminary studies to be effective for treatment of osteoporosis when given once or twice yearly at a dose of 4 mg. Improvements in BMD and suppression of biochemical markers comparable to the approved oral bisphosphonates were seen[104]. Fracture protection with zolendronate is being evaluated. Intravenous pamidronate is available for the treatment of Paget's disease and hypercalcemia of malignancy and has been used for prevention of osteoporosis.

## Nasal calcitonin

Nasal calcitonin is approved for treatment of osteoporosis in women who are 5 or more years postmenopausal but is not effective in preventing bone loss in early postmenopausal women[105,106]. Because there is no significant effect outside the spine, calcitonin is often reserved for women who cannot tolerate other therapies or who have significant pain. In a randomized, double-blind trial of approximately 230 postmenopausal women with osteoporosis in each group, the women received either placebo or three doses of nasal calcitonin (100, 200, and 400 IU/day) for 3 years. An increase of 1.0–1.5% over baseline in lumbar spine but not other skeletal sites was seen at the end of year 1 (significant), with no apparent dose response. Statistical significance over placebo was lost in years 2 and 3. Side effects of nasal calcitonin include rhinitis, nasal discomfort or ulceration, nausea, facial flushing and diarrhea. Injectable calcitonin does seem to have analgesic properties, which may be particularly useful in women with painful compression fractures[107].

*Fracture data*

Overgaard and colleagues[108] studied the effects of intranasal salmon calcitonin in a 2-year, double-blind, placebo-controlled trial of women aged 68–72 years randomized to receive 50, 100, or 200 IU calcitonin or placebo daily plus 500-mg calcium supplement. Among 162 women completing the study, spinal BMD increased by 1% in the placebo group and by 3% in the group receiving 200 IU calcitonin. Although a decreased number of fractures were seen, pooling of all doses was not preplanned and the small numbers of fractures leave uncertainty.

Four-year interim results[109] from the 5-year multicenter PROOF study (Prevent Recurrence of Osteoporotic Fractures) of 1255 postmenopausal women with established osteoporosis revealed a 36% reduction in relative risk of new fracture with 200 IU calcitonin compared to placebo ($p = 0.020$). The minimum intranasal dose needed for a significant effect on BMD was 200 IU. Reductions of 18% and 23% in new fractures were seen among those treated with 100 IU or 400 IU compared to placebo (not significant). The mean increments in BMD over baseline for placebo, 100 IU, 200 IU and 400 IU were 0.7, 1.2, 1.2 and 1.6%, respectively. The increases in lumbar spine BMD were statistically significantly increased in all treatment groups compared to placebo over baseline and at 2 years compared to placebo, and up to 3 years for the 400 IU dose. Despite modest increases in

BMD, the 200 IU dose of nasal calcitonin spray appeared to reduce the risk of new vertebral fractures in postmenopausal women with established osteoporosis. The study was not sufficiently powered to detect a reduction in hip fractures, and found no evidence of non-vertebral fracture protection. Because of the lack of a dose-response effect in this study and loss of 60% of individuals to follow-up, the authors of this review consider this to be level II evidence of efficacy.

## Selective estrogen receptor modulators and bone

Studies in postmenopausal (but not premenopausal) women using tamoxifen for prevention of breast cancer have shown average increases in BMD of 1-2% per year[110]. In the Tamoxifen Prevention Trial[111], a reduction in fractures of hip, spine, and other areas was observed which approached but did not reach statistical significance.

Raloxifene produced significant increases in bone mineral density in hip, spine and total body in large, randomized, placebo-controlled osteoporosis prevention trials[112,113]. Raloxifene acts as an antiresorptive agent in postmenopausal women, as does estrogen. Raloxifene increased total body bone mineral density from 1.8% to 2.5% over placebo after 24 months. This effect was similar to that seen with CEE and MPA or 5 mg of alendronate per day. In the total hip, the raloxifene group improved to a greater extent than those given placebo (1.8% to 2.3%). The effect was similar to that observed in women receiving 0.625 mg CEE/2.5 mg MPA or 5 mg of alendronate, and greater than effected by 200 IU of nasal calcitonin or tamoxifen.

*Fracture data with raloxifene*

The Multiple Outcomes of Raloxifene Evaluation (MORE) trial[112,113] was a double-blind, controlled study of 7705 recently postmenopausal (average 4.5-5 years) women with osteoporosis (mean age 66.5 years) treated with raloxifene (60 mg or 120 mg) or placebo, followed for 36 months. All received 500 mg of calcium and 400-600 IU vitamin D. Primary end-points were radiographic vertebral fractures and bone density[76,78]. Raloxifene at 60 mg showed significant reduction in vertebral fractures with 30% reduction (RR, 0.70; CI, 0.56-0.86) in women with prevalent fractures and 52% reduction (RR, 0.48; CI 0.29-0.71) in women without prior fractures. An insufficient number of hip fractures occurred to allow analysis of the effect of raloxifene on hip fracture reduction. These data are considered to represent level I evidence of efficacy of reduction of spine fracture with raloxifene.

*Extraskeletal benefits and risks of raloxifene*

The 4-year data from the MORE trial[114] of osteoporotic women revealed that raloxifene use was associated with a 72% risk reduction (RR, 0.28; CI 0.17-0.46) in invasive breast cancers with a reduction in estrogen receptor-positive breast cancer of 84% (RR, 0.16; CI 0.09-0.30). Raloxifene is currently being tested in women at high risk for breast cancer in the STAR trial (Tamoxifen vs. Raloxifene in women with Gail > 1.67) but has not been tested in breast cancer survivors following tamoxifen use. Concern exists that raloxifene may act differently in women who have previously received 5 years of tamoxifen. Recommendations cannot be made for breast cancer survivors who have been previously treated with tamoxifen until prospective studies have been performed.

Raloxifene increases the incidence of hot flushes; 9.7% of women noted this problem on raloxifene vs. 6.4% on placebo, with an average increase from one or two per day to only two to four per day. In the MORE trial, raloxifene caused a minimal increase in uterine thickness and no increase in incidence of endometrial cancer. Raloxifene is not associated with vaginal bleeding, which represents an advantage over HT. Side-effects included leg cramps and a 2.5 increased relative risk of deep vein thrombosis (similar to HT). Absolute risk of pulmonary embolism was 0.4% compared to 0.2% with placebo. No effect was seen on vaginitis, migraine, headache, anxiety or emotional lability. Limited data are available with respect to cognitive function, mood, or memory, but no decreases in memory or concentration have been found and no increases in depression.

## Parathyroid hormone

Parathyroid hormone (PTH) paradoxically stimulates bone formation when given by pulse injection and serves as the only agent which acts anabolically. A truncated form of parathyroid hormone, teriparatide (the 1-34 fragment ), was studied[115] for a median duration of 18-19 months in a level I double-blind, placebo-controlled trial. A total of 1637 postmenopausal women with prior vertebral fractures were randomized to receive either 20 or 40 μg of parathyroid hormone or placebo, administered subcutaneously daily. Bone mineral density increased significantly by 9-13% in lumbar spine and 3-6% in femoral neck, a larger increase than that seen with anti-resorptive therapies. More importantly, vertebral fracture risk was reduced by 65% and non-vertebral fracture risk by 53%. Ninety-six per cent of women responded with BMD increases. Decreased lumbar fracture risk persisted over a 50-month follow-up[115]. Unfortunately, the study was not powered for fractures of the hip. Because the efficacy of teriparatide appears to decrease after 2 years and long-term safety is not known, treatment beyond 2 years is not currently recommended.

PTH is indicated for patients with severe osteoporosis with fractures or for postmenopausal patients with osteoporosis who have failed to respond to other therapeutic alternatives. Teriparatide therapy is well tolerated, with slight increases in nausea, headache, dizziness and leg cramps. Effects on serum and urinary calcium were dose-dependent, small and transient. A concern is that very high doses of teriparatide caused sarcoma in Fisher rats; a finding considered unlikely to occur in patients.

## Phytoestrogens

Data on the effect of soy estrogens and ipriflavone (a synthetic isoflavone derivative) for prevention of postmenopausal bone loss are conflicting. A recent prospective, randomized, double-blind, 4-year trial[116] compared ipriflavone 200 mg tid vs. placebo in women receiving 500 mg/day of calcium. After 36 months of treatment, no significant difference occurred between groups with regards to BMD of lumbar spine, biochemical markers or vertebral fractures. In comparison, 24 weeks of 80.4 mg/day of soy protein isolate with isoflavones in a randomized, double-blind, controlled study showed increases in bone density in lumbar spine[117]. These inconsistent data do not allow recommendations regarding soy estrogens or ipriflavone in women with significant bone loss. Although diets rich in phytoestrogens appear to have bone-sparing effects, the magnitude and mechanism are currently unknown[118].

## Comparison data for different agents

Head-to-head comparisons of various agents in preventing fracture are non-existent and relative efficacy must be estimated by comparing results from different trials. The WHI study[4] demonstrated the efficacy of estrogen plus a progestin to reduce total fractures by 25% and hip and spine fractures by 34%. For alendronate, the decrease in lumbar spine and hip fractures is 50%[93], for risedronate 41%[99], for nasal calcitonin, the decrease in lumbar fractures is 36%[108], and for raloxifene the decrease in lumbar fractures was 38-52%[113]. Accordingly, one can conclude that alendronate, risedronate, nasal calcitonin, and raloxifene could serve as effective alternatives for estrogen for prevention and treatment of osteoporosis. As an additional benefit, raloxifene reduced the incidence of newly diagnosed breast cancer by up to 72% at 4 years when used to block bone resorption, as shown by the MORE trial[114]. The practical significance of this finding is that raloxifene might be chosen over the bisphosphonates or calcitonin in women with an increased risk of breast cancer.

## Combination therapy

Short-term, prospective, placebo-controlled studies of bisphosphonates and HT or raloxifene have shown slightly higher increases in BMD than with either treatment alone. Combined alendronate 10 mg daily and 0.625 mg CEE[119,120], risedronate 5 mg and 0.625 mg CEE[121], and alendronate 10 mg and raloxifene 60 mg[122] all showed the greatest reductions in bone marker turnover and greatest improvements in BMD in the combination groups, compared to the individual treatment groups. However, there is no evidence that combination therapy results in a greater reduction in the risk of fracture. Combination therapy is not recommended as routine therapy; it may be appropriate in individual patients.

Concomitant therapy with estrogen and PTH[123] does not seem to blunt the anabolic effects of PTH in postmenopausal women, but there is no evidence that the combination produces higher bone mass or greater bone strength than PTH alone. A recent, double-blind, randomized study of combined parathyroid hormone and alendronate, compared to parathyroid or alendronate alone, found that there was no evidence of synergy between parathyroid hormone and alendronate. The bone density increased in all treatment groups, with no significant difference in the increase between parathyroid hormone alone and the combination therapy. The increase in the parathyroid hormone group was about twice that found in either of the other two groups. Concurrent use of alendronate may reduce the anabolic effects of parathyroid hormone.

## PRIMARY PREVENTION OF CARDIOVASCULAR DISEASE

Previous observational data had suggested that hormone therapy might be beneficial for the primary prevention of heart disease in women. As reviewed below, the WHI trial demonstrated the opposite effect, namely that hormone therapy exerts an adverse effect on cardiac health. On this basis, one now needs to consider what to use in place of estrogen for cardiovascular prevention[124].

Physicians previously prescribed HT for the primary prevention of heart disease until the publication of the WHI study[4]. The rationale was based primarily on known effects on lipid level but also upon direct vascular effects[125–128]. When delivered transdermally, estrogen was believed to mediate its effects predominantly through non-lipid effects. On the other hand, hormone therapy is associated with increases in C-reactive protein in postmenopausal women, a potentially adverse, proinflammatory effect[126,127].

Evidence from over 30 epidemiological studies initially suggested a 35–50% decrease in the incidence of initial coronary events with estrogen replacement therapy[129–132]. However, level I evidence from the WHI now suggests that HT in the primary prevention setting is actually associated with an increased risk of heart disease within the first 6 months of use. This study reported an increase in cardiovascular events in women between the ages of 50 and 79 years (average age 63)[4]. Relative risk for heart attacks was 1.24 (CI, 1.00–1.54), for strokes was 1.41 (CI, 1.07–1.85), and for pulmonary embolism was 2.13 (CI, 1.39–3.25). The increase in myocardial infarction and stroke among patients randomized to HT was detected within the first 2 years and continued until the trial was stopped prematurely due to an unfavorable global benefit : risk score).

Despite the negative results above, some experts believe that there may be a critical stage at the time of menopause beyond which HT has no atheroprotective effect. In the Heart and Estrogen/progestin Study (HERS) and Estrogen Replacement and Atherosclerosis (ERA) trials, hormone therapy was initiated in older postmenopausal women after coronary artery disease was established. In the WHI study, the average age at entry was 63 years and these women also probably had subclinical coronary disease. Only one-third of participants in the WHI were less than 60 years of age, and over 20% were in their seventies.

The observational Nurses' Health Study[132] initially suggested an increased risk of stroke with doses of CEE greater than or equal to 0.625 mg/day (with and without progestin) but not with lower doses. Recent multiple randomized clinical trials support this finding[133]. The Women's Estrogen for Stroke Trial (WEST) suggested that estrogen use was associated with an increased risk for fatal stroke and more severe neurologic impairments. In the HERS trial, risk for venous throboembolism was increased three times compared to placebo[134]. In WHI, stroke was increased with a RR of 1.41. Attributable risk increases with age, as risk of stroke increases with age.

### Strategies to use in place of hormone therapy for primary prevention

The major risk factors for cardiovascular disease are the same in women and men: elevated serum lipids, hypertension, obesity, sedentary lifestyle and smoking. These factors are rationale targets for risk reduction strategies and are the first consideration for primary prevention (Tables 4 and 5).

*Lifestyle modifications*[135,136]

(1) Cessation of cigarette smoking and avoidance of passive smoke inhalation;

(2) Initiation of 30 min/day or more of moderate intensity physical activity, most days of the week;

(3) Choice of a heart-healthy diet with less than 30% fat, 8–10% saturated fat, < 300 mg/day of cholesterol;

(4) Limitation of salt to 6 g/day or less;

(5) Intake of 25–30 g/day total dietary fiber and five or more servings of fruit and vegetables per day;

(6) Achievement and maintenance of desirable weight with a target body mass index of 18.5–24.9 kg/m$^2$;

(7) Lipid management – in lower-risk women, low density lipoprotein (LDL) cholesterol < 150 mg/dl (optimal < 130 mg/dl); higher-risk women with two or more risk factors, LDL < 130 mg/dl, women with cardiovascular disease, < 100 mg/dl); high density lipoprotein (HDL) cholesterol > 40 mg/dl; triglycerides, < 150 mg/dl;

(8) Maintain blood pressure at 140/90 mmHg; optimal 120/80 mmHg.

**Table 5** The Adult Treatment Panel III LDL cholesterol goals

- *Patients with pre-existing CAD and CAD risk equivalents who are at highest risk for a CAD event*: CAD risk equivalents comprise other conditions, including peripheral artery disease, abdominal aortic aneurysm, diabetes, and multiple risk factors, which confer a 10-year CAD risk exceeding 20%. Patients in this category have the lowest LDL cholesterol goal (< 100 mg/dl)
- *Patients with two or more risk factors in whom the 10-year risk for CAD is ≤ 20% (i.e. annual absolute CAD risk > 2%)*. For this group, the LDL cholesterol goal is < 130 mg/dl
- *Patients having 0-1 risk factor (with a 10-year risk < 10%)*: the LDL cholesterol target for this group is < 160 mg/day

CAD, coronary artery disease

**Table 4** The Adult Treatment Panel III guidelines[135]

| |
|---|
| Determine fasting lipoprotein levels |
| Identify the presence of clinical atherosclerosis |
| Determine the presence of major risk factors |
| Calculate the global risk score |
| Determine the patient's CAD risk category and LDL-C goal |
| Institute TLC if the patient's LDL-C is above goal |
| Add lipid-lowering agents if the LDL-C continues to exceed initial levels |
| Identify the metabolic syndrome (insulin resistance, abdominal adiposity, hypertension, and dyslipidemia, i.e. low HDL, high triglycerides) and treat if present after 3 months of TLC |
| Treat elevated triglycerides (normal triglycerides < 50 mg/dl; borderline high 150–199 mg/dl; high 200–499 mg/dl and very high ≥ 500 mg/dl) |

CAD, coronary artery disease; LDL-C, low density lipoprotein cholesterol; TLC, therapeutic lifestyle changes; HDL, high density lipoprotein cholesterol

*Exercise and heart disease prevention*

Regular physical activity increases exercise capacity, endurance and skeletal muscle strength[137]. Exercise reduces the risk of chronic diseases such as type 2 diabetes, osteoporosis, obesity, depression, and cancer of the breast and colon. The reduced incidence of coronary artery disease occurs in the more physically active and fit subjects. Physically active subjects demonstrate coronary artery disease rates half those of the sedentary group[137]. It also helps other risk factors for coronary artery disease, including elevated blood pressure, insulin resistance and glucose intolerance, elevated triglycerides, low HDL cholesterol and obesity. In addition, several meta-analyses have shown that comprehensive exercise-based cardiac rehabilitation reduces mortality rates in patients after myocardial infarction. Vigorous physical activity increases the risk of sudden death (1/750 000) and myocardial infarction (1/220 000) in patients with heart disease[137].

*Statins*

The statins (HMG-CoA-reductase inhibitors) have an established role in the primary prevention of heart disease[138,139] and have replaced HT for this purpose in postmenopausal women. A key new 5-year study, comparing 40 mg of simvastatin to placebo, provides evidence of the efficacy of statins in women with or without elevations of lipid levels. This study, the Heart Protection Study[140], enrolled 20 536 primarily postmenopausal patients and included the largest number of women ($n = 5082$) ever studied in a prospective intervention trial with lipid-lowering therapy. The magnitude of benefit in women closely paralleled that observed in men and absolute benefit was greater in older patients. All-cause mortality was reduced by 12% with simvastatin vs. placebo ($p < 0.001$). Death from heart disease or related blood vessel disease was reduced by 17% ($p = 0.0002$). Simvastatin allocation was also associated with reductions of one-quarter in major coronary events ($p < 0.0001$), in strokes ($p < 0.0001$), in revascularizations ($p < 0.0001$), and in all such major vascular events (major coronary events, strokes, and revascularizations) ($p < 0.0001$). Approximately 3500 patients with an LDL cholesterol level of about 100 mg/dl or less entered the trial. Their relative risk reduction from lipid-lowering therapy was the same as that of those who started at high baseline levels. Thus, significant risk reductions were achieved with statin therapy regardless of baseline lipid levels. The target of therapy is an individual's risk, not their lipid levels.

The first primary prevention study that included women demonstrated the effectiveness of statins for primary prevention. The AFCAPs/TexCAPS study[141] examined the effect of 20 mg daily of lovastatin (or 40 mg per day if LDL cholesterol remained above 110 mg/dl) vs. placebo as primary prevention of acute coronary events. The study involved 5608 men and 997 women without a prior history of cardiovascular disease and with average LDL cholesterol and below average HDL cholesterol levels. Overall, the relative risk of first coronary event was 0.63 ($p < 0.001$) with a 33% reduction in revascularization procedures ($p = 0.002$) and a 40% reduction in incidence of fatal or non-fatal myocardial infarction ($p = 0.002$) after an average follow-up of 5.2 years in patients receiving lovastatin. The effect of treatment with lovastatin on the rate of first acute major coronary events was relatively greater in women than in men (46% vs. 37% reduction); however, the actual number of women who had a primary end-point was small (20 of 997) and there were no statistically significant differences in treatment effects between sexes.

*Beyond lipid-lowering benefits* Additional potential benefits from statin therapy beyond the known lipid-lowering benefits include inhibition of vascular smooth muscle proliferation and reduction in the number of inflammatory cells within the atherosclerotic lesions. Statins may also contribute to plaque stability by reducing plaque size, decreasing the number of inflammatory cells in the plaque, and reducing the production of collagen-degrading enzymes such as matrix metalloproteinases, and inhibition of tissue factor production[138].

*Side-effects of statins* In the large trial of 20 000 (Heart Protection Study[140]) patients, side-effects were exceedingly uncommon (i.e. < 0.01%). Dose-related abnormalities of liver function, often asymptomatic or clinically insignificant, may be seen. Other side-effects include myositis and, rarely, rhabdomyolysis[140].

*Selective estrogen receptor modulators*

*Tamoxifen and raloxifene* Tamoxifen exerts estrogenic effects on the liver and, thus, lowers LDL cholesterol levels. However, no reduction in cardiovascular events was observed in a large breast cancer prevention study involving more than 16 000 women[111]. In randomized studies on lipid effects in humans[142], raloxifene induced effects similar to those of estrogens on lipids but of somewhat smaller magnitude. Reductions in total cholesterol of 6.6% and LDL cholesterol by 10.9% were seen with no change in HDL cholesterol or triglycerides. Analysis of the MORE data[113] showed, overall, no cardiovascular or cerebrovascular risk and no early harm. Women in the MORE trial[143] were evaluated according to risk for heart disease using standard criteria for risk. In a subset analysis, those at high risk assigned to raloxifene had a significantly lower risk of cardiovascular events compared with placebo (RR, 60; CI, 0.38–0.95). A prospective study is currently in progress (RUTH, Raloxifene Use in The Heart) to study cardiovascular end-points during raloxifene treatment of postmenopausal women at risk for cardiovascular events.

*Phytoestrogens* Plant-derived isoflavones bind to estrogen receptors and exert both estrogen agonist and antagonist properties. A meta-analysis[144] of the effect of soy on cholesterol in humans revealed that 47 g daily of soy was associated with a 12.9% decrease in LDL cholesterol, 9.3% decrease in total cholesterol, and no change in HDL cholesterol. The amounts of total soy isoflavones which exert clinical effects approximate 40–80 mg per day. Recent data[145] in healthy postmenopausal women failed to show improvements in lipoprotein levels or endothelial function after 8 weeks of treatment with isoflavones (80 mg/day). Clinical end-point data from well-conducted trials are not yet available to make recommendations concerning the use of soy for prevention of cardiovascular disease.

## SECONDARY PREVENTION OF CARDIOVASCULAR DISEASE

### Estrogen

Non-randomized secondary prevention studies previously suggested that HT use in women with established cardiovascular disease reduces risk of death and future cardiovascular events. However, the randomized, prospective HERS trial[146] showed just the opposite result. This study involved 2763 women, mean age 66.7 years, with severe coronary heart disease who used CEE 0.625 mg/day and MPA 2.5 mg/day or placebo, with 4.1 years of follow-up. The HT group showed an increase in coronary heart disease and mortality at year 1 when compared to those using placebo. With continued use, it initially appeared that a beneficial effect of HT developed over time, with fewer deaths in years 4 and 5. However, at the end of 5 years on study, the number of deaths, heart attacks and coronary heart disease rates did not differ between the two groups.

HERS II[147] continues as a 4-year open-label extension of the original 4.1-year HERS trial, with a mean follow-up of 2.7 years to bring mean total overall for HERS to 6.8 years. A total of 2321 (93%) of the 2763 postmenopausal women in HERS consented to continue. When compared to placebo, no overall effect of HT on coronary heart disease, either primary or secondary was seen. The lower rates of coronary events observed in the HERS HT group during years 3–5 did not continue during the 2.7 years of follow-up. The overall relative risk during HERS II for coronary heart disease was 1.00.

A second randomized trial[148] for secondary prevention, the ERA trial compared the effects of placebo, estrogen (CEE 0.625 mg/day) alone, and estrogen/progestin (CEE 0.625 mg/day plus MPA 2.5 mg/day) after 3 years on the progression of atherosclerosis in postmenopausal women with documented coronary stenosis. Neither Premarin alone nor Premarin plus MPA resulted in a reduction of coronary narrowing as the study end-point when compared to the placebo group. Two other trials, the WELL-HART (17β-estradiol)[149] and ESPRIT (2 mg estradiol valerate)[150] trials, supported the evidence reported in the HERS and ERA trials that hormone therapy does not reduce the incidence of cardiovascular events[149,150].

Taken together, these data suggest again that therapeutic strategies for primary and secondary prevention of heart disease must be used in the place of hormone therapy and not as alternatives to it.

### Statins

Several statin trials reviewed below demonstrate the effectiveness of the HMG-CoA reductase inhibitors in preventing recurrent coronary disease events and indicate that coronary disease prevention is a class effect of the statins. The most significant advance in secondary heart disease protection is the evidence of benefit from aggressive LDL cholesterol lowering, regardless of baseline LDL cholesterol level, with larger decreases in the incidence of subsequent coronary events than seen with angioplasty. Statins lower coronary morbidity and mortality, along with total mortality[130,151]. Although the strongest evidence that coronary events can be lowered has been seen in middle-aged men, the results apply equally to both sexes when studied. A brief description of three pivotal trials (but not a comprehensive review of all trials) supporting these conclusions is provided below:

(1) In The Scandinavian Simvastatin Survival Study[152], a large, randomized trial of cholesterol lowering in 4444 patients with coronary heart disease cholesterol levels between 213 and 309 mg/dl, all-cause mortality was reduced by 30% ($p = 0.0003$), with a 42% reduction in risk of coronary death and 34% reduction in recurrent coronary events ($p < 0.00001$) and a 37% reduction in myocardial revascularization procedures ($p < 0.0001$).

(2) The Cholesterol and Recurrent Events (CARE) trial[153] showed that, in patients with average cholesterol levels, pravastatin therapy reduced the risk for coronary death or recurrent myocardial infarction by 24% ($p = 0.003$ and reduced the risk of fatal and non-fatal myocardial infarction by 25% ($p = 0.006$).

(3) The LIPID study[154] (Long-term Intervention with Pravastatin in Ischaemic Disease), a 6-year treatment resulted in 24% relative risk reduction in coronary heart disease ($p < 0.001$).

### Aspirin therapy

Antiplatelet therapy, most notably aspirin, has been documented to reduce the risks of cardiovascular disease, myocardial infarction and stroke, both in primary and secondary prevention. The US Preventive Services Task Force and the American Heart Association recommend aspirin use for women whose 10-year risks are greater than 10%[155]. Side-effects, especially bleeding, are dose-related.

*Additive benefits of pravastatin and aspirin to decrease risks of cardiovascular disease*

Individual trials and met-analyses[156] demonstrate additive benefits of pravastatin and aspirin on cardiovascular disease, with 31% significant reduction for myocardial infarction for pravastatin plus aspirin compared to aspirin alone, and 26% for pravastatin plus aspirin compared to pravastatin alone. Ischemic stroke was also reduced.

### Statins and stroke reduction

In addition to reduction in coronary artery disease morbidity and mortality, meta-analyses of cholesterol-lowering trials with statin therapy demonstrate a significant decline in stroke, similar to the decrease seen with coronary disease[151–155,157]. Interpretation of stroke data is limited because these studies were not designed with stroke as an end-point.

## PRACTICAL APPROACH TO USE OF ALTERNATIVES TO ESTROGEN

Options are now available for women who fear HT, discontinue HT or have relative contraindications such as a history of breast cancer. Participants in a consensus conference[19] recommended that breast cancer survivors be offered alternatives to HT as the initial approach to management of menopause. For menopausal women not taking HT, five specific areas need to be considered: vasomotor instability, urogenital atrophy, neurocognitive disturbances, treatment or prevention of osteoporosis, and prevention of cardiovascular disease. A sequential approach to treatment of each of these problems is recommended.

### Vasomotor symptoms

Lifestyle changes, such as avoidance of precipitating events and regular exercise, are beneficial in reducing hot flushes. Vitamin E at 800 IU daily is more effective than placebo, although of limited clinical efficacy. A trial of dietary isoflavones such as soy foods or supplements with black cohosh (40–80 mg/day) may be considered, as these are not associated with known serious side-effects. Safety is unknown for survivors of breast cancer. If hot flushes are persistent and hormone therapy contraindicated, we discuss with the patient other non-FDA approved therapies[158]. We utilize an SSRI, gabapentin, clonidine, and megestrol acetate sequentially and in the order listed. We find the SSRIs to be efficacious and well tolerated in low doses in most women. Preliminary experience indicates the beneficial effects of gabapentin. Treatment is only utilized if the severity of symptoms warrants, and after informed discussion of lack of long-term safety and efficacy data. Most recently, we have been using the SSRIs as the initial therapy. Paroxetine 20–40 mg daily, venlafaxine 37.5–75 mg daily and fluoxetine 20 mg daily are effective in small, randomized clinical trials. Hot flush relief is almost immediate, within 1–2 weeks. If no relief is experienced or if an SSRI is not indicated or desired, gabapentin is started at 300 mg per day for 1 week, 300 mg twice daily for week 2, and 300 mg three times daily the third week and thereafter. It is important to educate women about the side-effects, particularly drowsiness, dizziness and light-headedness and that these may resolve over time. Older patients or sensitive patients may need to start at much lower doses, such as 100 g/day, with slow increases. Clonidine may be started as one transdermal patch (TTS #1) for 1 week, followed by two patches for the second week, followed by three patches the third week, or until symptoms are relieved. Patients should not increase the number of patches if side-effects such as low blood pressure occur. During the fourth week, use of the TTS #1, #2, or #3 replaces the one, two or three patches needed for improvement in hot flushes during the induction phase. If hot flushes persist at night, supplementary night-time tablets of clonidine from 0.1 to 0.4 mg can be used. Only a percentage of patients respond to this regimen. Blood pressure should be monitored.

Progestins by themselves have demonstrated significant efficacy for hot flush reduction. Progestins have been linked to breast cancer and side-effects may be bothersome. Over-the-counter progesterone cream is probably not effective. Options include oral (5–20 mg daily) or intramuscular medroxyprogestone (150 mg every 3 months) and oral megestrol acetate (40 mg daily). Some women have an exacerbation of hot flushes for 1 week before diminution of this symptom. Weight gain and irregular bleeding are common complaints.

Some women will not have relief of menopausal symptoms despite full utilization of alternatives to estrogen. In such patients, we discuss the risks and benefits of HT with them. This includes patients with prior breast cancer who are at low risk of recurrence of breast cancer, based on clinical risk factors. After full discussion to provide informed consent regarding the use of HT, including increased risk of breast cancer seen in the WHI, early heart disease, stroke, dementia in those who initiate over age of 65, and thromboembolism, we prescribe and monitor this medication, using the lowest dose that relieves symptoms or maintains bone. The decision to continue HT is re-evaluated annually.

## Urogenital atrophy

The first approach for vaginal dryness and dyspareunia is vaginal moisturizers such as Replens or Vagisel and water-soluble vaginal lubricants such as KY Jelly or Astroglide. Women are cautioned not to use vaginal moisturizers just before intercourse but to apply three times weekly on a regular basis. Replens can be irritating when initially present in high concentration. The next step is either use of Vagifem 25 mg vaginal estradiol tablet, the Estring or 0.5 g of Premarin cream or 100 μg estradiol vaginal cream daily for 3 weeks followed by twice weekly thereafter. Estradiol cream can also be applied as a dime-sized amount externally 2–3 times per week. Potential risks exist from unopposed local vaginal estrogen.

## Neurocognitive dysfunction

For depression or anxiety associated with depression, we utilize standard SSRI therapy in conventional doses. Anxiety can be treated with anxiolytic medication, provided it is not a part of a syndrome with a predominance of depression. For problems with memory, we recommend rest, exercise and memory adjuncts. Decreased stress or number of involved activities or responsibilities may also help. Regular exercise is recommended as this may help menopausal depressive symptoms. Sleep aids are used on an intermittent basis.

## Prevention/treatment of osteoporosis

For women with osteopenia or osteoporosis, initial measures include a minimal calcium intake of 1500 mg daily and vitamin D of 400 IU daily. A 24-h urinary calcium ensures adequacy of calcium intake and absorption. Exercise against resistance is recommended, at least 30 min of weight-bearing exercise at least three times per week. Bone formation is stimulated by a combination of gravitational and weight-bearing forces such as the low repetitive muscle activity combined with weight load found in walking, jogging or low-impact aerobics. If the DEXA *T* score is −1.5 or higher (with one risk factor), we consider medical treatment. HT offers control of menopausal symptoms, builds bone mineral density and reduces both vertebral and non-vertebral fractures; however, concerns exist about the long-term risk/benefit profile. Reduced-dose estrogen has beneficial effects on bone, but long-term effectiveness and safety are not known. Bone-specific therapy is available, with the bisphosponates producing the best fracture protection. Both alendronate and risedronate are available as daily or weekly therapies. For women interested in vertebral fracture prevention and possible extraskeletal effects on breast cancer prevention or lowering of cholesterol, raloxifene may be the best choice. Women already on tamoxifen may not need additional bone-specific therapy as tamoxifen maintains bone density in postmenopausal women; periodic follow-up bone densities are necessary. Nasal calcitonin is reserved for patients with contraindications or side-effects from bisphosphonates or raloxifene, or with significant pain from compression fractures. Teriparatide is indicated for 2 years only and offered to women with severe osteoporosis, with osteoporotic fractures, multiple risk factors for fracture with low BMD, or intolerance to previous therapy.

## Prevention/treatment of heart disease

For patients with substantial risk of heart disease, we recommend a heart-healthy diet, cessation of smoking, exercise, and control of blood pressure. If there is no contraindication, aspirin therapy is discussed. If the LDL and HDL cholesterol levels meet criteria for treatment according to standard guidelines, we recommend use of a statin.

# CONCLUSIONS

Alternative therapies with varying efficacy are available for women for relief of menopause-related symptoms. A tailored treatment strategy which identifies the needs of each individual patient is recommended[2,19]. While several agents are available for the relief of vasomotor symptoms, none are as effective as HT, which remains the therapeutic standard. Efficacy of alternatives for vasomotor symptoms has been shown in small, short-duration, randomized clinical trials for the SSRIs, megestrol acetate and MPA. Clonidine is less effective and vitamin E marginal. Gabapentin appears effective in small trials but requires further study and side-effects may limit use. When moderate to severe vasomotor symptoms are not relieved sufficiently, then full discussion is needed regarding the benefits versus risks of short-term use of hormone replacement therapy.

Provision of low-dose estrogen to the vagina locally, via vaginal tablet, ring or cream, provides relief of symptoms of urogenital atrophy without increasing plasma estrogen levels substantially, although safety in breast cancer survivors is not determined. A potential risk of uterine cancer exists with unopposed local vaginal therapy.

Symptoms related to the effects of estrogen deficiency on the central nervous system may respond to central nervous system active agents such as antidepressants or anxiolytics. Bone-specific agents such as bisphosphonates and nasal calcitonin are available for prevention or treatment of osteoporosis. SERMS are available that offer benefits for osteoporosis, possible reduction in breast cancer but not relief of menopausal symptoms. Treatments such as 'statins' now exist for prevention of heart disease and have replaced the use of hormone therapy for both primary and secondary prevention.

# ACKNOWLEDGEMENT

Thanks to Sue Woodson, RN, CNP for review of this manuscript.

# References


1. Ganz PA, Greendale GA, Kahn B, O'Leary JF, Desmond KA. Are older breast carcinoma survivors willing to take hormone replacement therapy? *Cancer* 1999;86:814-20
2. Pinkerton JV, Santen R. Alternatives to the use of estrogen in postmenopausal women. *Endocr Rev* 1999;20:308-20
3. US Preventative Task Force Criteria. (http://odphp.osophs.dhhs.gov/pubs/guidecps/text/APP_A/(txt))
4. Rossouw JE, Anderson GL, Prentice RL, *et al.* Writing Group for the Women's Health Initiative Investigators. Risks and benefits of estrogen plus progestin in healthy postmenopausal women: principal results: From the Women's Health Initiative randomized controlled trial. *J Am Med Assoc* 2002;288:321-33
5. Chlebowski RT, Henrix SL, Langer RD, *et al.* for the WHI investigators. Influence of estrogen plus progestin on breast cancer and mammography in healthy postmenopausal women: the Women's Health Initiative randomized trial. *J Am Med Assoc* 2003;289:3243-53
6. The Women's Health Initiative Steering Committee. Effects of conjugated equine estrogen in postmenopausal women with hysterectomy. The Women's Health Initiative randomized controlled trial. *J Am Med Assoc* 2004;291:1701-12
7. Million Women Study Collaborators. Breast cancer and hormone-replacement therapy in the Million Women Study. *Lancet* 2003;362:419-27
8. Manson JE, Hsia J, Johnson KC, *et al.* Estrogen plus progestin and the risk of heart disease. *N Engl J Med* 2003;349:523-34
9. Santen RJ, Petroni GR. Relative versus attributable risk of breast cancer from estrogen replacement therapy. *J Clin Endocrinol Metab* 1999;84:1875-81
10. Wassertheil-Smoller S, Hendrix SL, Limacher M. Effect of estrogen plus progestogen on stroke in postmenopausal women: the Women's Health Initiative: a randomized trial. *J Am Med Assoc* 2003;289:2673-84
11. Shumaker SA, Legault C, Rapp SR, *et al.* for the WHIMS Investigators. Estrogen plus progestin and the incidence of dementia and mild cognitive impairment in postmenopausal women: the Women's Health Initiative Memory Study: a randomized, controlled trial. *J Am Med Assoc* 2003;289:2651-62
12. Breast cancer and hormone replacement therapy: collaborative reanalysis of data from 51 epidemiological studies of 52,705 women with breast cancer and 108,411 women without breast cancer. Collaborative Group on Hormonal Factors in Breast Cancer [published erratum appears in *Lancet* 1997;350:1484] *Lancet* 1997;350:1047-59
13. Schairer C, Lubin J, Troisi R, Sturgeon S, Brinton L, Hoover R. Menopausal estrogen and estrogen-progestin replacement therapy and breast cancer risk. *J Am Med Assoc* 2000;283:485-491
14. Colditz GA, Hankinson SE, Hunter DJ, *et al.* The use of estrogens and progestins and the risk of breast cancer in postmenopausal women. *N Engl J Med* 1995;332:1589-93
15. Ross RK, Paganini-Hill A, Wan PC, Pike MC. Effect of hormone replacement therapy on breast cancer risk: estrogen versus estrogen plus progestin. *J Nat Cancer Inst* 2000;92:328-32
16. Magnusson C, Baron JA, Correia N, Bergstrom R, Adami HO, Persson I. Breast-cancer risk following long-term oestrogen- and oestrogen-progestin-replacement therapy. *Int J Cancer* 1999;81:339-44
17. Feinleib M. Breast cancer and artificial menopause: a cohort study. *J Natl Cancer Inst* 1968;41:315-29
18. Trichopoulos D, MacMahon B, Cole P. Menopause and breast cancer risk. *J Natl Cancer Inst* 1972;48:605-13
19. Santen R, Pritchard K, Burger H. The consensus conference on treatment of estrogen deficiency symptoms in women surviving breast cancer. *Obstet Gynecol Surv* 1998;53(Suppl-8381):339-44
20. Dhodapkar MV, Ingle JN, Ahmann DL. Estrogen replacement therapy withdrawal and regression of metastatic breast cancer. *Cancer* 1995;75:43-6
21. Peters GN. Estrogen replacement therapy after breast cancer: a 12 year follow up. *Ann Surg Oncol* 2001;8:828-32
22. Decker DA, Pettinga JE, VanderVelde N, *et al.* Estrogen replacement therapy in breast cancer survivors: a matched-controlled series. *Menopause* 2003;10:277-85
23. Col NF, Hirota LK, Orr RK, Erban JK, Wong JB, Lau J. Hormone replacement therapy after breast cancer: a systematic review and quantitative assessment of risk. *J Clin Oncol* 2001;19:2357-63
24. Vassilopoulou-Sellin R, Asmar L, Hortobagyi GN, *et al.* Estrogen replacement therapy after localized breast cancer: clinical outcome of 319 women followed prospectively. *J Clin Oncol* 1999;17:1482-7
25. Position Statement. Treatment of menopause-associated vasomotor symptoms: position statement of the Northern American Menopause Society. *Menopause* 2004;11:11-33
26. Northern American Menopause Society. Estrogen and progestogen use in peri- and postmenopausal women. September 2003 Position Statement of

the North American Menopause Society. *Menopause* 2003;10:113–32

27. Anderson GL, Judd HJ, Kaunitz AM. Effects of estrogen and progestin on gynecologic cancers and associated diagnostic procedures The Women's Health Initiative Randomized Trial. *J Am Med Assoc* 2003;290:1739–48
28. Utian WH, Shoupe D, Bachmann G, *et al.* Relief of vasomotor symptoms and vaginal atrophy with lower doses of conjugated equine estrogens and medroxyprogesterone acetate. *Fertil Steril* 2001; 75:1065–79
29. Kronenberg F, Rugh-Berman A. Complementary and alternative medicine for menopausal symptoms: a review of randomized, controlled trials. *Ann Intern Med* 2002;137:805–13
30. McTiernan A, Kooperberg C, White E. Recreational physical activity and the risk of breast cancer in postmenopausal women: the Women's Health Initiative Cohort Study. *J Am Med Assoc* 2003;290:1377–9
31. Barton DL, Loprinzi CL, Quella SK, *et al.* Prospective evaluation of vitamin E for hot flashes in breast cancer survivors. *J Clin Oncol* 1998;16:495–500
32. Burke GL, Legault C, Anthony M, *et al.* Soy protein and isoflavone effects on vasomotor symptoms in peri- and postmenopausal women: the Soy Estrogen Alternative Study. *Menopause* 2003;10:147–53
33. Van Patten CL, Olivotto IA, Chamberrs GK, *et al.* Effect of soy phytoestrogens on hot flashes in postmenopausal women with breast cancer: a randomized, controlled clinical trial. *J Clin Oncol* 2002;20:1449–55
34. Han KK, Soares JM, Haidar MA, *et al.* Benefits of soy isoflavone therapeutic regimen on menopausal symptoms. *Obstet Gynecol* 2002;99:389–94
35. Nikander E, Kilkkinen A, Metsa-Heikkila M, *et al.* A randomized placebo-controlled crossover trial with phytoestrogens in treatment of menopause in breast cancer patients. *Obstet Gynecol* 2003; 101:1213–20
36. Fugh-Berman A, Kronenberg F. Red clover (*Trifolium pratense*) for menopausal women: current state of knowledge. *Menopause* 2001;8: 333–7
37. Tice JA, Ettinger B, Ensrud K, *et al.* Phytoestrogen supplements for the treatment of hot flashes: the Isoflavone Clover Extract (ICE): a randomized controlled trial. *J Am Med Assoc* 2003;290:207–14
38. Huntley AL, Ernst E. A systematic review of herbal medicinal products for the treatment of menopausal symptoms. *Menopause* 2003;10:58–64
39. Hirata JD, Swiersz LM, Zell B, Small R, Ettinger B. Does dong quai have estrogenic effects in postmenopausal women? A double-blind, placebo-controlled trial. *Fertil Steril* 1997;68:981–6
40. Wiklund IK, Mattsson LA, Lindgren R, *et al.* for the Swedish Alternative Medicine Group. Effects of a standardized ginseng extract on quality of life and physiological parameters in symptomatic postmenopausal women: a double-blind, placebo-controlled trial. *Int J Clin Pharm Res* 1999; 19:89–99
41. Chenoy R, Hussain S, Tayob Y, *et al.* Effect of oral gamolenic acid from evening primrose oil in menopausal flushing. *Br Med J* 1994;308:501–3
42. Wuttke W, Seidlova-Wuttke D, Gorkow C. The Cimifuga preparation BNO 1055 vs conjugated estrogens in a double-blind placebo-controlled study: effects on menopause symptoms and bone markers. *Maturitas* 2003;44(Suppl):S67–77
43. Jacobson JS, Troxel AB, Evans J, *et al.* Randomized trial of black cohosh for the treatment of hot flashes among women with a history of breast cancer. *J Clin Oncol* 2001;19:2739–45
44. Dog TL, Powell KL, Weisman SM. Critical evaluation of the safety of *Cimicifuga racemosa* in menopause symptom relief. *Menopause* 2003;10:299–313
45. Leonetti HB, Longo S, Anasti JN. Transdermal progesterone cream for vasomotor symptoms and postmenopausal bone loss. *Obstet Gynecol* 1999; 94:225–8
46. Wren BG, Champion SM, Willetts K, *et al.* Transdermal progesterone and its effect on vasomotor symptoms, blood lipid levels, bone metabolic markers, moods and quality of life for postmenopausal women. *Menopause* 2003;10: 13–18
47. Komesaroff PA, Black CV, Cable V, *et al.* Effects of wild yam extract on menopausal symptoms, lipids and sex hormones in healthy menopausal women. *Climacteric* 2001;4:144–50
48. Bertelli G, Venturini M, Del Mastro L, *et al.* Intramuscular depot-medroxyprogestereone acetate versus oral megestrol for the control of postmenopausal hot flashes in breast cancer patients: a randomized study. *Ann Oncol* 2002; 13:883–8
49. Quella SK, Loprinizi CL, Sloan JA, *et al.* Long term use of megestrol acetate by cancer survivors for the treatment of hot flashes. *Cancer* 1998; 82:1784–8
50. Loprinzi CL, Michalak JC, Quella SK, *et al.* Megestrol acetate for the prevention of hot flashes. *N Engl J Med* 1994;331:347–52
51. Loprinzi CL, Kugler JW, Sloan JA, *et al.* Venlafaxine in management of hot flashes in survivors of breast cancer: a randomized controlled trial. *Lancet* 2000;356:2059–63
52. Loprinizi CL, Sloan JA, Perez EA, *et al.* Phase III evaluation of fluoxetine for treatment of hot flashes. *J Clin Oncol* 2002;20:1578–83
53. Stearns V, Beebe KL, Iyengar M, *et al.* Paroxetine controlled release in the treatment of menopausal

hot flashes: a randomized controlled trial. *J Am Med Assoc* 2003;289:2827-34
54. Guttuso T Jr, Kurlan R, McDermott MP, *et al.* Gabapentin's effects on hot flashes in postmenopausal women: a randomized controlled trial. *Obstet Gynecol* 2003;101:337-45
55. Loprinzi L, Barton DL, Sloan JA, *et al.* Pilot evaluation of gabapentin for treating hot flashes. *Mayo Clin Proc* 2002;77:1159-63
56. Pandya KJ, Raubetas RF, Flynn PJ, *et al.* Oral clonidine in postmenopausal patients with breast cancer experiencing tamoxifen-induce hot flashes: a University of Rochester Cancer Center Community Clinical Oncology Program Study. *Ann Intern Med* 2000;132:788-93
57. Goldberg RM, Loprinzi CL, O'Fallon JR, Veeder MH, Miser AW. Transdermal clonidine for ameliorating tamoxifen-induced hot flashes [published erratum appears in *J Clin Oncol* 1996; 14:2411]. *J Clin Oncol* 1994;12:155-8
58. Loprinzi CL, Abu-Ghazaleh S, Sloan JA, *et al.* Phase III randomized double-blind study to evaluate the efficacy of a polycarbophil-based vaginal moisturizer in women with breast cancer. *J Clin Oncol* 1997;15:969-73
59. Nachtigall LE. Comparative study: Replens versus local estrogen in menopausal women. *Fertil Steril* 1994;61:178-80
60. Handa VL, Bachus KE, Johnston WW, Robboy SJ, Hammond CB. Vaginal administration of low-dose conjugated estrogens: systemic absorption and effects on the endometrium. *Obstet Gynecol* 1994;84:215-18
61. Henriksson L, Stjernquist M, Boquist L, Cedergren I, Selinus I. A one-year multicenter study of efficacy and safety of a continuous, low-dose, estradiol-releasing vaginal ring (Estring) in postmenopausal women with symptoms and signs of urogenital aging. *Am J Obstet Gynecol* 1996;174:t-92
62. Eriksen B. A randomized, open, parallel-group study on the preventive effect of an estradiol-releasing vaginal ring (Estring) on recurrent urinary tract infections in postmenopausal women. *Am J Obstet Gynecol* 1999;180:1072-9
63. Notelovitz M, Funk S, Nanavati N, Mazzeo M. Estradiol absorption from vaginal tables in postmenopausal women. *Obstet Gynecol* 2002;99: 556-62
64. Rioux JE, Devlin C, Gelfand MM, Steinberg WM, Hepburn DS. 17beta-estradiol vaginal tablet versus conjugated equine estrogen vaginal cream to relieve menopausal atrophic vaginitis. *Menopause* 2000;7:156-61
65. Santen RJ, Pinkerton JV, Conaway M, *et al.* Treatment of urogenital atrophy with low-dose estradiol: preliminary results. *Menopause* 2002;9: 179-87
66. Dessole S, Rubattu, Ambrosini G, *et al.* Efficacy of low-dose intravaginal estriol on urogenital aging in postmenopausal. *Menopause.* 2004;11:49-56
67. NIH Consensus Development Panel. Osteoporosis prevention, diagnosis and therapy. *J Am Med Assoc* 2001;285:785-95
68. National Osteoporosis Foundation. Physician's Guide to Prevention and Treatment of Osteoporosis 2003 www.nof.org/physguide, accessed 2/01/04
69. Lindsay R, Silverman SL, Cooper C, *et al.* Risk of new vertebral fracture in the year following a fracture. *J Am Med Assoc* 2001;285:320-3
70. Delmas P, Genant H, Crans G, *et al.* Prevalent vertebral fracture severity predicts subsequent vertebral and nonvertebral fracture risk in postmenopausal women with osteoporosis: results from the Multiple Outcomes of Raloxifene Evaluation (MORE) trial. *Osteoporos Int* 2002; 13:521
71. Cummings SR, Nevitt MC, Browner WS, *et al.* Risk factors for hip fracture in white women. *N Engl J Med* 1995;332:767-73
72. Lauritzen JB, Petersen MM, Lund B. Effect of external hip protectors on hip fractures. *Lancet* 1993;341:11-13
73. Shea B, Wells G, Cranney A, *et al.* Meta-analysis of calcium supplementation for the prevention of postmenopausal osteoporosis. *Endocr Rev* 2002;23:552-9
74. Riggs BL, Seeman E, Hodgson SF, *et al.* Effect of the fluoride/calcium regimen on vertebral fracture occurrence in postmenopausal osteoporosis. *N Engl J Med* 1982;306:446-50
75. Dawson-Huges B, Harris SS, Krall EA, *et al.* Vitamin D treatment effects on BMD have been inconsistent. Effect of calcium and vitamin D supplementation on bone density in men and women 65 years of age or older. *N Engl J Med* 1997;337:670-6
76. Chapuy MC, Pamphile R, Paris E, *et al.* Combined calcium and vitamin D3 supplementation in elderly women: confirmation of reversal of secondary hyperparathyroidism and hip fracture risk: the Decalyos II study. *Osteoporos Int* 2002; 13L:257-64
77. Lufkin EG, Wahner HW, O'Fallon WM, *et al.* Treatment of postmenopausal osteoporosis with transdermal estrogen. *Ann Intern Med* 1992; 117:1-9
78. Recker RR, Davies KM, Dowd RM, Heaney RP. The effect of low-dose continuous estrogen and progesterone therapy with calcium and vitamin D on bone in elderly women. A randomized, controlled trial. *Ann Intern Med* 1999;130: 897-904
79. Paganini-Hill A, Ross RK, Gerkins VR, Henderson BE, Arthur M, Mack TM. Menopausal

estrogen therapy and hip fractures. *Ann Intern Med* 1981;95:28–31

80. Cauley JA, Seeley DG, Ensrud K, Ettinger B, Black D, Cummings SR. Estrogen replacement therapy and fractures in older women. Study of Osteoporotic Fractures Research Group. *Ann Intern Med* 1995;122:9–16
81. Torgerson DJ, Bell-Shyer SE Hormone replacement therapy and prevention of nonvertebral fractures: a meta-analysis of randomized trials. *J Am Med Assoc* 2001;285:2891–7
82. Effects of hormone therapy on bone mineral density: results from the Postmenopausal Estrogen/Progestin Interventions (PEPI) trial. The Writing Group for the PEPI. *J Am Med Assoc* 1996;276:1389–96
83. Tremollieres FA, Pouilles JM, Ribot C. Withdrawal of hormone replacement therapy is associated with significant vertebral bone loss in postmenopausal women. *Osteoporos Int* 2001;12: 385–90
84. Greenspan SL, Emkey RD, Bone HG, *et al.* Significant differential effects of alendronate, estrogen, or combination therapy on the rate of bone loss after discontinuation of treatment of postmenopausal osteoporosis. A randomized, double-blind, placebo-controlled trial. *Ann Intern Med* 2002;137:875–83
85. Barrett-Connor E, Wehren LE, Siris ES, *et al.* Recency and duration of postmenopausal hormone therapy: effects on bone mineral density and fracture risk in the National Osteoporosis Risk Assessment ( NORA) study. *Menopause* 2003; 10:412–19
86. Boissier S, Ferreras M, Peyruchaud O, *et al.* Bisphosphonates inhibit breast and prostate carcinoma cell invasion, an early event in the formation of bone metastases. *Cancer Res* 2000; 60:2949–54
87. Hillner BE, Ingle JN, Chlebowski RT *et al.* American Society of Clinical Oncology (ASCO) 2003 update on the role of bisphosphonates and bone health issues in women with breast cancer. *J Clin Oncol* 2003;21:4042–57
88. Cranney A, Wells G, Willan A, *et al.* Meta-analysis of therapies for postmenopausal osteoporosis. II . Meta-analysis of alendronate for the treatment of postmenopausal women. *Endocr Rev* 2002;23: 508–16
89. Emkey R, Reid I, Mulloy A, *et al.* Ten-year efficacy and safety of alendronate in the treatment of osteoporosis in postmenopausal women. *J Bone Miner Res* 2002;17(Supp 1):S139
90. Hosking D, Chilvers CE, Christiansen C, *et al.* Prevention of bone loss with alendronate in postmenopausal women under 60 years of age. Early Postmenopausal Intervention Cohort Study Group. *N Engl J Med* 1998;338:485–92
91. Ravn P, Bidstrup M, Wasnich RD, *et al.* Alendronate and estrogen-progestin in the long-term prevention of bone loss: four-year results from the early postmenopausal intervention cohort study. A randomized, controlled trial. *Ann Intern Med* 1999;131:935–42
92. Bone HG, Downs RW Jr, Tucci JR, *et al.* Dose-response relationships for alendronate treatment in osteoporotic elderly women. Alendronate Elderly Osteoporosis Study Centers. *J Clin Endocrinol Metab* 1997;82:265–74
93. Liberman UA, Weiss SR, Broll J, *et al.* Effect of oral alendronate on bone mineral density and the incidence of fractures in postmenopausal osteoporosis. The Alendronate Phase III Osteoporosis Treatment Study Group. *N Engl J Med* 1995; 333:1437–43
94. Ensrud KE, Black DM, Palermo L, *et al.* Treatment with alendronate prevents fractures in women at highest risk: results from the Fracture Intervention Trial. *Arch Intern Med* 1997;157:2617–24
95. Black DM, Thompson DE, Bauer DC, *et al.* Fracture risk reduction with alendronate in women with osteoporosis: the Fracture Intervention Trial. FIT Research Group. *J Clin Endocrinol Metab* 2000;85:4118–24
96. Levis S, Quandt SA, Thompson D, *et al.* Alendronate reduces the risk of multiple symptomatic fractures: results from the Fracture Intervention Trial. *J Am Geriatr Soc* 2002;50:409–15
97. Cummings SR, Black DM, Thompson DE, *et al.* Effect of alendronate on risk of fracture in women with low bone density but without vertebral fractures: results from the Fracture Intervention Trial. *J Am Med Assoc* 1998;280:2077–82
98. Cranney A, Tugwell P, Adachi J, *et al.* Meta-analysis of therapies for postmenopausal osteoporosis. III. Meta-analysis of risedronate for the treatment of postmenopausal osteoporosis. *Endocr Rev* 2002;23:517–23
99. Harris ST, Watts NB, Genant HK, *et al.* Effects of risedronate treatment on vertebral and non-vertebral fractures in women with postmenopausal osteoporosis. *J Am Med Assoc* 1999;282: 1344–52
100. Reginster JY, Deroisy R, Lecart MP, *et al.* A double-blind, placebo-controlled, dose-finding trial of intermittent nasal salmon calcitonin for prevention of postmenopausal lumbar spine bone loss. *Am J Med* 1995;98:452–8
101. Watts NB, Josse RG, Hamdy RC, *et al.* Risedronate prevents new vertebral fractures in postmenopausal women at high risk. *J Clin Endocrinol Metab* 2003;88:542–9
102. Sorensen OH, Crawford GM, Mulder H, *et al.* Long-term efficacy of risedronate: a 5-year placebo-controlled clinical experience. *Bone* 2003;32:120–6

103. McClung MR, Geusens P, Miller PD, *et al.* Effect of risedronate on the risk of hip fracture in elderly women. Hip Intervention Program Study Group. *N Engl J Med* 2001;344:333–40
104. Reid IR, Brown JP, Burckhardt P, *et al.* Intravenous zolendronic acid in postmenopausal women with low bone density. *N Engl J Med* 2002;346:653–61
105. Reginster JY, Deroisy R, Lecart MP, *et al.* A double-blind, placebo-controlled, dose-finding trial of intermittent nasal salmon calcitonin for prevention of postmenopausal lumbar spine bone loss. *Am J Med* 1995;98:452–8
106. Ellerington MC, Hillard TC, Whitcroft SI, *et al.* Intranasal salmon calcitonin for the prevention and treatment of postmenopausal osteoporosis. *Calcif Tissue Int* 1996;59:6–11
107. Lyntis GP, Tsakalakos N, Magiasis B, *et al.* Analgesic effect of salmon calcitonin in osteoporotic vertebral fractures. A blind-blind placebo controlled trial. *Calcif Tissue Int* 1991;49:369–72
108. Overgaard K, Hansen MA, Jensen SB, Christiansen C. Effect of salcatonin given intranasally on bone mass and fracture rates in established osteoporosis: a dose-response study. *Br Med J* 1992;305:556–61
109. Chesnut CH, III, Silverman S, Andriano K, *et al.* A randomized trial of nasal spray salmon calcitonin in postmenopausal women with established osteoporosis: the prevent recurrence of osteoporotic fractures study. PROOF Study Group. *Am J Med* 2000;109:267–76
110. Powles TJ, Hickish T, Kanis JA, Tidy A, Ashley S. Effect of tamoxifen on bone mineral density measured by dual-energy x-ray absorptiometry in healthy premenopausal and postmenopausal women. *J Clin Oncol* 1996;14:78–84
111. Fisher B, Costantino JP, Wickerham DL, *et al.* Tamoxifen for prevention of breast cancer: report of the National Surgical Adjuvant Breast and Bowel Project P-1 Study. *J Natl Cancer Inst* 1998;90:1371–88
112. Ettinger B, Black DM, Mitlak BH, *et al.* Reduction of vertebral fracture risk in postmenopausal women with osteoporosis treated with raloxifene: results from a 3-year randomized clinical trial. Multiple Outcomes of Raloxifene Evaluation (MORE) Investigators. Erratum appears in *J Am Med Assoc* 1999;282:2124]. *J Am Med Assoc* 1999;282:637–45
113. Delmas PD, Ensrud KE, Adachi JD, *et al.* Efficacy of raloxifene on vertebral fracture risk reduction in postmenopausal women with osteoporosis: four-year results from a randomized clinical trial. *J Clin Endocrinol Metab* 2002;87:3609–17
114. Cauley JA, Norton L, Lippman ME, *et al.* Continued breast cancer risk reduction in postmenopausal women treated with raloxifene: 4 year results from the MORE trial. *Breast Cancer Res Treat* 2001;65:125–34
115. Neer RM, Arnaud CD, Zucchetto JR, *et al.* Effect of parathyroid hormone (1-34) on fracture and bone mineral density in postmenopausal women with osteoporosis. *N Engl J Med* 2001;344:1434–41
116. Alexandersen P, Toussaint A, Christiansen C, *et al.* Ipriflavone in the treatment of postmenopausal osteoporosis – a randomized controlled trial. *J Am Med Assoc* 2001;285:1482–8
117. Alekel DL, Germain AS, Peterson CT, Hanson KB, Stewart JW, Toda T. Isoflavone-rich soy protein isolate attenuates bone loss in the lumbar spine of perimenopausal women. *Am J Clin Nutr* 2000;72:844–52
118. Setchell KD, Lydeking-Olsen D. Dietary phytoestrgoens and their effects on bone: evidence from in vitro and in vivo, human observational, and dietary intervention studies. *Am J Clin Nutr* 2003; 78:593S–609S
119. Bone HG, Greenspan SL, McKeever C, *et al.* Alendronate and estrogen effects in postmenopausal women with low bone mineral density. *J Clin Endocrinol Metab* 2000;85:720–6
120. Lindsay R, Cosman F, Lobo RA, *et al.* Addition of alendronate to ongoing hormone replacement therapy in the treatment of osteoporosis: a randomized, controlled clinical trial. *J Clin Endocrinol Metab* 1999;84:3076–81
121. Harris D, Eriksen EF, Davidson M, *et al.* Effect of combined risedronate and HT on BMD of postmenopausal women. *J Clin Endocrinol Metab* 2001;86:1890–7
122. Johnell O, Scheele WH, Lu Y, *et al.* Additive effects of raloxifene and alendronate on bone density and biochemical markers of bone remodeling in postmenopausal women with osteoporosis. *J Clin Endocrinol Metab* 2002;87:985–92
123. Black DM, Greenspan SL, Ensrud KE, *et al.* The effects of parathyroid hormone and alendronate alone or in combination in postmenopausal osteoporosis. *N Engl J Med* 2003;349:1207–15
124. Pearson TA, Blair SN, Daniels SR, *et al.* AHA Guidelines for Primary Prevention of Cardiovascular Disease and Stroke: 2002 Update: Consensus Panel Guide to Comprehensive Risk Reduction for Adult Patients Without Coronary or Other Atherosclerotic Vascular Diseases. American Heart Association Science Advisory and Coordinating Committee. *Circulation* 2002; 106:388–91
125. Effects of estrogen or estrogen/progestin regimens on heart disease risk factors in postmenopausal women. The Postmenopausal Estrogen/Progestin Interventions (PEPI) Trial. The Writing Group for the PEPI Trial. [erratum appears in *J Am Med Assoc* 1995;274:1676] *J Am Med Assoc* 1995;273:199–208

126. Cushman M, Legault C, Barrett-Connor E, *et al.* Effect of postmenopausal hormones on inflammation-sensitive proteins: the Postmenopausal Estrogen/Progestin Interventions (PEPI) Study. *Circulation* 1999;100:717-22
127. van Baal WM, Kenemans P, van der Mooren MJ, Kessel H, Emeis JJ, Stehouwer CD. Increased C-reactive protein levels during short-term hormone replacement therapy in healthy postmenopausal women. *Thrombosis Haemostasis* 1999;81:925-8
128. Ylikorkala O, Cacciatore B, Paakkari I, Tikkanen MJ, Viinikka L, Toivonen J. The long-term effects of oral and transdermal postmenopausal hormone replacement therapy on nitric oxide, endothelin-1, prostacyclin, and thromboxane. *Fertil Steril* 1998;69:883-8
129. Barrett-Connor E, Grady D. Hormone replacement therapy, heart disease, and other considerations. *Ann Rev Pub Health* 1998;19:55-72
130. Mendelsohn ME, Karas RH. The protective effects of estrogen on the cardiovascular system. *N Engl J Med* 1999;340:1801-11
131. Grodstein F, Stampfer MJ, Manson JE, *et al.* Postmenopausal estrogen and progestin use and the risk of cardiovascular disease. [erratum appears in *N Engl J Med* 1996;335:1406]. *N Engl J Med* 1996;335:453-61
132. Grodstein F, Manson JE, Colditz GA, Willett WC, Speizer FE, Stampfer MJ. A prospective, observational study of postmenopausal hormone therapy and primary prevention of cardiovascular disease. *Ann Intern Med* 2000;133:933-41
133. Viscoli CM, Brass LM, Kernan WN, Sarrel PM, Suissa S, Horwitz RI. A clinical trial of estrogen-replacement therapy after ischemic stroke. *N Engl J Med* 2001;345:1243-9
134. Hulley S, Grady D, Bush T, *et al.* Randomized trial of estrogen plus progestin for secondary prevention of coronary heart disease in postmenopausal women. Heart and Estrogen/progestin Replacement Study (HERS) Research Group. *J Am Med Assoc* 1998;280:605-13
135. American Heart Association 2001. Heart and Stroke Statistical Update, Dallas Texas, American Heart Association, 2002
136. Third Report of the Expert Panel on Detection, Evaluation, and Treatment of High Blood Cholesterol in Adults (Adult Treatment Panel). www.nhlbi.nih.gov/guidelines/cholesterol; accessed 2/02/04
137. Thompson PD, Buchner D, Pina IL. Exercise and Physical Activity in the Prevention and Treatment of Atherosclerotic Cardiovascular disease. A statement from the Council on Clinical Cardiology. (Subcommittee on Exercise, Rehabilitation, and Prevention) and the Council on Nutrition, Physical Activity, and Metabolism (Subcommittee on Physical Activity). AHA scientific statement *Circulation* 2003;107:3109-16
138. Moghadasian MH. Statins and menopause. *Drug* 2002;62:2421-31
139. Paternak RC, Smith SC Jr, Bairey-Merz CN. ACC/AHA/NHLBI Clinical Advisory on the Use and Safety of Statins. *Circulation* 2002;106: 1024-8
140. Heart Protection Study Collaborative Group. MRC/BHF Heart Protection Study of cholesterol lowering with simvastatin in 20,536 high risk individuals: a randomized placebo controlled trial. *Lancet* 2002;360:7-22
141. Downs JR, Clearfield M, Weis S, *et al.* Primary prevention of acute coronary events with lovastatin in men and women with average cholesterol levels: results of AFCAPS/TexCAPS. Air Force/ Texas Coronary Atherosclerosis Prevention Study. *J Am Med Assoc* 1998;279:1615-22
142. Delmas PD, Bjarnason NH, Mitlak BH, *et al.* Effects of raloxifene on bone mineral density, serum cholesterol concentrations, and uterine endometrium in postmenopausal women. *N Eng J Med* 1997;337:1641-7
143. Barrett-Connor E, Grady D, Sashegyi A, *et al.* for the MORE Investigators (Multiple Outcomes of Raloxifene Evaluation). Raloxifene and cardiovascular events in osteoporotic postmenopausal women: four-year results from the MORE (Multiple Outcomes of Raloxifene Evaluation) randomized trial. *J Am Med Assoc* 2002;287: 847-57
144. Anderson JW, Johnstone BM, Cook-Newell ME. Meta-analysis of the effects of soy protein intake on serum lipids. *N Eng J Med* 1995;333: 276-82
145. Simons LA, von Konigsmark M, Simons J, Celermajer DS. Phytoestrogens do not influence lipoprotein levels or endothelial function in healthy, postmenopausal women. *Am J Cardiol* 2000;85:1297-301
146. Hulley S, Grady D, Bush T, *et al.* Randomized trial of estrogen plus progestin for secondary prevention of coronary heart disease in postmenopausal women. Heart and Estrogen/progestin Replacement Study (HERS) Research Group. *J Am Med Assoc* 1998;280:605-13
147. Grady D, Herrington D, Bittner V, *et al.* HERS Research Group. Cardiovascular disease outcomes during 6.8 years of hormone therapy: Heart and Estrogen/progestin Replacement Study follow-up (HERS II). *J Am Med Assoc* 2002;288: 49-57
148. Herrington DM, Reboussin DM, Brosnihan KB, *et al.* Effects of estrogen replacement on the progression of coronary-artery atherosclerosis. *N Eng J Med* 2000;343:522-9
149. Hodis, HN, Lobo RA, Faxon DP, *et al.* Hormone therapy and the progression of coronary-artery atherosclerosis in postmenopausal women. *N Engl J Med* 2003;349:535-45

150. Cherry N, Gilmour K, Hannaford P, *et al.* Oestrogen therapy for the prevention of reinfarction in postmenopausal women: a randomized placebo-controlled trial. *Lancet* 2002;360:2001–8
151. LaRosa JC. What do the statins tell us? *Am Heart J* 2002;144:S21–6
152. Pedersen TR, Olsson AG, Faergeman O, *et al.* Lipoprotein changes and reduction in the incidence of major coronary heart disease events in the Scandinavian Simvastatin Survival Study (4S). *Circulation* 1998;97:1453–60
153. Sacks FM, Pfeffer MA, Moye LA, *et al.* The effect of pravastatin on coronary events after myocardial infarction in patients with average cholesterol levels. Cholesterol and Recurrent Events Trial Investigators. *N Engl J Med* 1996;335: 10001–9
154. The Long-term Intervention with Pravastatin in Ischemic Disease (LIPID) study group. *N Engl J Med* 1998;339:1349–57
155. Hennekens CH. Update on aspirin in the treatment and prevention of cardiovascular disease. *Am J Managed Care* 2002;8:S691–700
156. Hebert PR, Gaziano M, Chan KS, *et al.* Cholesterol lowering with statin drugs, risks of stroke and total mortality: an overview of randomized trials. *J Am Med Assoc* 1997;278:313–21
157. Hennekens CH, Sacks FM, Tonkin A *et al.* Additive benefits of pravastatin and aspirin to decrease risks of cardiovascular disease. Randomized and observational comparisons of secondary prevention trials and their meta-analyses. *Arch Intern Med* 2004;164;40–4
158. Mayo Clinic Proceedings article (Fitzpatrick LA. Santen RJ. Hot flashes: the old and the new, what is really true? [Editorial] *Mayo Clinic Proc* 2002;77:1155–8

# Women's perspectives of hormone replacement therapy in Europe: country-specific aspects

9

*A. Strothmann and H. P. G. Schneider*

## INTRODUCTION

The findings of the Women's Health Initiative (WHI), but also from other studies such as the Heart and Estrogen/progestin Replacement Study (HERS)[1], a secondary prevention trial reporting multiple outcomes, the recent meta-analysis of hormone replacement therapy (HRT) trials[2], or the actual British Million Women Study[3], resulted in a broad scientific discussion on the benefits and risks of HRT. This, together with the rather alarming media coverage, has made many women and their health-care professionals feel uncertain about HRT use.

In the light of the recent epidemiological data, recommendations for clinical practice from past years might appear to be outdated and are, at least partly, being re-evaluated. As the majority of women actively take part in the decision-making for or against HRT[4], an investigation of patterns of HRT use in Europe seemed mandatory[5]; moreover, this would provide a better insight into the market's reaction towards the late scientific debate.

Between February and April 2003, a cross-sectional survey was conducted in four European countries (Germany, Great Britain, France and Spain) to ascertain the current profile of the menopausal women. A stratified sample of 8012 women aged 45–75 years (Table 1) was interviewed via standardized computer-aided telephone interviewing. Quota were used as to age, regional distribution and educational level to ensure that representative samples of women were drawn in the four different survey countries.

## AWARENESS OF HRT AND ITS BENEFITS AND RISKS

A total of 73% of all interviewed women were aware of HRT as a treatment option for menopausal symptoms, with this percentage varying from 41% in Spain to 90% in Great Britain (Figure 1). Among non-HRT users, the proportion of women who had heard of HRT was, on average, 60%.

Women were well informed about two of the most widely discussed benefits and risks of HRT, osteoporosis prevention and breast cancer. Among HRT ever-users, 69% knew that the risk of losing bone mass density decreased by using HRT, and 52% were aware of an increased risk of breast

**Table 1** Number of interviewed women

| Country | Total number of interviewed women | Number of current HRT users *n* | Number of current HRT users % | Number of former HRT users *n* | Number of former HRT users % | Number of never-HRT users *n* | Number of never-HRT users % |
|---|---|---|---|---|---|---|---|
| Germany | 1997 | 386 | 19 | 419 | 21 | 1192 | 60 |
| Great Britain | 2012 | 376 | 19 | 407 | 20 | 1229 | 61 |
| France | 2004 | 454 | 23 | 324 | 16 | 1226 | 61 |
| Spain | 1999 | 101 | 5 | 129 | 7 | 1769 | 89 |

HRT, hormone replacement therapy

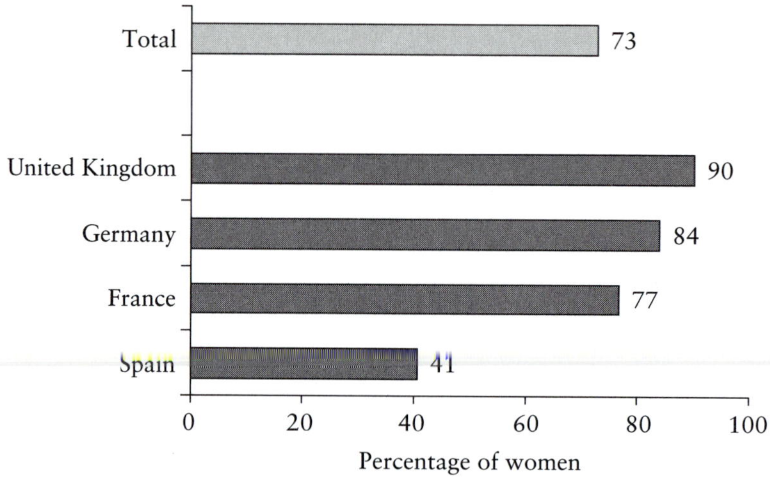


**Figure 1** Awareness of hormone replacement therapy amongst all interviewed women

cancer. Among non-users, these percentages were 49% and 43%, respectively.

Nevertheless, when it comes to less well-known risks such as uterine or colon cancer, the majority of HRT ever-users, as well as never-users, do not appear to be adequately informed about the effects of HRT, e.g. more ever-users (9%) thought that HRT increases the risk of colon cancer rather than decreases it (7%). This was also the case regarding cancer of the uterus (23% vs. 13%).

Regarding the effect of HRT on heart diseases, the opinion of two-thirds of the women rather reflected uncertainty. This could either be due to inadequate counselling in the European countries investigated, or might have been reinforced by the ongoing scientific debate on this topic. One-fifth of HRT ever-users answered that the risk of falling ill with heart diseases decreased with HRT usage. Only 18% stated that the risk increased.

In general, higher proportions of Spanish women stated that they did not to know about HRT's effect on the questioned benefits and risks than in the other three survey countries.

## REASONS FOR REFRAINING FROM HRT USE

Interestingly, HRT never-users do not appear to be scared away from HRT usage by one special/certain risk, but refrain from usage for more general reasons such as having no need for an HRT medication (29%), no recommendation to use HRT from their doctor (16%), or the doctor advised against the usage of HRT (10%).

## ACCEPTANCE RATES OF HRT

Country-specific awareness of HRT being a treatment option for menopausal symptoms is also reflected in the HRT acceptance rates of the survey countries. In the age group 45–75 years, only 12% of Spanish women reported HRT experience. In the remaining three countries of this survey (Germany, Great Britain and France), on average, more than three times as many women (39%) aged 45–75 years have HRT experience and 20% are current HRT users.

The prevalence of current use was highest in the 50–54-year (24%) and the 55–59-year (27%) age bands, which was particularly evident in France and Germany. Among women 70 years or older, on average 6% were still using HRT, the proportions in France and Germany being as high as 13%.

## REASONS TO START HRT USE

European women do not only start HRT usage for present symptom relief, although 70% of the users state that this was one of the main reasons to initiate therapy. They also greatly value the possibility of preventing postmenopausal osteoporosis. The effectiveness of HRT in the relief of hot flushes and protection from postmenopausal osteoporosis is well established and remains unchallenged by the results of WHI[6]. To HRT users, maintenance or improvement of general well-being also seems to be closely linked to HRT usage (Figure 2).

These three main reasons stated for commencing usage of HRT were similar to those mentioned most frequently and spontaneously as HRT benefits in the four survey countries.

Although there is some variability in the ranking of the main reasons to start HRT use among the survey countries, e.g. French HRT users putting highest weight on the prevention of osteoporosis instead of relief of hot flushes, the three main reasons to start HRT are consistent from country to country. Only in Britain do women also put high weight on the relief from depressive mood, anxiety and irritability; therefore, osteoporosis prevention is named only in fourth place, but closely following the psychological factors mentioned above.

On average, women started HRT usage at the age of 49 years (95% confidence interval (CI) = 48.5–48.96 years) showing that women from the four European countries started HRT use at a much younger age (mean age of 49 years) when compared to the vast majority of women who entered the study population of the WHI trial. Women in the WHI trial were, on average, 14 years older (63 years) at inclusion in the trial and 73% of the women in the estrogen + progestin arm of the trial started on HRT at this advanced age[6,7]. Naturally, women in their sixties present more relative risks of frailty and disabilities than women in their high forties or early fifties. The relevance of the WHI trial results for early menopausal women must consequently remain subject to debate.

## PRODUCT CHANGES AND TREATMENT BREAKS

About half of all HRT users never change their HRT product during their entire treatment period

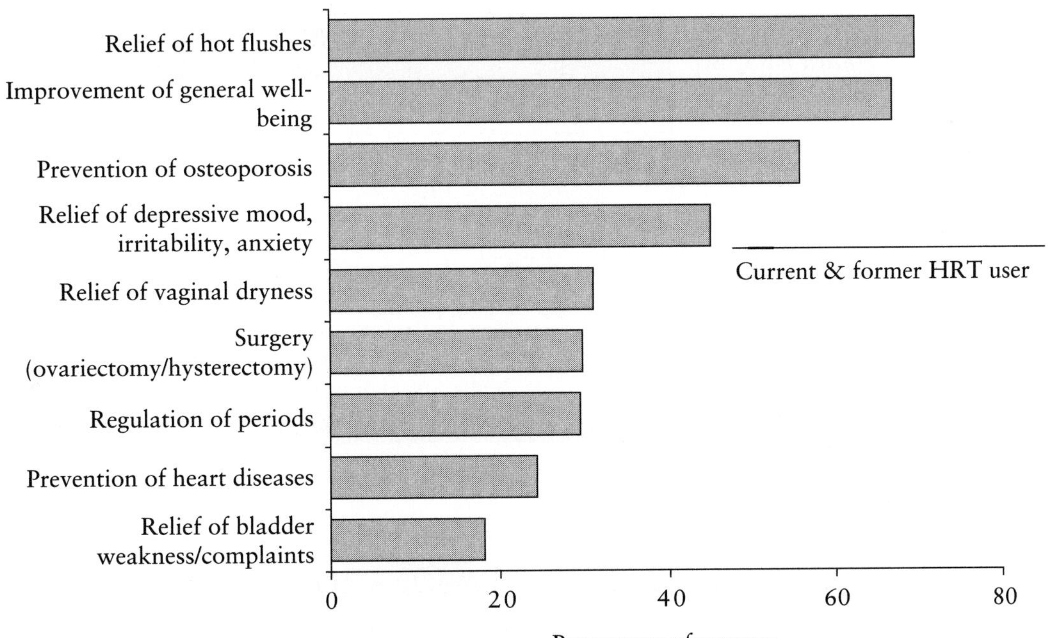


**Figure 2** Main reasons to start hormone replacement therapy use (more than one answer possible); results for all four survey countries

with HRT. If they do so, they mostly change because they are not satisfied with the relief from menopausal symptoms achieved with their current product (36%), or because they think the product has caused them to gain weight (26%). Another reason frequently given was bleeding problems (25%), which might at least partly be due to the therapeutic regimen that the women were on (Figure 3).

Also, only a few women take breaks from HRT usage. Roughly about 70% of women using HRT stated that they had never interrupted intake and, if they did so, the longest break was on average only 3.5 months (Figure 3).

## REASONS TO DISCONTINUE HRT USE

Apart from discontinuing HRT use because their menopausal symptoms have disappeared, to women, breast cancer is the central topic of concern. A large number of respondents stated that breast cancer was the major risk factor of HRT and information about increased risk of breast cancer associated with HRT led 26% to discontinue their treatment. This finding is consistent with results from previous studies[6–10] and reflects a continuous and widespread cancer phobia that has only been further stimulated by

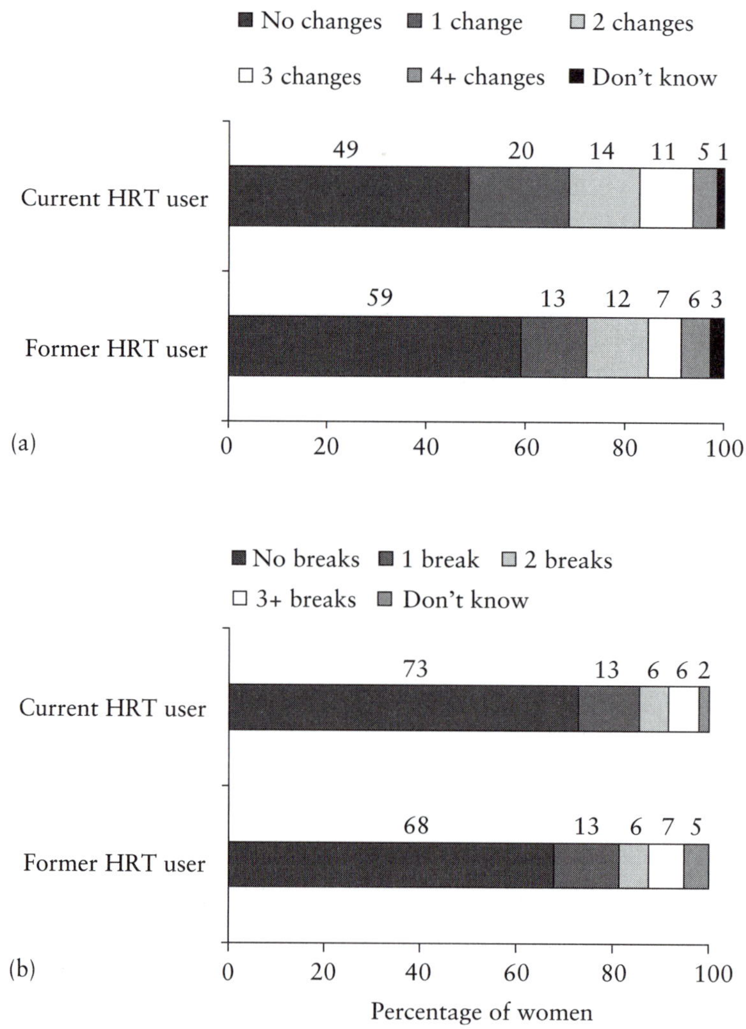


**Figure 3** Treatment changes (a) and breaks (b); results for all four survey countries

the way in which the media, and especially the lay press, have covered recent results.

European women were also concerned with weight gain whilst using HRT. Consequently, a quarter (25%) of the women discontinued therapy for this reason (Figure 4). In particular, French women (29%) perceived weight gain as a major problem with HRT. Weight gain attributed to HRT is a frequently mentioned reason for discontinuing HRT treatment in other studies, although clinical trials have not given evidence that estrogen causes weight gain[11-13].

In Germany, compared to the remaining survey countries, the highest proportion of women stated that a principal reason to discontinue HRT use was information about increased risk of heart diseases (18%). In France and Great Britain, only 11% and 9%, respectively discontinued therapy for this reason; in Spain, none of the former HRT users stopped therapy because of information about an increased risk of heart diseases.

## TREATMENT DURATION

Results from past publications have suggested that women discontinue HRT use after menopausal symptoms have disappeared[4,14]. In contrast, more than half of the current HRT users in our survey continued to use their HRT for more than 5 years, when, since the results of the WHI, it is seriously recommended to reconsider HRT use.

Among all participants who reported current HRT use, 43% were using it for up to 5 years and 27% for 6–10 years. The remaining 30% of current users had already continued their HRT for more than 10 years (Figure 5). Thereby the mean duration of therapy for current users amounts to 8.1 years (CI = 7.8–8.5 years), ranging from 4.8 (CI = 3.99–5.7) years in Spain to 9.7 (CI = 8.98–10.5) years in Germany. As anticipated, the treatment duration by women who had already ceased HRT use was less, with 64% usage below 5 years, 20% using it for 6–10 and 16% for longer than 10 years. Once again, Spain had the shortest mean duration of therapy (3.5 years, CI = 2.8–4.2 years), and France had the longest (7.6 years, CI = 5.8–7.3 years). Current users were also asked for how long they would be willing to continue their HRT. In response, 11% of the participants had not yet decided on a certain time period. One-third (33%) of the current HRT users answered that they would rely on their doctor to tell them when to cease treatment, and 6% of the woman were willing to discontinue treatment when their menopausal symptoms disappeared.

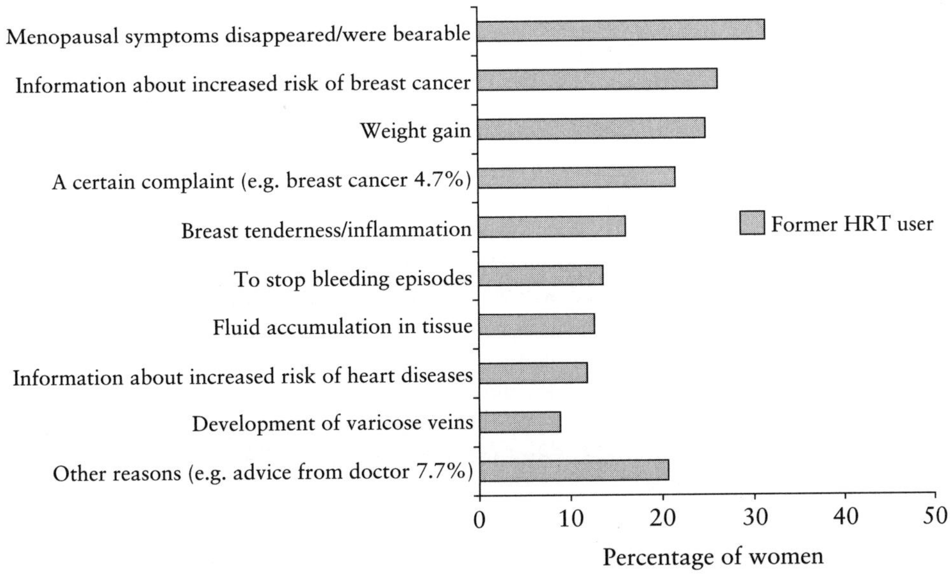


**Figure 4** Main reasons to discontinue hormone replacement therapy use (more than one answer possible); results for all four survey countries

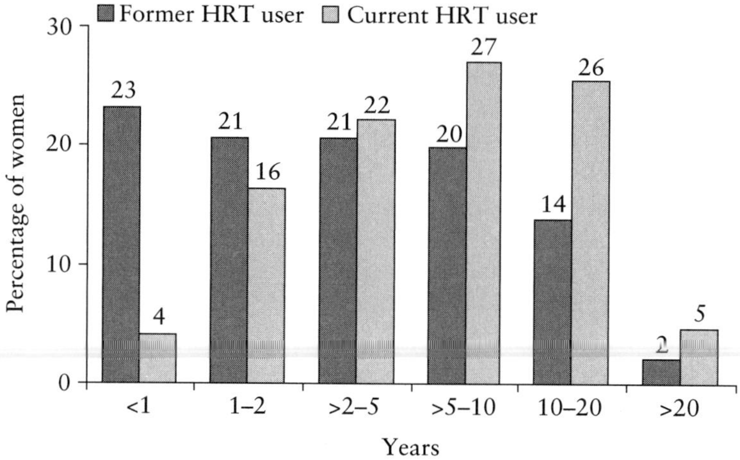


**Figure 5** Treatment duration for hormone replacement therapy (HRT); results for all four survey countries

Of those HRT users who gave a time estimate, 27% were willing to continue their HRT treatment for up to 5 years and 14% for more than 5 years. Another 10% intended to use HRT for the rest of their lives. Among the latter, British and German women most frequently predicted life-long HRT usage (13% and 12% respectively, vs. 7% of Spanish and 5% of French women). More than every other Spanish (60%) woman would rely on her doctor to take this decision, whilst only 24% of the German women would leave this decision to their physician.

A large proportion (84%) of current HRT users expressed their satisfaction with the HRT that they received (Figure 6).

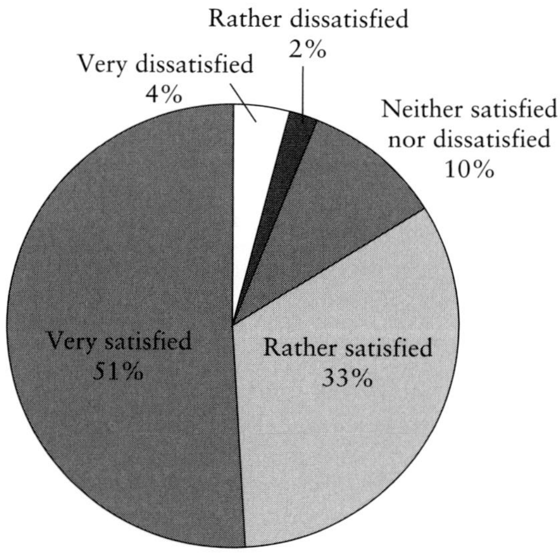


**Figure 6** Satisfaction with current hormone replacement therapy product; results for all four survey countries

## AWARENESS ABOUT RECENT SCIENTIFIC DEBATE

To investigate the awareness of women regarding the new epidemiology on HRT, the women were questioned whether they had heard any information about benefits and risks of HRT since July 2002.

Among current and former HRT users, about two-thirds (68% and 60%, respectively) stated that they had received information, either about benefits, risks or both during the past half year. As could be anticipated, never-users were less aware of the current discussion. More than half of the women in this group (52%) had not heard any news about HRT since July 2002.

When comparing the data for the four survey countries, it seems that German and French women were most knowledgeable of new information on HRT, with up to 78% of the current users stating that they had received new information during the past half year. At the lower end, British and Spanish women appear to be least informed about the recent scientific news regarding HRT.

## CONCLUSION

There are still major differences in the knowledge of HRT's benefits and risks among women in the four surveyed countries. Expectations of this therapy also vary according to the different cultural backgrounds.

In addition, the scientific uncertainties around HRT present a challenge to women and their health-care providers. It is thus crucial to offer women accurate information about the benefits and risks of HRT and it is the responsibility of health-care professionals to assist them in their individual risk assessment.

There is, however, unanimous agreement among Europeans that proper counseling and individual care offered by clinically experienced physicians will provide the type of assistance women deserve during the climacteric age.

## ACKNOWLEDGEMENT

This work forms part of the doctoral thesis of A. Strothmann, Humboldt-University Berlin, Germany.

# References

1. Hulley S, Grady D, Bush T, *et al.* Randomized trial of estrogen plus progestin for secondary prevention of coronary heart disease in postmenopausal women. Heart and Estrogen/progestin Replacement Study (HERS) Research Group. *J Am Med Assoc* 1998;280:605–13
2. Beral V, Banks E, Reeves G. Evidence from randomised trials on the long-term effects of hormone replacement therapy. *Lancet* 2002;360: 942–4
3. Million Women Study Collaborators. Breast cancer and hormone replacement therapy in the Million Women Study. *Lancet* 2003;362:419–27
4. Schneider HPG. Cross-national study of women's use of hormone replacement therapy (HRT) in Europe. *Int J Fertil Womens Med* 1997;42(Suppl 2): 365–75
5. Strothmann A, Schneider HPG. Hormone replacement therapy: the European women's perspective. *Climacteric* 2003;6:337–46
6. Rossouw JE, Anderson GL, Prentice RL, *et al.* Writing Group for the Women's Health Initiative Investigators. Risks and benefits of estrogen plus progestin in healthy postmenopausal women: principal results from the Women's Health Initiative randomized controlled trial. *J Am Med Assoc* 2002;288:321–33
7. The Women's Health Initiative Study Group. Design of the Women's Health Initiative clinical trial and observational study. *Control Clin Trials* 1998;19:61–109
8. Castel-Branco C, Figueras F, Sanjuan A, *et al.* Long-term compliance with estrogen replacement therapy in surgical postmenopausal women: benefits to bone and analysis of factors associated with discontinuation. *Menopause* 1999;6:307–11
9. Li C, Samsioe G, Lidfelt J, Nerbrand C, Agardh CD; Women's Health in Lund Area (WHILA) Study. Important factors for use of hormone replacement therapy: a population-based study of Swedish women. The Women's Health in Lund Area (WHILA) Study. *Menopause* 2000;7:273–81
10. Vihtamaki T, Savilahti R, Tuimala R. Why do postmenopausal women discontinue hormone replacement therapy? *Maturitas* 1999;33:99–105
11. Jensen LB, Vestergaard P, Hermann AP, *et al.* Hormone replacement therapy dissociates fat mass and bone mass, and tends to reduce weight gain in early postmenopausal women: a randomized controlled 5-year clinical trial of the Danish Osteoporosis Prevention Study. *J Bone Miner Res* 2003;18:333–42
12. Guthrie JR, Dennerstein L, Dudley EC. Weight gain and the menopause: a 5-year prospective study. *Climacteric* 1999;2:205–11
13. Davies KM, Heaney RP, Recker RR, Barger-Lux MJ, Lappe JM. Hormones, weight change and menopause. *Int J Obes* 2001;25:874–9
14. Groeneveld FP, Bareman FP, Barentsen R, Dokter HJ, Drogendijk AC, Hoes AW. Duration of hormonal replacement therapy in general practice; a follow-up study. *Maturitas* 1998;29:125–31

# Recent clinical data and the role of menopausal hormone therapy today

10

*J. H. Pickar*

The Women's Health Initiative (WHI) is composed of a clinical trial and an observational study. The clinical trial consists of three components, hormone replacement therapy (HRT), dietary modification, and calcium/vitamin D supplementation. The HRT component consists of two arms, estrogen plus progestin and unopposed estrogen. On July 17, 2002 the Writing Group for the WHI Investigators published the principal results from the estrogen plus progestin arm of that study[1].

The WHI study protocol indicates that the outcomes for the clinical trial are divided into primary, subsidiary and composite outcomes. Primary outcomes are those with significant power for detection, subsidiary outcomes are of interest but not necessarily with adequate power, and composite outcomes are combinations of primary and subsidiary outcomes. The primary outcome for the HRT component is coronary heart disease (CHD)[2]. Secondary outcomes consist of the subsidiary and composite outcomes[3]. Table 1, obtained from the WHI protocol, lists the outcomes for the HRT arm of the WHI clinical trial. There is one primary outcome, CHD, with multiple secondary outcomes including breast cancer. Subsequently, The Guidelines for the Statistical Monitoring of the WHI Clinical Trial indicated that, within the secondary outcomes, breast cancer would be designated as a primary adverse outcome[3]. Hence, the publication of the principal results lists CHD (CHD death and non-fatal myocardial infarction) as the primary outcome and breast cancer as a primary adverse outcome[1]. The primary outcomes listed in the protocol for the dietary modification and calcium/vitamin D supplementation components were breast cancer and colorectal cancer (dietary modification), and hip fracture (calcium/vitamin D supplementation).

**Table 1** Outcomes for the WHI HRT clinical trial. '1' indicates primary outcomes; '2' subsidiary and composite outcomes; 'X' ascertained

| *Outcome* | *HRT* |
|---|---|
| *Cardiovascular* | |
| Coronary heart disease | 1 |
| Stroke | 2 |
| Congestive heart failure | 2 |
| Angina | 2 |
| Peripheral vascular disease | 2 |
| Coronary revascularization | 2 |
| Total cardiovascular | 2 |
| *Cancer* | |
| Breast cancer | 2 |
| Endometrial cancer | 2 |
| Colorectal cancer | X |
| Ovarian cancer | 2 |
| Total cancers | 2 |
| *Fractures* | |
| Hip | 2 |
| Other fractures | 2 |
| Total fractures | 2 |
| *Venous thromboembolic disease* | |
| Pulmonary embolism | 2 |
| Deep vein thrombosis | 2 |
| Diabetes mellitus requiring therapy | 2 |
| Death from any cause | 2 |

The publication of the principal results was based on outcomes adjudicated by clinical center physicians (local adjudication); subsequent publications were to be based on centrally adjudicated outcomes. The hazard ratio for the primary outcome was presented with two confidence intervals (CI) and was stratified by clinical center, age, prior disease, and randomization status in the low-fat diet trial. The nominal 95% CI is unadjusted and hence has a probability greater than 0.05 of a type I error (falsely concluding that the confidence interval does not include 1). The adjusted 95% CI uses a group sequential method to correct for multiple analyses over time; however, for the primary outcome, the primary adverse outcome, and the global index, a correction for multiple outcomes was not performed. For other outcomes the adjusted 95% CI also included a Bonferroni correction for multiple outcomes, the seven specifically monitored outcomes other than breast cancer (CHD, stroke, pulmonary embolus, colorectal cancer, endometrial cancer, hip fracture, and death due to other causes).

## PRIMARY OUTCOME

The initial publication of the principal results, with a mean of 5.2 years of follow-up, reported a hazard ratio for the primary outcome of 1.29, nominal 95% CI (1.02–1.63), adjusted 95% CI (0.85–1.97). This was based on the local adjudication of events used for trial monitoring purposes. At that time the agreement between local and central adjudication for myocardial infarction was 84%[1]. Slightly over 1 year later, the final results of the estrogen plus progestin arm of WHI on the risk of CHD were published with an average of 5.6 years of follow-up[4]. An adjusted hazard ratio and nominal 95% CI were presented, adjusting for the presence or absence of a history of coronary revascularization (coronary-artery bypass grafting or percutaneous transluminal coronary angioplasty). This was based on the fact that the only baseline variable that differed significantly between the groups was a history of coronary revascularization ($p = 0.04$). The adjusted hazard ratio and nominal 95% CI were stratified as in the previous publication. In addition, the adjusted 95% CI for the primary outcome also controlled for sequential monitoring. For CHD, the adjusted hazard ratio was 1.24, nominal 95% CI (1.00–1.54), adjusted 95% CI (0.97–1.60). In this report, acute myocardial infarctions and deaths due to CHD were confirmed by central physician-adjudicators. The rate of concordance between local and central reviews was 90% for myocardial infarction and 97% for death due to atherosclerotic CHD.

Following publication of the final CHD results, an article in *The Wall Street Journal* noted 'The confidence interval – a key number that every statistician uses to show that a result is meaningful and unlikely to have happened simply by chance – had slipped. Suddenly, the biggest and most shocking data in the study – that hormone users had a 24% increase in heart risk – no longer met the threshold for statistical significance'[5]. *Ob Gyn News* reported, 'The definitive study on the risks and benefits of hormone therapy may not be so definitive after all'[6].

The critical period hypothesis: 'What if older women and younger women react differently to hormones? What if the timing of hormone therapy – whether it's given just at the time the body stops producing estrogen or whether it's started years later – makes a difference?' has been succinctly stated[5]. However, it has been pointed out that, 'With so few women in the 50–54-year-old age group, could the study (WHI) provide any meaningful conclusions about younger women, the age group most likely to be taking hormone for menopausal symptoms in the first place?'[5]. Per protocol, only 10% of randomized women were to be in the 50–54-year age range[2]. There is good reason, based on data from non-human primates, to conclude that the timing of intervention is critical on the effect of estrogen on atherogenesis and needs to be initiated close to the time of menopause or the effect may be lost[7–10]. Hazard ratios for CHD based on years since menopause reported from the estrogen plus progestin arm of WHI are consistent with this finding. Manson and colleagues report hazard ratios of 0.89, 1.22 and 1.71 for women less than 10, 10–19, and equal to or greater than 20 years since menopause, respectively[4]. The failure to demonstrate a significant interaction may reflect the small number of participants within a few years of menopause. The data clearly show a trend suggesting the fewer years since menopause, the lower the hazard ratio for CHD.

## BREAST CANCER

Among the secondary outcomes, breast cancer was designated as a primary adverse outcome. Hazard ratios for invasive breast cancer are reported with nominal 95% CIs. Adjusted CIs were not reported in the updated analysis, based on centrally adjudicated breast cancers and a mean follow-up of 5.6 years. The hazard ratios and nominal 95% CIs for total, invasive, and *in situ* breast cancer are 1.24 (1.02–1.50), 1.24 (1.01–1.54), and 1.10 (0.77–1.82), respectively. *In situ* breast cancer was not significantly increased, while the Kaplan–Meier plot for invasive breast cancer suggests a separation in the curves for estrogen plus progestin and for placebo between years 3 and 4[11]. Among women with and without prior menopausal hormone use, more than 97% in the estrogen plus progestin and the placebo groups did not develop invasive breast cancer. When invasive breast cancer outcomes were reported by prior menopausal hormone use and by year from study entry, the hazard ratios and lower limit of the nominal 95% CIs exceeded unity only in year 5 and then only in the subgroup with prior menopausal hormone use, not in the subgroup without prior menopausal hormone use. Based on the initial publication of WHI results, it would be anticipated that adjusted 95% CIs for invasive breast cancer analyses would have lower limits less than one.

## WHI GLOBAL INDEX

'When the global index was defined, it really was for the purpose of monitoring the trial (WHI) . . .'[12]. When the principal results of the WHI estrogen plus progestin arm were published, they noted that 'Procedures for monitoring the trial involved semi-annual comparisons of the estrogen plus progestin and placebo groups with respect to each of the elements of the global index and to the overall global index'[1]. The global index was never a primary or secondary outcome of the clinical trial.

The components of the global index, with the exception of invasive breast cancer, accounted for the seven major outcomes specifically monitored which made up the Bonferroni correction[1]. However, the number of major outcomes specifically monitored, that is, the components of the global index, changed during the course of the trial. For example, in 1997, the index included CHD, hip fracture, other fracture, breast cancer, ductal carcinoma *in situ*, stroke, deep vein thrombosis, pulmonary embolism, endometrial cancer, and death due to other causes; vertebral fractures were separated from other fractures. In 1998, ductal carcinoma *in situ*, deep venous thrombosis, and vertebral and other fractures were removed from the specifically monitored outcomes. Ultimately, the global index was changed to include CHD, stroke, colorectal cancer, endometrial cancer, pulmonary embolism, hip fracture, death due to other causes, and invasive breast cancer. Additionally, in 1996, a weighted global index was proposed and, in 1998, an unweighted version with a time-to-first-event analysis[3]. Hence, changing the global index of specifically monitored outcomes not only affected the Data Safety and Monitoring Board and their analyses, but also affected the magnitude of the statistical adjustment made to the overall study analysis.

## SUBGROUP ANALYSES

The testing of increasing numbers of questions increases the chance of obtaining incorrect or false-positive results (type I error) unless appropriate statistical corrections are made[13]. For example, performing 20 independent comparisons, each at the 0.05 level of significance, has a 64% chance of producing at least one false-positive result. There are a number of approaches for dealing with this. The first approach would be not to perform subgroup or post hoc analyses. This has obvious limitations. The second approach would be to adjust the level of significance for each of the subgroups, for example using a Bonferroni approach. However, since different outcomes add to the multiplicity in the same manner as additional subgroups and the variation in the patient population is considerable, the number of comparisons will be large and the required $p$ value nearly impossible to reach[13]. In the Heart and Estrogen/progestin Replacement Study (HERS) trial, 172 subgroup analyses were performed to evaluate treatment effect in 86 subgroups after 1 year and the entire follow-up. The adjusted significance level after a Bonferroni correction for the 172 comparisons would be about 0.0003[14]. The third approach would be simply to use the subgroup analyses for hypothesis generating and not consider them to be definitive, but rather to be tested in additional studies.

In the estrogen plus progestin arm of WHI, there were a very large number of comparisons or analyses performed. Aside from CHD, there were 18 outcomes listed in the protocol[2]. Additionally, for most of those outcomes, multiple additional analyses were performed. For example, in the publication of the final CHD results, reference is made to at least 36 subgroups for that endpoint; the paper states 'The results should be interpreted with caution, since some significant findings (at least one or two, based on a 0.05 nominal level of statistical significance) could have occurred by chance alone'[4].

There is little question that many more comparisons were made in WHI than in HERS.

For similar reasons, Browner and Hulley stated, 'It is essential to regard all apparent interactions sceptically and proposed 'Criteria for evaluating the possibility of an interaction in subgroups in a clinical trial'. They are:

(1) Do observational results conform to the expected results based on previous studies?

(2) Is the difference in relative benefit between subgroups substantial?

(3) Is the interaction biologically plausible?

(4) Is the interaction seen consistently in other studies?[15]

## CONCLUSIONS

The WHI estrogen plus progestin study arm represents an important contribution to the total body of data on hormone therapy accumulated over many decades. However, it is important to fully understand how the study was designed and conducted in order to fully appreciate the implications of the data. Appropriate consideration of the manner in which the primary and secondary outcomes, the WHI global index, as well as the many subgroups, were analyzed is important to this understanding.

Some years ago, Lee and colleagues wrote, 'In assessing therapeutic claims, the doctor must consider the adequacy of the experimental design and conduct of the study, the adequacy of the analyses and presentation of results, the strength of the conclusion and how the findings relate to his clinical experience and to clinical knowledge'[16]. Continued discussion among members of the scientific community regarding the WHI estrogen plus progestin arm is necessary to fully understand the study results and their implications.

# References

1. Writing Group for the Women's Health Initiative Investigators. Risks and benefits of estrogen plus progestin in healthy postmenopausal women: Principal results from the Women's Health Initiative randomized controlled trial. *J Am Med Assoc* 2002;288:321–33
2. WHI Manuals: Volume 1 – Study protocol and policies. September 1, 1994
3. Freedman L, Anderson G, Kipnis V, *et al.* Guidelines for the statistical monitoring of the Women's Health Initiative clinical trial. April 1, 1998
4. Manson JE, Hsia J, Johnson KC, *et al.* Estrogen plus progestin and the risk of coronary heart disease. *N Engl J Med* 2003;34:523–34
5. Parker-Pope T. The case for hormone therapy: Menopause hormones have been battered by recent studies highlighting their potential dangers. Here's why women might still want to take them. *The Wall Street Journal* October 21, 2003
6. Sullivan MG. Doctors rethink impact of WHI on clinical practices: Research suggests that timing

may be key to treatment success, fewer adverse events. *ObGyn News* 2003;38(20)

7. Clarkson TB, Anthony MS, Jerome CP. Lack of effect of raloxifene on coronary artery atherosclerosis of postmenopausal monkeys. *J Clin Endocrinol Metab* 1998;83:721-6
8. Adams MR, Register TC, Golden DL, Wagner JD, Williams JK. Medroxyprogesterone acetate antagonizes inhibitory effects of conjugated equine estrogens on coronary artery atherosclerosis. *Arterioscler Thromb Vasc Biol* 1997;17:217-21
9. Clarkson TB, Anthony MS, Morgan TM. Inhibition of postmenopausal atherosclerosis progression: a comparison of the effects of conjugated equine estrogens and soy phytoestrogens. *J Clin Endocrinol Metab* 2001;86:41-7
10. Williams JK, Anthony MS, Honore EK, *et al.* Regression of atherosclerosis in female monkeys. *Arterioscler Thromb Vasc Biol* 1995;15:827-36
11. Chlebowski RT, Hendrix SL, Langer RD, *et al.* Influence of estrogen plus progestin on breast cancer and mammography in healthy postmenopausal women: The Women's Health Initiative randomized trial. *J Am Med Assoc* 2003;289: 3243-53
12. Garnet Anderson. FDA Endocrinologic and Metabolic Drugs Advisory Committee Meeting, October 7, 2003
13. Friedman LM, Furberg CD, CeMets DL. *Fundamentals of Clinical Trials.* New York: Springer, 1998
14. Furberg CD, Vittinghoff E, Davidson M, *et al.* Subgroup interactions in the Heart and Estrogen/progestin Replacement Study: Lessons learned. *Circulation* 2002;105:917-22
15. Browner WS, Hulley SB. Effect of risk status on treatment criteria: implications of hypertension trials. *Hypertension* 1989;13(Suppl I): I-51-6
16. Lee KL, McNeer F, Starmer F, Harris PJ, Rosati RA. Clinical judgment and statistics: lessons from a simulated randomized trial in coronary artery disease. *Circulation* 1980;61:508-15

# Impact on current clinical practice in Spain 11

*S. Palacios*

## INTRODUCTION

After the interruption of the estrogen-progestin arm of the Women's Health Initiative (WHI) and the subsequent subanalysis of that study[1-6], some changes have been generated in relation to the clinical practice of hormone therapy (HT)[7].

The Spanish Menopause Society has created a study group to analyze what is now happening in the climacteric period of Spanish women, with the objective of improving information and performance in three areas of climacteric management (physicians, patients and mass media)[8,9]. All these play an important role in creating a strategy for improving the quality of life in the climacterium.

The first step of the project, named PRISMA (Programme for the Integral Revision of the Menopause Situation), consists of analyzing the three different areas, and then elaborating the most convenient strategies. In this paper, I shall analyze one of these areas, that of the physicians, and establish their current clinical practice for managing the climacteric.

## MATERIAL AND METHODS

This is a survey with statistical significance from the universal sample of Spanish gynecologists. With the idea of a quantitative survey, a phone call interview was used, with a semi-structured questionnaire. The statistical system used for recording and data processing was SPSS-Win 8.5.

A preliminary selection was made of 1650 physicians. A representative sample was chosen, taking into account the number of gynecologists per province. The field work required that a final sample of 500 should be obtained, as shown in Table 1. The error was 1.47% (95% confidence interval). Participation in this study required that gynecologists accept and attend menopausal women in their daily practice (Table 1).

## RESULTS

The doctors had an average age of 47 years, the majority being men (60%), and all had extensive professional experience, 46% of more than 20 years and 34% between 10 and 20 years; the majority worked in the national health service (70%).

Women in the climacteric period comprised a large proportion of the total number of clinic appointments for each doctor, with an average of 32%. The reasons for these appointments were, first, the women were concerned about their health and decided themselves to visit the doctor (58%), and, second, the women were sent by their primary-care physicians (35%).

Their reason for consultation was a gynecological check-up (65%), with only 35% giving symptoms as the reason. The most frequent symptoms were hot flushes, followed by genital and urinary disorders. In Table 2, the principal reasons why the physicians prescibed treatment are shown.

The three most important factors for prescribing HT were women's opinion, sociocultural factors and sexual activity. In relation to the question as to the choice of bleeding profile, the physicians answered that patients preferred no bleeding (65.6%), followed by regular bleeding (34.4%). The percentages of women who received some form of treatment after their consultation were 54% in the symptomatic group and 21% in the asymptomatic group. The types of treatment preferred by the Spanish gynecologists are shown in Table 3.

**Table 1** Field work

| | |
|---|---|
| Total number of interviews given | 500 |
| Confidence interval | 95.5% |
| Margin of error | 4.5% |
| Margin of variability | $p = q = 50$ |
| Total number of professionals contacted | 1270 |

**Table 2** Prescription profile: principal reasons for prescribing hormone therapy

| *Reason* | *1st place* (%) | *2nd place* (%) | *3rd place* (%) |
|---|---|---|---|
| Relief of climacteric symptoms | 41 | 32 | 9 |
| Prevention of osteoporosis | 23 | 30 | 19 |
| Alleviation of irregular bleeding | 25 | 14 | 16 |
| Reduction of genital/urine symptoms | 3 | 11 | 20 |
| Cardiovascular prevention | 3 | 4 | 18 |

When the physicians prescribe HT, they prefer the continuous regimen (53%) and sequential regimen (44%); the preferred delivery routes are transdermal (45%), oral (39%), vaginal (7%), and percutaneous (7%). The type of estrogen preferred is 17β-estradiol by 53%, estradiol valerate by 31%, and conjugated equine estrogens by 12%. The preferred type of progestin is progesterone by 50%, and medroxyprogesterone acetate by 20%. The recommended length of HT is 5 years in the majority of cases (57.4%) (Figure 1). The principal reasons for physicians withdrawing treatment were bleeding irregularities, side-effects, and women quitting treatment. The main reasons given by women for quitting were fear of cancer (42%), negative media information (23%), and bleeding irregularities (19%).

**Table 3** Prescription profile: type of treatment

| *Treatment* | *Women with symptoms* (%) | *Women without symptoms* (%) |
|---|---|---|
| Estrogen + progestin | 39 | 28 |
| Estrogen only | 17 | 16 |
| Phytoestrogens | 15 | 22 |
| Tibolone | 14 | 21 |
| Raloxifene | 16 | 14 |

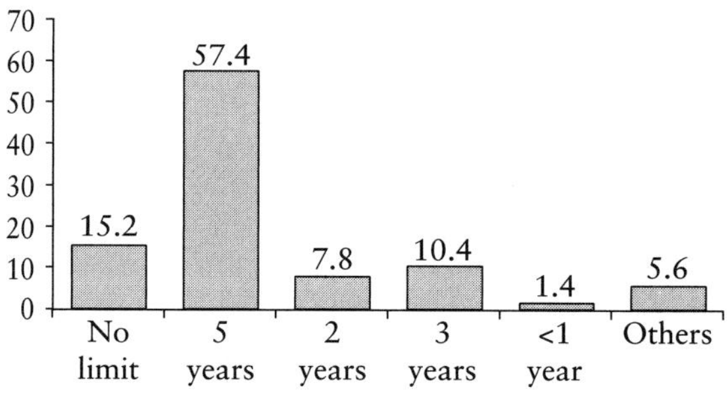


**Figure 1** Prescription profile: period of hormone therapy recommended by physicians

## DISCUSSION

After the WHI study, there have been some changes in physicians' clinical decisions and in women's perception of HT; as a result, current clinical practice for the menopausal woman is changing. However, the usual type of woman in Spain using HT, the type of estrogen–progestin used and the delivery route used by Spanish physicians are quite different from those used in the WHI study. The HT indications in Spain, which are the same as those before the WHI, are for the relief of climacteric symptoms (hot flushes and genito-urinary atrophy) and osteoporosis prevention. But now, after the WHI study, the most important reason which influences HT prescription is the preconceived idea that women have of HT. Only half of the women (54%) suffering from climacteric symptoms are prescribed HT. This fact gives an idea of the low prescribing rate now seen in patients with climacteric symptoms, which is undoubtedly produced by the results of the WHI study.

The most common type of estrogen recommended in Spain is 17β-estradiol, followed by estradiol valerate. The most recommended delivery route is the transdermal route, which is more popular than the oral route. The most recommended progestin is progesterone (50%). Clearly, the type of estrogen–progestin used and the route are completely different to those used in the WHI study.

There are clear differences in the reasons for recommending or abandoning treatment. For physicians, they are bleeding disorders and side-effects, and for patients it is the fear of breast cancer and the negative information received through the mass media.

Finally, we can conclude that there are clear changes in Spain in the use of HT after the WHI study. Nevertheless, current clinical practice and recommendations for our gynecologists are the same as before the WHI. We would like to emphasize that we can not extrapolate the results of the WHI study in the normal population that use HT in Spain, since treatment is for symptomatic patients and the type of estrogen-progestin and route are completely different.

## References


1. Writing Group for the Women's Health Initiative Investigators. Risk and benefits of estrogen plus progestin in healthy postmenopausal women. Principal results from the Women's Health Initiative randomized controlled trial. *J Am Med Assoc* 2002;288:321–33
2. Shumaker SA, Legault C, Rapp SR, *et al.* for the WHIMS Investigators. Estrogen plus progestin and the incidence of dementia and mild cognitive impairment in postmenopausal women: the Women's Health Initiative Memory Study: a randomized controlled trial. *J Am Med Assoc* 2003;289:2651–62
3. Rapp SR, Espeland MA, Shumaker SA, *et al.* Effect of estrogen plus progestin on global cognitive function in postmenopausal women: the Women's Health Initiative Memory Study: a randomized controlled trial. *J Am Med Assoc* 2003; 289:2663–72
4. Chlebowski RT, Hendrix SL, Langer RD, *et al.* Influence of estrogen plus progestin on breast cancer and mammography in healthy postmenopausal women: the Women's Health Initiative Randomized Trial. *J Am Med Assoc* 2003;289:3243–53
5. Cauley JA, Robbins J, Chen Z, *et al.* Effects of estrogen plus progestin on risk of fracture and bone mineral density: the Women's Health Initiative randomized trial. *J Am Med Assoc* 2003;290: 1729–38
6. Anderson GL, Judd HL, Kaunitz AM, *et al.* Effects of estrogen plus progestin on gynecologic cancers and associated diagnostic procedures: the Women's Health Initiative randomized trial. *J Am Med Assoc* 2003;290:1739–48
7. Hersh AL, Stefanick ML, Stafford RS. National use of postmenopausal hormone therapy: annual trends and response to recent evidence. *J Am Med Assoc* 2004;291:47–53
8. Palacios S, Calaf J, Cano A, Parrilla JJ, for the Spanish Menopause Society (AEEM). Relevant results of the WHI study for the management of the menopause in Spain. *Maturitas* 2003;44:83–6
9. Palacios S, Quereda F, Cancelo MJ. Hormone therapy: a survey of Spanish physicians' change in prescribing practices after the WHI study. *Menopause* 2003;10:593

# A clinician's response to the WHI 12

*L. Speroff*

## INTRODUCTION

Clinicians are unique in bringing a special personal relationship with patients to the process of utilizing their store of knowledge. The process requires individualization, the application of knowledge in a modified form based upon the clinician's experience and the clinician's familiarity and understanding of the individual patient. Decision-making in this clinician–patient interaction is called 'medical judgment'. Medical judgment is always based upon a foundation of knowledge, the accumulated information and understanding acquired through experience, education, and appraisal of the literature. It is never static, but medical judgment is constantly evolving and changing in the effort to be clinically appropriate. The final impact on a patient is never the result of single, solitary fact or one scientific study. The entire process is the art *and* science of medicine. It is the fundamental reason that clinicians enjoy being clinicians and why clinicians are so valued by patients.

The challenge for clinicians is to make medical judgments that are suitable and correct for individual patients. The publicity generated by the Women's Health Initiative (WHI) publications has made decision-making regarding postmenopausal hormone therapy more difficult than ever. This situation was enhanced by the absence of a critical response from academicians and medical organizations. Indeed, the immediate commentaries included adjectives such as 'definitive', 'unequivocal', and 'solid'. But, in my view, there are problems and unanswered questions with the epidemiological data that should influence contemporary clinical decisions. Decision-making in the wake of the WHI has been most influenced by two medical conditions, cardiovascular disease and breast cancer.

## CARDIOVASCULAR DISEASE

The published results of the WHI trial agree with more than 20 years of case-control and cohort data, with the exception of the cardiovascular data. The critical clinical question is the following: are the small increases in cardiovascular events reported by the WHI real or are there other explanations for the reported results? This is a very important question because the reported increases were not large, and a shift in a small number of cases can change the conclusions.

It is relevant to note that, in the Heart and Estrogen/progestin Replacement Study (HERS), statins and aspirin protected against venous thromboembolism, and, most importantly, the reported increase in arterial events in the first year of the trial was no longer significant when adjusted for statin and aspirin treatment[1]. A higher prevalence of new statin and aspirin treatment in the placebo arm of the WHI could have produced lower event rates, giving the false impression of higher rates in the treatment arm; this is an important analysis yet to be provided. In my view, the HERS did not have the statistical power to provide this important analysis – the impact of new statin and aspirin treatment per year of the trial – because of the high drop-out rate.

Consider also the possibility of diagnostic bias. Of the treated group in the WHI, 40.5% (nearly 5000 of the 8500 in the treated group), in contrast to 6.8% of the placebo group, was unblinded because of vaginal bleeding. What was the impact on the clinicians' final management and diagnosis when told the patient is in the WHI study and experiencing vaginal bleeding? This problem affects the data not only in regards to cardiovascular disease, but also to breast cancer.

The initial published results from the canceled arm of the WHI trial depended upon cardiovascular diagnoses made 'in the field'. Central adjudication of the cardiac diagnoses revealed disagreement with 10% of the diagnoses for myocardial infarction and 3% for death due to coronary heart disease[2]. This small disagreement resulted in a shift of a critical number of cases, and the final overall hazard ratio for coronary heart disease was no longer statistically significant. In the subgroup analyses, only the women who were 20 or more years distant from menopause had a statistically significant increased risk of coronary heart disease (1.71; confidence interval (CI) 1.20–2.50). Subtracting this group from the rest of the participants, coronary heart disease now was observed in an identical prevalence comparing the treated and placebo groups. It is inappropriate to conclude that hormone therapy increases the risk of coronary clinical events in all postmenopausal women; this conclusion can only be applied to a specific older group of women.

Will postmenopausal hormone therapy begun at or near the time of the menopause, and maintained for a relatively long duration of time, provide protection against coronary artery disease (primary prevention)? The design of the canceled arm of the WHI did not allow an answer to this question. Women with significant menopausal symptoms were excluded from the study to avoid an exceedingly high drop-out rate in the placebo group. The WHI investigators address this problem by pointing out that the ratios of cardiovascular events in the treated and placebo arms were the same when assessed by decades of age, fifties, sixties, seventies. However, this is not the critical analysis. By excluding women with menopausal symptoms, it is very likely that a small number of the participants were close to their age of menopause (only 250 in the treated group were aged 50–59 years, and it is likely that even these women were relatively distant from their menopause). Until the results are analyzed according to years from menopause, perhaps forthcoming, the cardiovascular results in the WHI cannot be viewed as the product of a primary prevention trial. Even with the appropriate analysis according to years from menopause, the results are likely to be limited by very small numbers of women in their early postmenopausal years.

The WHI concluded (and many individuals and organizations did as well) that hormone therapy is not a viable intervention for primary prevention. I am comfortable in accepting the conclusion that postmenopausal hormone therapy does not reduce or slow the progression of established coronary heart disease. However, the WHI did not study the appropriate population in the appropriate time period to establish that hormone therapy does not exert a primary preventive effect on the risk of coronary heart disease.

## BREAST CANCER

For nearly a decade, we have been teaching that the lack of a uniform, consistent conclusion in more than 60 case-control and cohort studies on breast cancer and postmenopausal hormone therapy means that any effect has to be a small one. The WHI results do not change that teaching. The most important unanswered question is whether postmenopausal hormone therapy initiates the growth of new breast cancers or whether the epidemiological results reflect an impact on pre-existing tumors. Observations that favor an impact on pre-existing tumors include:

(1) The return of the hazard risk in the WHI study almost to 1.0 in year 6;

(2) No difference in non-invasive breast cancers in the treatment and placebo arms;

(3) The large body of literature documenting lower grade and stage disease in hormone users, resulting in better survival rates.

The WHI did agree with convincing evidence that postmenopausal hormone therapy does not increase the risk of breast cancer beyond that already associated with recognized risk factors, such as a positive family history.

The updated report on breast cancer after adjudication of the WHI diagnoses resulted in little change in the hazard ratios[3]. The WHI detected no differences in the histological types of breast cancer, disagreeing with case-control studies that estrogen-progestin therapy is associated with mainly an increase in invasive lobular tumors[4,5]. How does this correlate with national statistics that indicate a rise in lobular tumors and an unchanging incidence of ductal cancers[6]?

Abnormal mammograms were reported at a greater rate in the treated group compared with the placebo group. The mammography findings are very important, suggesting that the greater rate of abnormal mammograms in women treated with estrogen-progestin represents an unwanted and expensive effect of hormone therapy. As noted above, nearly 5000 of the 8506 women in the treated group were unblinded because of vaginal bleeding. Is it possible that this unblinding introduced diagnostic bias into the mammography findings? The WHI believes this is unlikely because mammography findings were managed by the participants' local clinicians, separately from the WHI study reports. However, the most important individual unblinded was the patient. What influence is there on that management when the patient reports to her clinician that she is experiencing vaginal bleeding? Surely the clinician, knowing the patient is a WHI participant, would conclude that she is receiving hormonal treatment.

The updated WHI results on breast cancer indicate an earlier appearance of worse tumors than previously reported in case-control and cohort studies[3]. The authors point out in their discussion that the results (both the invasive breast cancers and the mammography findings) are consistent with stimulation of growth in established breast cancers, but at the same time a delay in diagnosis. This certainly challenges the idea that hormone users have better outcomes because of earlier detection. The authors suggest that this disagreement could be because of a difference of mammography use in the observational studies. However, even in studies that examine tumor characteristics and outcome in users and non-users who have equally used mammography, lower grade and stage disease with a better outcome is identified in the users[7-9]. In addition, a prospective cohort study found little impact of hormone use on mammography specificity[10].

Does hormone therapy impair mammographic screening? The literature is mixed on this question. A review of seven studies concluded that six of the seven studies indicated decreased mammographic sensitivity in hormone users, with a slight increase in false-positive recalls[11]. A French study found a lower incidence of interval cancers in non-users, but a prospective American study concluded that recall rates were essentially the same comparing hormone users and non-users, and that hormone therapy rarely causes a diagnostic dilemma[12,13]. However, overall, studies have suggested a decrease in mammographic sensitivity with little impact on specificity (false recall rates). The studies are based on small numbers of interval cancers, and it is uncertain how real or how large this effect is because of the difficulty in controlling for confounding factors (for example, age, age at menopause, and time since menopause). If the effectiveness of breast cancer screening is reduced by postmenopausal hormone therapy, one would expect an adverse impact on breast cancer mortality. Instead, a study that indicated a reduction in mammographic sensitivity also reported smaller, more differentiated (grade I) tumors among the users compared with the non-users[14], and most of the studies that have examined the breast cancer mortality rates of women who had used postmenopausal hormone therapy have documented improved survival rates[7,8,15-23]. Evidence indicates that hormone users develop smaller, better differentiated (lower grade) tumors, evidence that is consistent with effects on pre-existing tumors, and that surveillance/detection bias is not the only explanation for better survival[24-29]. Lower-grade tumors are present even when there is no difference in the prevalence of mammography comparing hormone users and non-users, or when the data are adjusted for the method of detection[7,8,29].

An analysis of the breast cancers in our own institution revealed that more tumors in hormone users were detected by screening mammography, but, when assessing outcomes in all cancers detected by mammography, hormone users had more ductal *in situ* tumors, more node-negative cancers, smaller tumors, and less invasive disease; thus survival rates were better[9].

Women with a greater mammographic breast density have a higher risk of breast cancer, and about 25% of women on estrogen-progestin therapy have an increase in their breast density. However, it is not certain that the short-term increase in density with hormone therapy changes an individual's risk of breast cancer. The increase in breast density associated with postmenopausal hormone therapy appears to be a transient, reversible change, a change not consistent with a persistent effect on cellular proliferation. After discontinuing hormone therapy, breast density rapidly decreases[30-32]. In a retrospective analysis, regression of hormone-induced abnormalities was found to occur within 2 weeks of cessation of treatment[32]. In the 12 patients who exhibited no change after discontinuing therapy, eight were biopsied after ultrasonography, revealing one cancer and one case of atypical hyperplasia. Larger and better studies of this approach are needed, but it suggests the following clinical recommendation. The older a postmenopausal patient is, the greater the risk of developing an increase in breast density with hormone therapy. Therefore, there is a good reason to recommend the discontinuation of hormone therapy for 2 weeks prior to mammography in women older than age 65 years who have dense breasts. In younger women who are recalled for a suspicious or difficult-to-read mammogram, it would be worthwhile to discontinue hormone treatment for 2 weeks prior to the repeat evaluation.

There may be a small increase in breast cancers with estrogen–progestin therapy or this treatment stimulates pre-existing tumors to grow. There is a large body of literature indicating that tumors in hormone users are better differentiated, of lower grade and stage disease, with better outcomes. The contrary finding in the WHI may reflect the older age of its participants. This older population is more likely to have pre-existing occult tumors that would become detectable quickly after hormonal stimulation. In addition, breast tissue in older postmenopausal women may respond differently to hormone stimulation than breast tissue in women close to their menopause.

## MEDICAL JUDGMENTS

The following clinical judgments are my own, based upon the large body of epidemiological and biological research accumulated over the last 20 years, and directed toward making informed decisions to translate the accumulated knowledge into effective and appropriate clinical practice.

(1) The results of secondary prevention trials and the WHI provide a reasonably solid basis not to recommend postmenopausal hormone therapy for women with existing atherosclerosis, in the anticipation of preventing future cardiovascular events.

(2) Results from multiple studies indicate that postmenopausal hormone therapy increases the risk of venous thromboembolism, mostly in the first year or two of treatment. This is a risk that is reduced with the use of statins and aspirin, although it is not known whether statin and aspirin use would completely protect against the increased risk associated with hormone therapy. Appropriate prophylactic anticoagulant treatment is recommended when hormone users are anticipating immobility with hospitalization, and hormone therapy should be discontinued 4 weeks prior to major surgery.

(3) Postmenopausal hormone therapy is either associated with a small increase in the risk of breast cancer or it affects pre-existing tumors. Of course, even a small increase in risk for breast cancer is frightening for patients to contemplate. I find it helpful to remind patients of the risk of lung cancer associated with smoking (a relative risk of 10–20), a risk magnitude that provides perspective on the possible risk associated with hormone therapy. It is also worth pointing out that the reported risk with hormone therapy is even smaller than that associated with recognized risk factors such as a positive family history, being overweight after menopause, and alcohol intake. Finally, clinicians should emphasize that the evidence uniformly indicates that a positive family history of breast cancer is not a contraindication for hormone therapy.

(4) Long-term postmenopausal hormone therapy is not precluded by the results reported by the WHI. There continues to be good reason to believe that there are benefits associated with treatment, including improvement of quality of life beyond the relief of hot flushes, maximal protection against osteoporotic fractures, a reduction in colorectal cancers,

maintenance of skin turgor and elasticity, and the possibility of primary prevention of coronary heart disease and Alzheimer's disease. Of course, this should not detract or subtract from efforts to apply proven therapies (such as statins) and to support beneficial lifestyle modifications.

(5) I believe a theme has emerged from the epidemiological confusion of the last few years: it takes healthy tissue to allow effective response to estrogen and maintenance of health. Experimental evidence in monkeys and women indicates that, as endothelial cells become involved with atherosclerosis and neurons become affected with the pathological process of Alzhemier's disease, beneficial responses to estrogen diminish[33-35]. Maximal benefit, therefore, may require early onset of treatment, near the time of menopause.

(6) The most effective and appropriate method to help in decision-making is to identify the specific goals and objective of the individual patient. Once identified, choices from multiple treatment options can be reviewed. This is at least an annual decision, incorporating new knowledge as it appears. Approached in this fashion, the terms 'short-term' and 'long-term' and the imposition of time limits for therapy become meaningless. Clinician and patient together make a clinical judgment that is appropriately directed to accomplishing the individual patient's goals.

## CONCLUSION

The most disturbing development since the initial publication of the WHI results is the emotional and political polarization of postmenopausal hormone therapy. On the one side are those who believe hormone therapy is harmful, and that harm is a consequence of physicians with vested interests and the pharmaceutical industry. On the other side are clinicians and patients who continue to believe that hormone therapy has important benefits. The challenge is for clinicians, academicians, the scientists in the field, and our organizations to find the middle ground. In my view, we should focus on how and why the studies disagree. For example, clinicians want to know *why* the WHI breast cancer results disagree in regards to stage of disease with a large number of reports in the medical literature. I believe that the discovery and understanding of the differences will allow us to find the middle ground and establish the appropriate place for postmenopausal hormone therapy.

# References


1. Herrington DM, Vittinghoff E, Lin F, *et al.* Statin therapy, cardiovascular events, and total mortality in the Heart and Estrogen/Progestin Replacement Study (HERS). *Circulation* 2002;105:2962–7
2. Manson JE, Hsia J, Johnson KC, *et al.* Estrogen plus progestin and the risk of coronary heart disease. *N Engl J Med* 2003;349:523–34
3. Chlebowski RT, Hendrix SL, Langer RD, *et al.* Influence of estrogen plus progestin on breast cancer and mammography in healthy postmenopausal women. The Women's Health Initiative Randomized Trial. *J Am Med Assoc* 2003; 289:3243–53
4. Li CI, Weiss NS, Stanford JL, Daling JR. Hormone replacement therapy in relation to risk of lobular and ductal breast carcinoma in middle-aged women. *Cancer* 2000;88:2570–7
5. Li CI, Malone KE, Porter PL, *et al.* Relationship between long durations and different regimens of hormone therapy and risk of breast cancer. *J Am Med Assoc* 2003;289:3254–63
6. Li CI, Anderson BO, Daling JR, Moe RE. Trends in incidence rates of invasive lobular and ductal breast carcinoma. *J Am Med Assoc* 2003;289:1421–4
7. Schairer C, Gail M, Byrne C, *et al.* Estrogen replacement therapy and breast cancer survival in a large screening study. *J Natl Cancer Inst* 1999;91:264–70
8. Jernström H, Frenander J, Fernö M, Olsson H. Hormone replacement therapy before breast cancer diagnosis significantly reduces the overall death

rate compared with never-use among 984 breast cancer patients. *Br J Cancer* 1999;80:1453-8
9. Cheek J, Lacy J, Toth-Fejel S, Morris K, Calhoun K, Pommier RF. The impact of hormone replacement therapy on the detection and stage of breast cancer. *Arch Surg* 2002;137:1015-19
10. Carney PA, Miglioretti DL, Yankaskas BC, *et al.* Individual and combined effects of age, breast density, and hormone replacement therapy use on the accuracy of screening mammography. *Ann Intern Med* 2003;138:168-75
11. Banks E. Hormone replacement therapy and the sensitivity and specificity of breast cancer screening: a review. *J Med Screen* 2001;8:29-35
12. Séradour B, Estève J, Heid P, Jacquemier J. Hormone replacement therapy and screening mammography: analysis of the results in the Bouches du Rhône programme. *J Med Screen* 1999;6:99-102
13. Moy L, Slanetz PJ, Yeh ED, Moore RH, Rafferty EA, Kopans DB. Hormone replacement therapy rarely complicates or alters interpretation on screening mammography: a prospective analysis. *Radiology* 2000;217:446 (Abstr)
14. Sendag F, Terek MC, Özsener S, *et al.* Mammographic density changes during different postmenopausal hormone replacement therapies. *Fertil Steril* 2001;76:445-50
15. Bergkvist L, Adami H-O, Persson I, Bergstrom R, Krusemo UB. Prognosis after breast cancer diagnosis in women exposed to estrogen and estrogen-progestogen replacement therapy. *Am J Epidemiol* 1989;130:221-7
16. Hunt K, Vessey M, McPherson K. Mortality in a cohort of long-term users of hormone replacement therapy: an updated analysis. *Br J Obstet Gynaecol* 1990;97:1080
17. Henderson BE, Paganini-Hill A, Ross RK. Decreased mortality in users of estrogen replacement therapy. *Arch Intern Med* 1991;151:75-8
18. Persson I, Yuen J, Bergkvist L, Schairer C. Cancer incidence and mortality in women receiving estrogen and estrogen-progestin replacement therapy - long-term follow-up of a Swedish cohort. *Int J Cancer* 1996;67:327-32
19. Willis DB, Calle EE, Miracle-McMahill HL, Heath Jr CW. Estrogen replacement therapy and risk of fatal breast cancer in a prospective cohort of postmenopausal women in the United States. *Cancer Causes Control* 1996;7:449-57
20. Grodstein F, Stampfer MJ, Colditz GA, *et al.* Postmenopausal hormone therapy and mortality. *N Engl J Med* 1997;336:1769-75
21. Sellers TA, Mink PJ, Cerhan JR, *et al.* The role of hormone replacement therapy in the risk for breast cancer and total mortality in women with a family history of breast cancer. *Ann Intern Med* 1997; 127:973-80
22. Fowble B, Hanlon A, Greedman G, *et al.* Postmenopausal hormone replacement therapy: effect on diagnosis and outcome in early-stage invasive breast cancer treated with conservative surgery and radiation. *J Clin Oncol* 1999;17:1680-8
23. Nanda K, Bastian LA, Schulz K. Hormone replacement therapy and the risk of death from breast cancer: a systematic review. *Am J Obstet Gynecol* 2002;186:325-34
24. Bonnier P, Romain S, Giacalone PL, Laffargue F, Martin PM, Piana L. Clinical and biologic prognostic factors in breast cancer diagnosed during postmenopausal hormone replacement therapy. *Obstet Gynecol* 1995;85:11
25. Magnusson C, Holmberg L, Norden T, Lindgren A, Persson I. Prognostic characteristics in breast cancers after hormone replacement therapy. *Breast Cancer Res Treat* 1996;38:325-34
26. Holli K, Isola J, Cuzick J. Low biologic aggressiveness in breast cancer in women using hormone replacement therapy. *J Clin Oncol* 1998;16:3115-20
27. O'Connor IF, Shembekar MV, Shousha S. Breast carcinoma developing in patients on hormone replacement therapy: a histological and immunohistological study. *J Clin Pathol* 1998;51:935-8
28. Salmon RJ, Ansquer Y, Asselain B, Languille O, Lesec G, Remvikos Y. Clinical and biological characteristics of breast cancers in post-menopausal women receiving hormone replacement therapy for menopause. *Oncol Rep* 1999;6:699-703
29. Bilimoria MM, Winchester DJ, Sener SF, Motykie G, Sehgal UL, Winchester DP. Estrogen replacement therapy and breast cancer: analysis of age of onset and tumor characteristics. *Ann Surg Oncol* 1999;6:200-7
30. Rutter CM, Mandelson MT, Laya MB, Seger DJ, Taplin S. Changes in breast density associated with initiation, discontinuation, and continuing use of hormone replacement therapy. *J Am Med Assoc* 2001;285:171-6
31. Berkowitz JE, Gatewood OMB, Goldblum LE, Gayler BW. Hormonal replacement therapy: mammographic manifestations. *Radiology* 1990; 174:199-201
32. Harvey JA, Pinkerton JV, Herman CR. Short-term cessation of hormone replacement therapy and improvement of mammographic specificity. *J Natl Cancer Inst* 1997;89:1623-5
33. Herrington DM, Espeland MA, Crouse JR 3rd, *et al.* Estrogen replacement and brachial artery flow-mediated vasodilatation in older women. *Arterioscl Thromb Vasc Biol* 2001;21:1955-61
34. Mikkola TS, Clarkson TB. Estrogen replacement therapy: atherosclerosis, and vascular function. *Cardiovasc Res* 2002;53:605-19
35. Zandi PP, Carlson MC, Plassman BL, *et al.* Hormone replacement therapy and incidence of Alzheimer disease in older women. The Cache County Study. *J Am Med Assoc* 2002;288:2123-9

# Pharmacology during the menopausal transition

13

*M. Notelovitz*

## INTRODUCTION

The menopause is a biological fulcrum around which the quality of postmenopausal life revolves. Central to this issue is the alteration in the synthesis and metabolism of androgens and estrogens, and the effect that this change may have on hormone-associated conditions, other than those related to reproductive function. The appropriate use of pharmacological agents, including postmenopausal hormone therapy, is predicated by an understanding of the pathogenesis of conditions requiring pharmacological intervention. This, in turn, will govern the principles of the treatment objective: health promotion and disease prevention, or curative (post-event) therapy. The pathogenesis of relevant conditions, such as osteoporosis, cardiovascular disease, Alzheimer's disease and breast cancer, commences well before the menopause (Figure 1) and varies between and among women of different ages, racial and ethnic backgrounds. Due to advances in

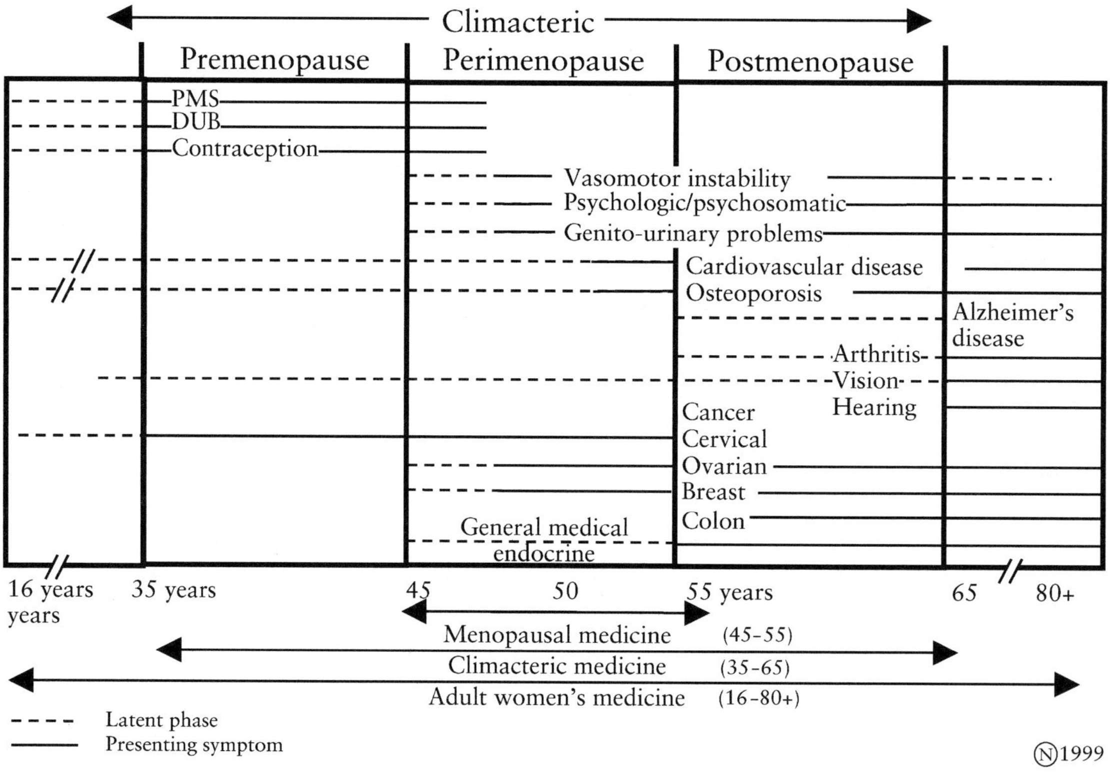


**Figure 1** Health-care needs by life stage. PMS, premenstrual syndrome; DUBS, dysfunctional uterine bleeding

technology, it is now possible to individualize therapy by determining the age-specific health-care needs of women across their life cycle. For example, as reflected by the concept template (Figure 2), the *primary prevention* of cardiovascular disease and osteoporosis should be initiated at the menarche and will involve good nutrition, exercise and a healthy lifestyle; *disease-specific* treatment for those conditions (e.g. bisphosphonates for osteoporosis, statins for atherothrombosis) is relevant to women with evidence of latent or established disease (usually after age 65 years), while hormonal therapy is appropriate during the climacteric years (age 35–65 years). In this context, peri- and postmenopausal hormone therapy is best regarded as *secondary preventive* therapy, provided that the condition being treated has a biologically plausible hormonal basis. In short, individualized postmenopausal hormone therapy is governed by three criteria: definition of the need for treatment (clinical diagnosis), tailoring the treatment to the individual, and monitoring the safety and efficacy of the prescribed therapy (yearly re-evaluation). This chapter is restricted to the principles of postmenopausal hormone therapy, primarily estrogen therapy.

## THE SYNTHESIS AND METABOLISM OF ESTROGEN

All naturally menopausal women are estrogen- and androgen-deficient relative to their premenopausal cohorts. They are not hormonally depleted. The source of estrogen in postmenopausal women is primarily from androgens of adrenal origin (dehydroepiandrosterone and dehydroepiandrosterone sulfate), and, to a lesser extent, the ovarian stroma, which are aromatized in adipose tissue and muscle to estrone (from androstenedione) and to estradiol (from testosterone). Additional bioavailable estradiol is synthesized from estrone (via 17β-hydroxysteroid dehydrogenase activity), while the liver metabolizes both estrone and estradiol into metabolites that are highly estrogenic and potentially carcinogenic (such as 4-hydroxyestradiol, 16α-hydroxysterone) or to

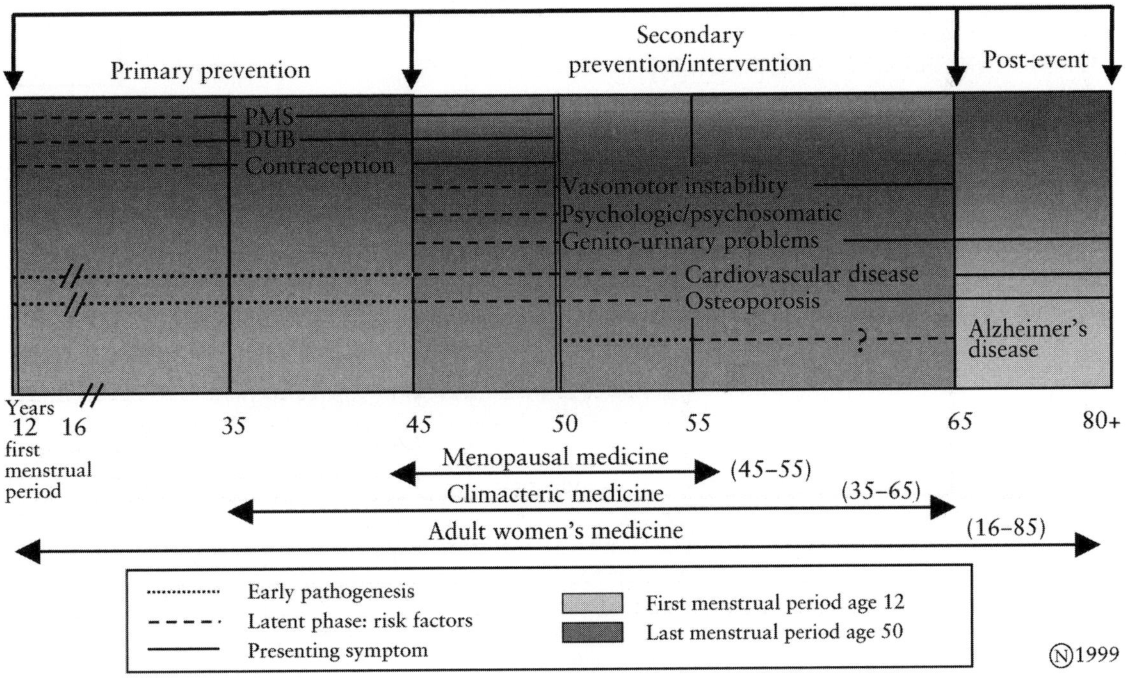


**Figure 2** The climacteric and menopause: 'window of therapeutic opportunity' for hormone therapy. PMS, premenstrual syndrome; DUBS, dysfunctional uterine bleeding

other competitive metabolites with low estrogenicity (anticarcinogenic) such as 2-hydroxy and 2-methoxyestradiol[1,2].

The pathways described in Figure 3 result in only two biological estrogens, estrone and estradiol. Each step in this pathway is dependent on genetically determined (CYP 17, CYP 19, CYP1-A-1, CYP 1-B-1) enzymes (sulfatase, aromatase, 17β-OH steroid dehydrogenase, catechol-o-methyl transferase) that are present in target organs such as the breast, bone, coronary artery and brain. The local tissue synthesis of estradiol is greater than that measured in peripheral blood samples. Tissue estrogen sensitivity is dependent on *free* estradiol binding to an estrogen receptor (ER) and the interaction between the estrogen response elements and the estrogen receptor co-activators and co-repressors. Transcription, the organ tissue functional response, may occur through this genomic mechanism via the cell membrane or via an estrogen-independent second messenger system. Additional variables influencing a target organ's estrogen response include: the distribution of ERα and ERβ (ERβ down-regulates ERα[3]); the co-localization of the androgen receptor (AR) and its modulation of ER activity (testosterone up-regulates ERβ in breast tissue[4]); the hepatic synthesis of sex hormone binding globulin (SHBG) and hence the bioavailability of endogenous and exogenous estrogen and androgen. This is of particular importance to the brain, since SHBG-bound estrogen and androgen do not cross the blood–brain barrier[5].

*Clinical message*

The genetically determined complexity of estrogen and androgen steroidogenesis is further compounded by the amount of endogenous

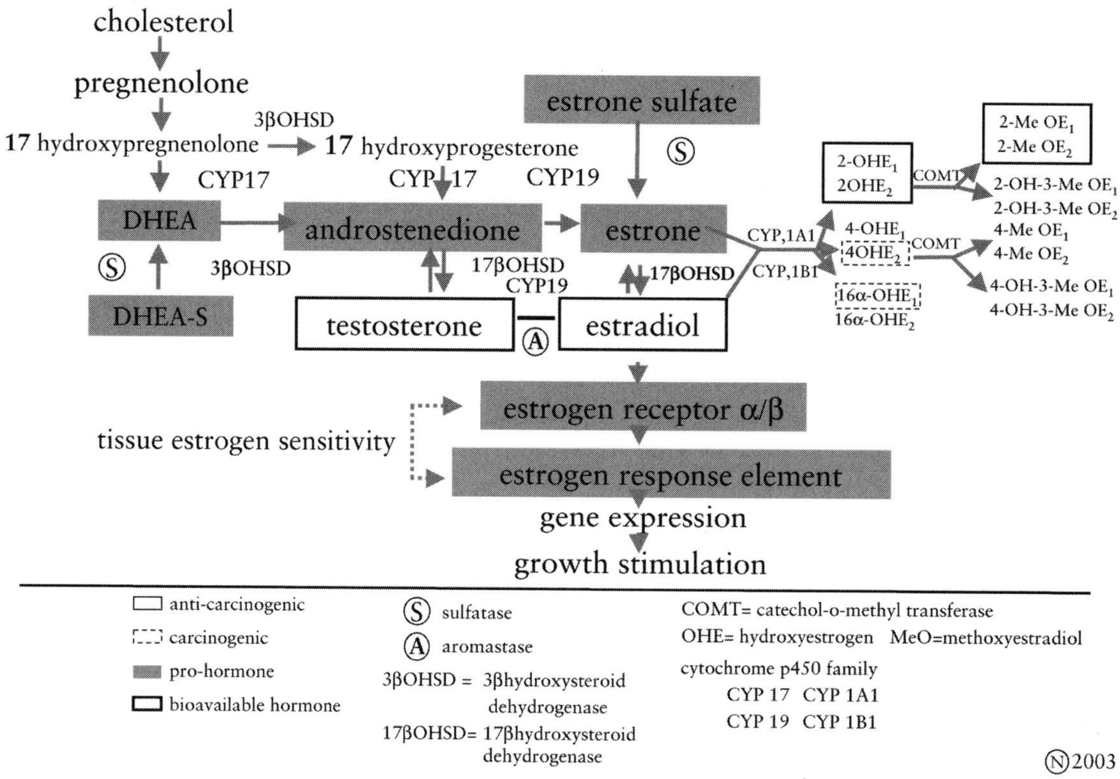


**Figure 3** Synthesis and metabolism of estrogen

estrogen produced (this increases with age) and the variability in the *hormone threshold* needed for normal functioning of individual organ systems. This differs within the same woman, and between women. Although the menopause is generic to all women, the variations above account for both the individualized presentation of women to the menopausal transition and their response to hormone therapy. There is no *one* menopause nor is there *one* hormonal therapy.

## SYMPTOMATIC MENOPAUSE

The most prevalent menopausal symptoms - hot flushes, atrophic vaginitis and certain mood disorders are causally related to alterations in estrogen biosynthesis and usually respond to appropriate estrogen therapy. These symptoms are not experienced by all menopausal women and may even occur premenopausally. In a recent community study[6], approximately 20% of still menstruating women reported typical menopausal hot flushes. Hot flushes that occur during the luteal/menstrual phase of the cycle are responsive to low-dose estrogen therapy. Although these women produce estrogen in amounts adequate for endometrial stimulation, the relative cyclic decline in estradiol is apparently insufficient to maintain thermoregulatory stability of the hypothalamus and the vasomotor center. Conversely, there are many menopausal women who remained completely asymptomatic throughout the menopausal transition. The majority of symptomatic women report hot flushes, but these are of differing severity. The dose of estrogen needed to relieve women of these symptoms, and the duration of estrogen therapy required for symptom control are variable[7]. Doses as low as 0.3 mg of conjugated equine estrogen, 0.5 mg of oral 17β-estradiol or 25 μg of transdermal estrogen have been shown to reduce the frequency and intensity of hot flushes. Approximately 2–4 weeks of estrogen therapy are needed before significant relief is reported; hot flushes persist for 15 or more years in about 20% of women.

The presence of symptoms in estrogen-replete women, such as reduced libido, loss of energy, diminished mood, reduced affect and depression, are indicators of female androgen insufficiency. These symptoms are often coupled with osteopenia/osteoporosis and muscle weakness/wasting. Normal free testosterone blood levels have not been established for menopausal women. The most practical confirmatory test is the free testosterone index (total testosterone/SHBG). Values below the lower quartile of normal for reproductive women are indicative of female androgen insufficiency. Treatment is with estrogen/androgen therapy[8].

Urogenital aging and its associated conditions - atrophic vaginitis, urethral syndrome, recurrent cystitis, reduced urethral closure pressure-related incontinence - are most prevalent and affect the majority of postmenopausal women, especially the elderly. Apart from clinical examination, routine testing of the pH of the lateral vaginal wall is recommended. Values greater than 4.5 are indicative of urogenital estrogen deficiency. Treatment is with locally applied estrogen vaginal creams, estradiol vaginal rings or low-dose estradiol vaginal matrix tablets[9].

## HORMONE THERAPY AND 'SECONDARY PREVENTION'

Timing the initiation of hormone therapy for optimal secondary prevention of osteoporosis, cardiovascular disease and, in all probability, Alzheimer's disease is determined by validated pathophysiological and pharmacological scientific evidence. As with the management of the symptomatic menopause, there are variables that can only be based on the assessment of the *total* woman. This will influence the type, dose and route of hormonal therapy.

### Osteoporosis

Bone mineral density is an accurate marker of bone mass, but not necessarily of bone strength. The latter is dependent upon the integrity of the microarchitecture of bone; in the trabecular compartment of bone, for example, the maintenance of the anatomical continuity of the vertical and horizontal trabecular plates determines the response of the bone to compression and torsional stress, and the risk of fracture[10].

Bone remodeling is complex, but is basically dependent on the balance between three cell types that *control* bone resorption and bone formation. The osteoclasts are the cells involved in the absorption of *'old bone'*; the osteoblasts fill the microscopic resorption cavities that result and synthesize bone matrix - *'new bone'*. Osteocytes are osteoblast-derived cells that chemically modulate bone remodeling by inhibiting and stimulating osteoclast and osteoblast activity, respectively. The osteocytes are the bone's mechanico-receptors and are stimulated by gravitational force and by exercise (mechanical loading). All of these cell types have estrogen and androgen receptors and are responsive to exogenous hormonal therapy[11].

*Clinical application*

Loss of bone mineral is a normal consequence of aging, and is accelerated postmenopausally. The regional bone mineral density (as measured by dual X-ray absorptiometry, DEXA) and the rate at which bone mineral is lost (serum and/or urinary collagen cross-link excretion) are surrogate determinants of bone health and the risk for future fracture. Studies utilizing these technologies have confirmed the ability of hormone therapy to improve bone mineral density, restore bone marker patterns to premenopausal levels, and, in both observational and randomized clinical trials, to prevent/reduce the risk of vertebral and hip fractures[10]. Two additional clinical caveats: the dose of estrogen needed to maintain bone mineral density lessens with aging; stopping hormone therapy will restore bone remodeling to its pretreatment level of activity[10].

*Clinical messages*

Hormone therapy (for osteoporosis prevention) needs to be started in the early menopause (before significant microarchitectural damage); to maintain its efficacy, hormone therapy needs to be prescribed on a long-term basis; the dose of estrogen therapy can be titrated downwards over time. Monitoring with DEXA testing and the measurement of bone marker activity are the only means of objectively determining an individual's response to a given dose and regimen of hormone therapy. The frequency and type of tests used vary with regional standards of practice. Women with documented osteoporosis - clinically and/or radiologically determined fracture(s) - are also eligible for hormone therapy but are candidates for alternative antiresorptive drugs such as bisphosphonates (alendronate, risedronate) and selective estrogen receptor modulators (SERMS, e.g. raloxifene)[12].

## Cardiovascular disease

Cardiovascular disease (CVD) is a multifactorial syndrome. Some of the factors involved in the dynamics of atherothrombosis are summarized in Figure 4. As with bone, there is a strong biological plausibility to support the role of estrogen therapy for the secondary prevention of CVD. Estrogen receptors (ER$\alpha$, ER$\beta$) are present in target tissues relevant to cardiovascular protection: coronary artery endothelium and smooth muscle, liver, muscle and adipose tissue[18]. Early intervention is essential: animal[14] and human clinical studies[15] have shown that plaque formation can be stabilized and, in some instances, reduced by appropriately timed hormone therapy. This is mediated by the favorable action of estrogen on lipid and lipoprotein metabolism, insulin resistance and blood pressure[16]. Distinction must be made between the proven efficacy of estrogen in modulating the menopause/age-related changes in lipid and carbohydrate metabolism from dyslipidemia, diabetes and hypertension - diseases that are not hormone-related and which need disease-specific therapies: statins, hypoglycemic agents and antihypertensives, respectively.

*Clinical application*

A fasting blood profile that measures glucose, cholesterol, triglycerides and high density lipoprotein (HDL) cholesterol will differentiate healthy women at low risk for CVD from those with latent or overt (but asymptomatic) disease. In addition, the results will determine the optimal type and route of hormone therapy: women with endogenously low levels of HDL cholesterol will benefit from the hepatic induced increase in HDL cholesterol following oral estrogen therapy; women with hypertriglyceridemia are best treated

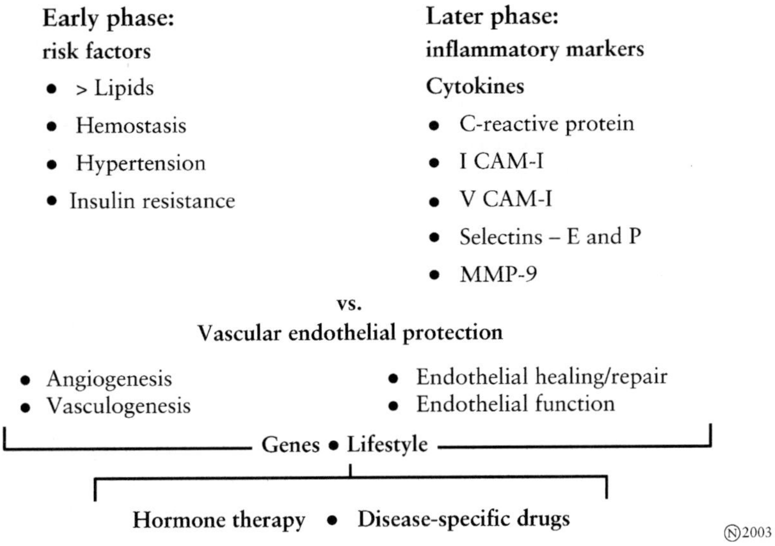


**Figure 4** The dynamics of atherothrombosis and endothelial health

with low-dose transdermal estrogen, since the oral route of estrogen therapy (especially with conjugated equine estrogen) may increase triglyceride levels significantly. Low-dose estrogen therapy (oral or transdermal) improves insulin sensitivity; high-dose estrogen therapy may increase insulin resistance. Improvement of the above biochemical parameters in recently menopausal women may be indicative of future CVD protection[16].

Improvement of the same biochemical profile in women with established disease on estrogen therapy - post-myocardial infarction and stroke - is not necessarily reflective of protection against *future* CVD events. Indeed, women who respond to oral hormone therapy with the greatest increase in HDL cholesterol may be more vulnerable to recurrent plaque rupture and thrombosis[13]. It is in the later phase of atherothrombosis that estrogen therapy may increase the risk - albeit low when measured in absolute terms - of rupturing the fibrin capsule of lipid-rich soft core atheromatous plaques. This may be mediated via a variety of cytokines and inflammatory agents (Figure 4), especially the matrix metalloproteinases (MMP-9)[18]. These adverse estrogen therapy-induced events are probably secondary to an underlying *pretreatment* abnormality in synthesis of these factors[19].

*Clinical application*

Women with known or suspected significant atheromatous disease should have levels of C-reactive protein and possibly MMP-9 in blood measured prior to estrogen therapy. Technology that non-invasively detects unstable atherosclerotic plaques is available but is not cost-effective for routine clinical practice. Estrogen receptor distribution and activity are also negatively impacted by the presence and degree of atherosclerotic disease. Reduced ER expression in the vascular endothelium and smooth muscle may be further compromised by the known progestin-induced down-regulation of the ER.

*Clinical message*

When hormone therapy is indicated in women with established CVD, prescribe transdermal estradiol (to lessen SHBG and enhance bioavailable estrogen levels) and cyclic progestins with short half-lives (to reduce inhibition of ER activity).

## Cognition and Alzheimer's disease

Estrogen has proven neuronal functions that provide brain protection and correct certain aspects of neuronal dysfunction[20]. These include reduction of neuronal atrophy and damage via a number of mechanisms including stimulation/induction of nerve growth factors, improvement in neurotransmitting activity, neurite branching and cerebral blood flow and metabolism. The brain is rich in ER$\alpha$, ER$\beta$ and androgen receptors, especially in regions associated with cognition and memory[3].

Timing of estrogen therapy, and the presence of latent or overt disease are critical to the benefit that may accrue from estrogen therapy (and androgen therapy). Relevant clinical issues include:

(1) Discriminating between the *normal* age-related deterioration of memory (benign senescent forgetfulness) from mild cognitive impairment, a pre-condition to *late-onset* Alzheimer's disease. The latter must be differentiated from early-onset Alzheimer's disease, a genetically distinct and less common condition;

(2) Bioavailability of endogenous and prescribed estrogen. The cognitive decline in aging women is increasingly proportional to the levels of non-protein bound and bioavailable estrogen[21]. Improvement in visual memory and vigilance in non-demented healthy menopausal women is similarly related to the type, dose and route of estrogen therapy[22];

(3) Long-term observational studies confirming cell culture and animal studies demonstrating neuroprotection against Alzheimer's disease, provided the intervention is *early* and *sustained*[23].

*Clinical message*

A number of questionnaires and validated tests are available for the early screening and identification of cognitive decline. Where relevant, specific genotyping for Alzheimer's disease and various brain imaging technologies could be used to determine the risk for/and the presence of Alzheimer-related disease. When estrogen therapy is indicated, 17$\beta$-estradiol (oral or transdermal) is the estrogen of choice since it is least likely to increase SHBG levels and thereby enhance estrogen bioavailability in the central nervous system.

## HORMONE THERAPY AND BREAST CANCER

Long-term exposure to endogenous and exogenous estrogen is associated with a significant, yet in absolute terms, modest increase in breast cancer[24]. This is true for women with a predisposition to estrogen-related breast cancer, and is different from early- versus later-onset breast cancer. Women who develop breast cancer before age 50 are more likely to have a genetically determined high penetrance but low prevalence form of cancer (BRCA 1, BRCA 2, $\rho$53); cancer due to abnormalities in breast tissue estrogen synthesis and hepatic estrogen metabolism occurs at a later age and is associated with lower penetrance but a higher prevalent genetic polymorphism (CYP 17, CYP 19, CYP 1 A 1, CYP 1 B 1)[25]. Studies have confirmed an increased risk of breast cancer in women with excess enzyme activity (sulfatase, aromatase and 17$\beta$-dehydrogenase) controlled by these genes.

Excess local breast tissue estradiol synthesis has been correlated with both an increase in mammographic breast density[26] and breast cancer[27]. The correlation between breast density and breast cancer is only present in pretreatment mammograms.

*Clinical message*

Mammograms can be used as a means of identifying women with a *predisposition* to breast cancer. High-sensitivity estradiol blood values above 10–15 pg/ml are an additional indication of an increased risk of breast cancer. These women need to be carefully monitored; hormone therapy (when indicated) should be limited to the lowest effective dose, and consideration given to treatment with a SERM (raloxifene) or to a tissue-specific hormone such as tibolone. Advances in genomic medicine will, in the foreseeable future, provide clinicians with a more specific diagnosis and the ability to treat the underlying abnormality with specific therapeutic agents, e.g. sulfatase, aromatase or 17$\beta$-OH steroid dehydrogenase inhibitors. If down-regulation of the breast's ER$\alpha$ activity by ER$\beta$ is shown to reduce the breast cancer risk, androgen therapy (which up-regulates ER$\beta$) should be added to all long-term estrogen therapy regimens.

## CONCLUSION

Premenopausal estrogen steroidogenesis and function are the foundation on which the health and well-being of postmenopausal women depend. The contribution of postmenopausal estrogen synthesis, although much reduced, plays a pivotal role in maintaining health and reducing the morbidity of diseases prevalent in postmenopausal women, such as osteoporosis. Appreciation of differences in pre- and postmenopausal estrogen biosynthesis and function and the physiology/ pathology of bone, coronary arteries, breast and the brain, allows for the selective choice of appropriate estrogen therapy for a given individual, at a given point in time, based on sound biological and pharmacological principles. Postmenopausal hormone therapy is pharmacological. However, based on the pharmacokinetics and the pharmacodynamics of estrogen therapy, it is possible to adjust the type of therapy to the physiological needs of menopausal women. Thus, for women who experience a premature menopause (natural or surgical), it is possible to replicate (replace) the premenopausal estrogen milieu with transdermal or percutaneous estradiol therapy; the normal estrone : estradiol ratio of estrogen in postmenopausal women can be maintained but increased (replenished) via oral estrogen therapy. The *physiological* approach can only be achieved by adjusting the dose prescribed to pretreatment estradiol levels by the use of *simple* estrogen compounds such as estradiol. A similar pharmacological response can be achieved with *complex* estrogens (such as conjugated equine estrogen) which have estrogen activity, but are not native to women. The route and type of estrogen therapy will vary with the chronological and menopausal age of the

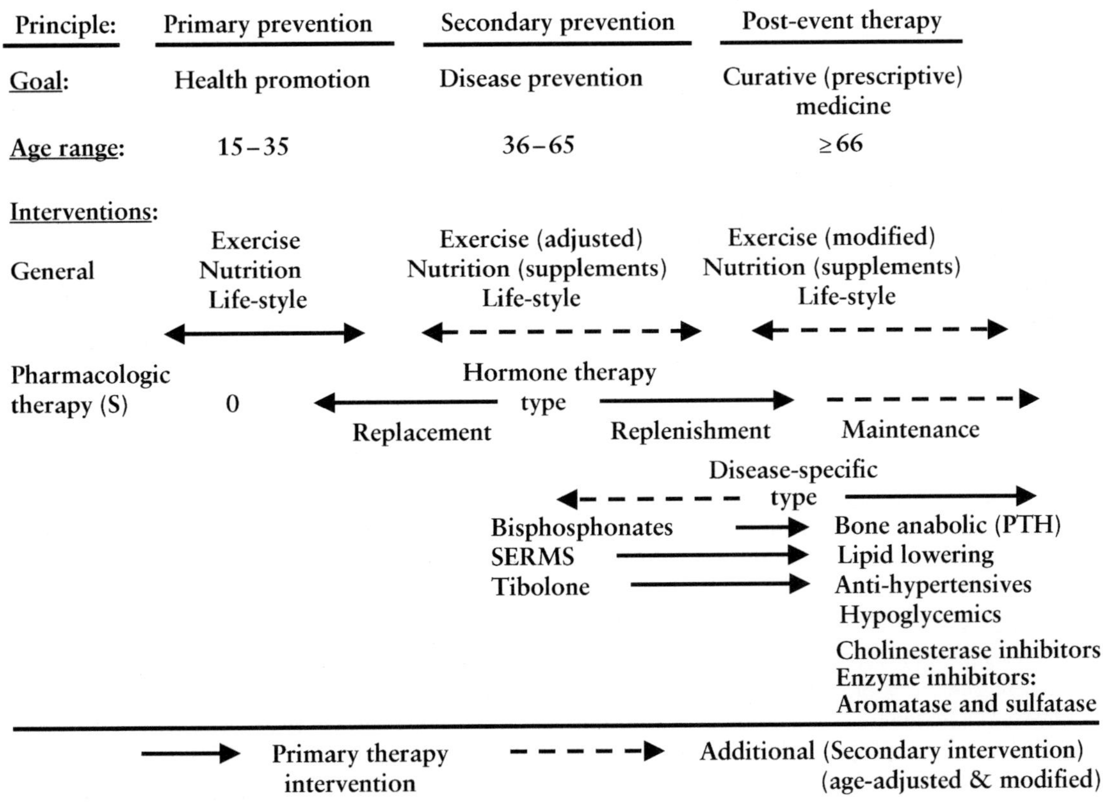


**Figure 5** Pharmacology during the menopausal transition: applied clinical principles

individual and her clinical preferences and needs. This will necessitate testing of surrogate biomarkers such as fasting lipid profile, glucose, C-reactive protein (in older women), bone density (bone markers), mammography (breast density), vaginal pH, and, selectively, serum estradiol (total and free) and follicle stimulating hormone (FSH)/SHBG levels. Three biological approaches may be considered (Figure 5):

(1) Estrogen replacement therapy: to meet the physiological hormonal requirement of younger menopausal women (< 50 years);

(2) Estrogen replenishment therapy: the pharmacological addition of estrogen to ensure quality of life and maintenance of tissue integrity and health (50–65 years);

(3) Estrogen maintenance therapy: continuation of previously prescribed and well-tolerated estrogen therapy (65 years and above).

All of the above approaches are subject to the following clinical caveats: prescribe the lowest effective dose of estrogen; adjust the dose over time to meet the dual objectives of efficacy and safety; monitor annually. Conditions such as dyslipidemia, diabetes, or hypertension require disease-specific therapy. Estrogen therapy enhances the quality of life for menopausal women.

# References


1. Gruber CJ, Tschugguel W, Schneeberger C, Huber JC. Production and action of estrogens. *N Engl J Med* 2002;346:340–52
2. Clemmons M, Goss P. Estrogen and risk of breast cancer. *N Engl J Med* 2001;344:276–85
3. Ishunina TA, Kruijver FPM, Balesar R, Swaab DF. Differential expression of estrogen receptor α and β immunoreactivity in human supraoptic nucleus in relation to sex and aging. *J Clin Endocrinol Metab* 2000;85:3283–91
4. Dimitrakakis C, Zhou J, Wang J, *et al.* A physiologic role for testosterone in limiting estrogenic stimulation of the breast. *Menopause* 2003;10:292–8
5. Hobb CJ, Jones RE, Plymate SR. The effect of sex hormone binding globulin (SHBG) in testosterone transport into the cerebrospinal fluid. *J Steroid Biochem Molec Biol* 1991;42:629–35
6. Oldenhave A, Jaszmann IJ, Haspels AA, *et al.* Impact of climacteric on well-being. A survey based on 5313 women 39 to 60 years old. *Am J Obstet Gynecol* 1993;168:772–80
7. Stearns V, Ullmer L, Lopez JF, *et al.* Hot flushes. *Lancet* 2002;360:1851–61
8. Braunstein GD. Androgen insufficiency in women: summary of critical issues. *Fertil Steril* 2002;Suppl 4:594–9
9. Notelovitz M. Urogenital atrophy and low-dose vaginal estrogen therapy. *Menopause* 2000;7:140–2
10. Notelovitz M. Estrogen therapy and osteoporosis: principles and practice. *Am J Med Sci* 1999;213: 2–12
11. Smit TH, Burger EH. Is BMU-coupling a strain-regulated phenomenon? A finite element analysis. *J Bone Miner Res* 2000;15:301–7
12. Cranney A, Guyatt G,Griffith L, I. Meta-analysis of therapies for post-menopausal osteoporosis. IX. Summary of meta-analysis of therapies for post-menopausal osteoporosis. *Endocr Rev* 2002;23: 570–8
13. Mendelsohn ME, Karas RH. The protective effects of estrogen on the cardiovascular system. *N Engl J Med* 1999;340:1801–11
14. Clarkson TB. The new conundrum: do estrogens have any cardiovascular benefits. *Int J Fertil* 2002; 47:61–8
15. Hodis HN, Mack WJ, Lobo RA, *et al.* Estrogen in the prevention of atherosclerosis: a randomized, double blind, placebo-controlled trial. *Ann Intern Med* 2001;135:929–53
16. Davidson M, Maki KC, Marx P, *et al.* Effect of continuous estrogen and estrogen-progestin replacement regimens on cardiovascular risk markers in post-menopausal women. *Arch Intern Med* 2000;160:3315–25
17. Herrington DM, Howard TD, Hawkins GA, *et al.* Estrogen-receptor polymorphisms and effects of estrogen replacement on high-density lipoprotein cholesterol in women with coronary disease. *N Engl J Med* 2003;346:967–74
18. Zanger D, Yang BK, Ardans J, *et al.* Divergent effects of hormone therapy on serum markers of inflammation in postmenopausal women with

coronary artery disease on appropriate medical management. *J Am Coll Cardiol* 2000;36:1797–802
19. Pradham D, Mannon JE, Roussouw JE, *et al.* Inflammatory biomarkers, hormone replacement therapy and incident coronary heart disease. *J Am Med Assoc* 2002;28:980–7
20. McEwen BS, Alves BS. Estrogen actions in the central nervous system. *Endocr Rev* 1999;20: 279–307
21. Yaffe K, Lui L-Y, Grady D, *et al.* Cognitive decline in women in relation to non-protein bound estradiol concentrations. *Lancet* 2000;356:708–12
22. Le Blanc ES, Janowsky J, Chan BKS, Nelson HD. Hormone replacement therapy and cognition. Systemic review and meta-analysis. *J Am Med Assoc* 2001;285:1489–99
23. Zandi PP, Carlson MC, Plassman BL, *et al.* Hormone replacement therapy and incidence of Alzheimer's disease in older women. *J Am Med Assoc* 2002;288:2123–9
24. Collaborative Group on Hormone Factors in Breast Cancer. Familial breast cancer: collaborative re-analysis of individual data from 52 epidemiological studies including 58,209 women with breast cancer and 101,986 women without disease. *Lancet* 2001;358:1389–99
25. Armstrong K. Genetic susceptibility to breast cancer. *J Am Med Assoc* 2001;285:2907–9
26. Speroff L. The meaning of mammographic breast density in users of postmenopausal hormone therapy. *Maturitas* 2002;41:171–5
27. Cummings SR, Duong T, Kenyon E, *et al.* Serum estradiol level and risk of breast cancer during treatment with raloxifene. *J Am Med Assoc* 2002; 287:216–20

# Some background considerations relevant to the evaluation of the effects of hormone therapy

14

*S. Shapiro*

The publication of findings from the Women's Health Initiative Randomized Controlled Trial[1], soon followed by those reported from the Million Women Study[2], has raised major issues as to how the evidence from these and other studies should be interpreted. Those issues are examined in detail in the body of this book. But, before getting to those issues, it is helpful to consider in a general way the weight that should be given to evidence derived from sources such as randomized controlled trials and observational studies, and from clinical and biological research.

Kuhn has defined a 'paradigm' as a universally accepted set of assumptions under which scientific enquiry and inference proceeds; he has defined a 'paradigm shift' as a radical change in those assumptions, a phenomenon that occurs from time to time. In the present context, in inferring causality, the currently prevailing paradigm is that the greatest validity is to be accorded to evidence derived from randomized controlled trials, such as the Women's Health Initiative, followed by evidence from observational studies, particularly follow-up (cohort) studies, and particularly if they are massive, such as the Million Women Study. Beyond that, the evidence derived from other forms of epidemiological research is regarded as having less intrinsic validity.

Randomized controlled trials are given pride of place because randomization is assumed to eliminate or reduce the likelihood of confounding, while 'double-blinding' eliminates or reduces the likelihood of bias. Follow-up studies, especially if they are large, rank next because they produce statistically robust and precise data.

Are these assumptions always correct, or has the time come for a paradigm shift? It is certainly the case that, if any given study can truly remain randomized and double-blind, a randomized controlled trial is likely to afford the most valid evidence. This objective can commonly be achieved in relatively short-term studies, but less commonly in complex long-term studies, especially if one of the arms in a given trial is a placebo. If a substantial proportion of the study subjects become unblinded for one or another reason, bias may not only become a possibility, but, because the study participants become aware that they are participating in an experiment, bias may become an even stronger possibility than in an observational study. If, in the course of follow-up, a substantial proportion of the subjects do not adhere to their assigned treatments, confounding also becomes possible, despite randomization at baseline – a problem that becomes further compounded if, in addition, cross-overs occur at all commonly. In addition, while analysis according to intention-to-treat may be an effective way to deal with such confounding in a short-term study, in a long-term and complex study, it cannot be assumed to have been controlled by the use of that approach. In short, such a study takes on the characteristics of an observational study; it needs to be analyzed as such, and it has to be recognized as having most or all of the limitations intrinsic to observational research.

What about the validity of massive follow-up studies? Possible sources of bias and confounding are acknowledged to be problems that can never entirely be eliminated in observational research, and their possible existence imposes limits on the interpretability of any association identified in such research. In that circumstance, if, in a well-conducted study, an association is large (say, a relative risk well in excess of 3.0), it may be reasonable to conclude that any residual sources of bias or confounding are unlikely to fully account for it. However, if an association is small, it may not be possible to discriminate among bias, confounding and causation as alternative explanations. In that circumstance, it is a common fallacy to interpret a highly statistically significant association as a causal one. However, once a bias is present, all that a large study accomplishes, relative to a small one, is to set narrower confidence limits around the magnitude of that bias. In short, once a study is biased, increasing its magnitude may make it more statistically robust, but robustness does not equate with validity.

A further consequence of according the greatest validity to randomized controlled trials and massive follow-up studies is that the underlying perspective in the conduct and interpretation of such studies can tend to be governed by statistical reasoning, at the expense of clinical and biological insight. To be sure, the proper use of statistics is essential to the proper manipulation and interpretation of numerical data. However, causation is always ultimately a biological phenomenon, not a statistical one. In the ultimate analysis, insight as to whether an association is causal must give due weight to clinical and biological considerations and the ranking of such considerations as being of lesser validity may not be justified. Optimally valid causal research in population studies should incorporate the complementary roles of clinical medicine, biology, and statistics, with the latter serving as the servant rather than the master.

There is also a common misunderstanding of the respective roles played in causal research by epidemiology, clinical medicine, and biological research. Epidemiology can be informative about effects in populations, and its strength is that it can identify causal associations that may not be readily apparent in clinical or biological studies. A weakness, however, is that, in order to do so, it must necessarily be reductionist in its definition of exposures and outcomes. Clinical medicine can be informative about effects in individual patients, and it can sometimes document details and subtleties in the causation and evolution of disease that may not be accessible to epidemiology. Some of its weaknesses are that causal associations may be missed, and that clinical observations can be susceptible to bias. Biological research can identify mechanisms and raise hypotheses. But a weakness is that the findings from such research may not be generalizable to human populations.

Based on the foregoing considerations, it is clear that causal research is likely to be most valid when the different approaches are all taken into account, and considered to be complementary. I suggest that the paradigm of giving the highest validity ranking to randomized controlled trials, followed by observational studies, and then by clinical medicine and biology is not valid. Each approach has strengths and weaknesses, and a paradigm shift is required in which no single approach is considered to be superior to any other.

I hope that this brief overview will be helpful to readers as they read the Proceedings of this Workshop.

## References


1. Writing Group for the Women's Health Initiative Investigators. Risks and benefits of estrogen plus progestin in healthy postmenopausal women: principal results from the Women's Health Initiative randomized controlled trial. *J Am Med Assoc* 2002;288:321–33
2. Million Women Study Collaborators. Breast cancer and hormone-replacement therapy in the Million Women Study. *Lancet* 2003:362:419–27

# Menopausal medicine and its potential drug development opportunities 15

*V. V. Ragavan and F. T. Kawakami*

## INTRODUCTION

Estrogens given with or without progestins have been prescribed to women for treatment of menopausal symptoms and prevention of osteoporosis for over 60 years. However, the results of the Women's Health Initiative (WHI)[1] altered dramatically the perception of the benefit/risk relation of the hormonal therapy for postmenopausal women, and made clear that further research would be needed to demonstrate the long-term effects of different estrogens given by different routes in younger women in the pre-, peri- and early postmenopause. However, the feasibility of conducting any new randomized, prospective studies of such magnitude is now reduced dramatically.

But the need to find new treatments for the serious and quality-of-life ailments of the postmenopausal woman has become even more urgent with the loss of the wide use of estrogens. In order to adequately meet these new needs, the pharmaceutical companies must seriously consider conducting research which is oriented to understanding the factors that regulate estrogen action at the cellular level, in order to find new drugs that are targeted to specific tissues, such as those of the skeleton, breast, reproductive tract, central nervous and cardiovascular systems. In the postmenopausal woman, improving the balance between the positive effects of estrogens on suppression of hot flushes and in the preservation of the bone density and the negative effects on the breast, uterus and cardiovascular system is an important unmet medical need.

Understanding estrogen's action at the molecular level is crucial to developing organ-specific targeted drugs for the future. The approach taken in this paper is to re-examine the biological actions of estrogen on some organ systems as an example to potential drug development targets and to speculate about potential drug development pathways.

## SELECTIVE ESTROGEN RECEPTOR MODULATORS

Estrogens belong to a class of hormones that are unique due in their ability to bind to nuclear receptors that then interact with locations on the DNA, resulting in the transcriptional effect of the gene post-binding. To date, much is known about the interactions between the estrogen receptor and estrogens and other ligands. The knowledge regarding the role of different co-factors which activate or suppress the estrogen action at the gene level is also progressing rapidly. However, much remains to be discovered about post-receptor events that modify the biology of estrogen action and that are also specific to the organ of interest.

Molecules with specific positive/negative affinity for the estrogen receptor have been derived and are called selective estrogen receptor modulators (SERMs) because of their differing binding affinities and post-receptor events in different organ systems[2]. Tamoxifen belongs to the first generation of such compounds and has anti-mitogenic effects on the breast. It exerts, however, estrogenic effects on the endometrium and is associated with an increased risk of endometrial hyperplasia and cancer. Raloxifene seems to be devoid of proliferative effects on the uterus, while it is effective in the prevention and treatment of osteoporosis. Both SERMs, however, are neutral on, or worsen, hot flushes and carry a similar risk of deep vein thrombosis as estrogens.

**Table 1** The search for the ideal selective estrogen receptor modulator (SERM). Adapted from Riggs and Hartmann[4]

| *Risk/benefit* | *Estrogen* | *Tamoxifen* | *Toremifene* | *Raloxifene* | *Ideal SERM* |
|---|---|---|---|---|---|
| Hot flushes | ↓↓↓ | ↑ | ↑ | ↑ | ↓↓↓ |
| Uterine bleeding | ↑↑↑ | ↑ | ↑ | ↔ | ↔ |
| Risk of endometrial cancer | ↑↑ | ↑ | ? | ↔ | ↔ |
| Prevention of postmenopausal bone loss | ↑↑↑ | ↑ | ↔ | ↑↑ | ↑↑↑ |
| Risk of breast cancer | ↑↑ | ↓↓ | ↓↓ | ↓↓ | ↓↓ |
| Favorable pattern of serum lipids | ↑↑↑ | ↑ | ↑↑ | ↑ | ↑↑↑ |
| Venous thrombosis | ↑↑ | ↑↑ | ? | ↑↑ | ↔ |

The search for the ideal SERM[3] is still ongoing, as noted in Table 1.

The desirable and undesirable effects of estrogens and SERMs are related to their interaction with the estrogen receptor (ER). Two different estrogen receptors have been identified: ER$\alpha$ and ER$\beta$[5]. Both receptors share a highly conserved DNA-binding domain and a moderately conserved ligand-binding domain, but a divergent N-terminal A/B domain that contains a transactivation factor (AF-1) which interacts with the genomic proteins prior to activation. The estrogen receptors are known to form different conformations on binding to various ligands and it is these varying conformations which may be responsible for specific effects in different organ systems[6].

## SERMS AND BONE

Estrogen deficiency is the most common cause of osteoporotic fractures and the recent WHI study showed that estrogens and progestins given continuously are protective of fractures, with a 34% reduction in vertebral and hip fractures[1].

Postmenopausal bone loss effects due to estrogen deficiency are thought to be due to an increase in bone resorption which outpaces bone formation[7]. Estrogen action in bone has been extensively studied[8]. Estrogen has been shown to inhibit several cytokines, interleukin-1 (IL-1), IL-6, IL-11, tumor necrosis factor (TNF), macrophage colony stimulating factor (M-CSF) and granulocyte/macrophage colony stimulating factor (GM-CSF).

Although not clearly confirmed, estrogen seems to act primarily through IL-6, a cytokine thought to be responsible for an early stage of osteoclastogenesis, which results in an increase in osteoclasts and increase in bone breakdown. Estrogen is thought to suppress IL-6 activation in the bone[9].

Further understanding of estrogen action on the bone can lead to drugs which target inactivation of IL-6 or other cytokine candidates and must be ideally delivered to the skeleton preferentially without systemic effects, since many of these cytokines are also known to have effects on many other systems, including their beneficial effects on the immune system. Raloxifene is a SERM which is approved for the treatment and prevention of postmenopausal osteoporosis, but, in comparative studies, it has been shown to increase bone density to a lesser effect than estrogen and also has not been shown to prevent hip fractures in a fashion similar to estrogen, as found in the WHI[10,11]. The reason for the lower protection of bone density with raloxifene is not known, but this type of research could result in the discovery of a more potent SERM that can prevent postmenopausal osteoporosis while not affecting other organ systems adversely.

## SERMS AND THE BREAST

Tamoxifen was the first known and approved SERM for the treatment of estrogen receptor-positive breast cancer and its use is now well established. Other SERMs, such as toremifene and raloxifene, are also known, or thought, to have a similar functional utility for breast cancer. Interestingly and perhaps based on receptor function, different SERMs seem to affect differing aspects of estrogen action on the breast cancer tissues. Clinical data such as the WHI have shown that estrogen (and progestins) can have a modulatory effect on breast cancer cells, but as to whether there is an active promotion or a 'potentiation' of underlying cells with carcinogenic potential still remains to be identified.

Tamoxifen has been best studied for its effect on breast cancer cells and is thought to work on several mechanisms. Such actions include inhibition of protein kinase C[12], upregulation of c-myc expression[13], and other mechanisms[14,15]. However, tamoxifen is also associated with an increase in the risk of endometrial cancer, which limits its use in prevention of breast cancer in high-risk populations. A sub-analysis of a large clinical trial with raloxifene has shown a potential reduction in the risk of breast cancer in postmenopausal women with osteoporosis[16]. Also, raloxifene[17] and tamoxifen[18] were found to decrease Ki67, an immunohistochemical marker of proliferation. A large study (STAR) is ongoing to evaluate the comparative efficacy of tamoxifen and raloxifene in prevention of breast cancer in high-risk patients.

Given the potential for various pathways of action of SERMs on normal breast and breast cancer tissue, it is possible that understanding of specific pathways will lead to the discovery of SERMs that can have positive effects on the breast but no effects on the uterus and other organs.

## SERMS AND THE UTERUS

Protecting the endometrium against endometrial cancer or hyperplasia is a desired effect of a SERM and would differentiate it from estrogen. As mentioned before, although tamoxifen is approved for treatment of breast cancer, it is also known to increase the incidence of endometrial cancer[19]. So far, raloxifene does not seem to appear to carry the same risk, although the mechanism of this protective effect is not known and warrants further investigation[20].

## SERMS AND HOT FLUSHES

Estrogen relieves hot flushes in a dose-dependent manner and is more effective than any other alternate therapies, such as clonidine, selective serotonin reuptake inhibitors, gabapentin, etc. The mechanism of the hot flush and estrogen's actions to relieve hot flushes is still not clearly understood and certainly any molecular mechanisms relating to this action is still unclear. It is thought that declining hormone levels lead to instability of the thermoregulatory mechanism in the brain, which may be potentially related to estrogen-induced imbalances of various neurotransmitters[21,22]. The current SERMs are known to induce hot flushes and this provides a significant drawback for their use in younger postmenopausal women[23].

## SERMS AND THROMBOEMBOLIC EVENTS

Estrogen agonist properties of all the SERMs on the market are thought to be responsible for the increase in thromboembolic events, with a similar relative risk of 3–4 : 1. Estrogens[24], tamoxifen[25], and raloxifene[16,26] have all been shown to increase the risk of thromboembolic disorders. However, the mechanism of this adverse effect is not well known and hence it is still a difficult task to find a SERM that can prevent this problem.

## CONCLUSION

There are many challenges to menopausal medicine in the future. The concept, that one molecule, namely estrogen, can help to cure all the hormone-related aging problems, is a concept that has come under increasing disfavor. So, although this molecule is a very old one, its function and cellular mechanisms continue to be a source of interesting science. Further understanding of the molecular mechanism of action of estrogen can help to provide the basis of future drug development.

# References


1. Writing Group for the Women's Health Initiative Investigators: risks and benefits of estrogen plus progestin in healthy postmenopausal women: principal results from the Women's Health Initiative randomized controlled study. *J Am Med Assoc* 2002;288:321-3
2. Lonard DM, Smith CL. Molecular perspective on selective estrogen receptor modulators (SERMs): progress in understanding their tissue-specific agonist and antagonist actions. *Steroids* 2002;67: 15-24
3. Arun B, Dunn A, Dunn B. The search for the ideal SERM. *Expert Opin Pharmacother* 2002;3:681-91
4. Riggs BL, Hartmann LC. Selective estrogen-receptor modulators - mechanism of action and application to clinical practice. *N Engl J Med* 2003: 348:618-29
5. Mueller ST. Molecular determinants of the stereoselectivity of agonist activity of estrogen receptors (ER) α and β. *J Biol Chem* 2003;278:12255-62
6. Paech K, Webb P, Kuiper GG, *et al.* Differential ligand activation of estrogen receptors ER α and β at AP-1 sites. *Science* 1997;277:1508-10
7. Riggs BL, Khosla S, Melton LJ. A unitary model for involutional osteoporosis:estrogen deficiency causes both type 1 and type II osteoporosis in postmenopausal women and contributes to bone loss in aging men. *J Bone Min Res* 1998;13:763-73
8. Rickard DJ, Subramaniam M, Spelsberg TC. Molecular and cellular mechanisms of estrogen action on the skeleton. *J Cell Biochem* 1999;32/33 (Suppl):123-32
9. Manolagas SC, Jilka RL. Bone marrow, cytokines, and bone remodeling. *N Engl J Med* 1995;332: 305-11
10. Delmas PD, Bjarnason NH, Mitlak BH, *et al.* Effects of raloxifene on bone mineral density, serum cholesterol concentrations and uterine endometrium in postmenopausal women. *N Engl J Med* 1997;337:1641-7
11. Lufkin EG, Whitaker MD, Nickelsen T, *et al.* Treatment of established postmenopausal osteoporosis with raloxifene: a randomized trial. *J Bone Miner Res* 1998;13:1747-54
12. Issandou M, Faucher C, Bayard F, *et al.* Opposite effects of tamoxifen on in vitro protein kinase C activity and endogenous protein phosphorylation in intact MCF-7 cells. *Cancer Res* 1990;50:5845-50
13. Kang Y, Cortina R, Perry RR, *et al.* Role of c-myc in tamoxifen induced apoptosis in estrogen-independent breast cancer cells. *J Natl Cancer Inst* 1996;88:279-84
14. Cuzcick J. Chemoprevention of breast cancer with tamoxifen. *IARC Sci Publ* 1996;136:95-105
15. Jordan VC, Lababidi MK, Mirecki DM, *et al.* Anti-oestrogenic and anti-tumour properties of prolonged tamoxifen therapy in CH3/OUJ mice. *Eur J Cancer* 1990;26:718-21
16. Cummings SR, Eckert S, Krueger KA, *et al.* The effect of raloxifene on risk of breast cancer in postmenopausal women. Results from the MORE trial. *J Am Med Assoc* 1999;281:2189-97
17. Dowsett M, Bundred NJ, Derensi A, *et al.* Effect of raloxifene on breast cancer cell Ki67 and apoptosis: a double-blind, placebo-controlled, randomized clinical trial in postmenopausal patients. *Cancer Epidemiol Biomarkers Prev* 2001;10:961-6
18. Clarke RB, Laidlaw IJ, Jones LJ, *et al.* Effect of tamoxifen on Ki67 labelling index in human breast tumours and its relationship to oestrogen and progesterone receptor status. *Br J Cancer* 1993; 67:606-11
19. Fisher B, Costantino JP, Wickerham DL, *et al.* Tamoxifen for prevention of breast cancer: report of the National Surgical Adjuvant Breast and Bowel Project P-1 Study. *J Natl Cancer Inst* 1998;90: 1371-98
20. Fugere P, Scheele WH, Shah A, *et al.* Uterine effects of raloxifene in comparison with continuous-combined hormone replacement therapy in postmenopausal women. *Am J Obstet Gynecol* 2000;182: 568-74
21. Freedman RR. Hot flushes and mechanisms. *Menopause* 2002:9:151-2
22. Stearns V, Ullimer L, Lopez JF, *et al.* Hot flushes. *Lancet* 2002;360:1851-61
23. Davies GC, Huster WJ, Lu Y, *et al.* Adverse events reported by postmenopausal women in controlled trials with raloxifene. *Obstet Gynecol* 1999; 93:558-65
24. Daly E, Vessey MP, Hawkins MM, *et al.* Risk of venous thromboembolism in users of hormone replacement therapy. *Lancet* 1996;348:977-80
25. Pritchard KI, Paterson AH, Paul NA, *et al.* Increased thromboembolic complications with concurrent tamoxifen and chemotherapy in a randomized trial of adjuvant therapy for women with breast cancer. National Cancer Institute of Canada Clinical Trials Group Breast Cancer Site Group. *J Clin Oncol* 1996;14:2731-7
26. Ettinger B, Black DM, Mitlak BH, *et al.* Reduction of vertebral fractures risk in postmenopausal women with osteoporosis treated with raloxifene: results from a 3-year randomized clinical trial. Multiple Outcomes of Raloxifene Evaluation (MORE) Investigators. *J Am Med Assoc* 1999; 282:637-45

# Clinical background of prescribing tibolone 16

*F. A. Helmond*

## INTRODUCTION

Tibolone (Livial®) is indicated for the relief of climacteric symptoms and prevention of osteoporosis in postmenopausal women. Tibolone expresses estrogenic effects in a tissue-selective manner, resulting in desired estrogenic effects on tissues such as the brain, bone and vagina, while avoiding the undesired estrogenic effects on the endometrium and breast[1].

The effect on climacteric symptoms and on bone is due to the conversion of tibolone into two estrogenic 3-OH metabolites. These two metabolites can fully activate the estrogen receptor (ER) and have a high preference for ERα[2]. Although the two estrogenic metabolites have a lower intrinsic activity than estradiol, they are present in sufficient quantities in the circulation to generate a full estrogenic response. Tibolone and its metabolites cannot be metabolized into compounds with an aromatic A-ring, which would increase their intrinsic estrogenic activity, because they are not a substrate for the enzyme aromatase[3].

Increased estrogenic activity is not seen in the endometrium or the breast during tibolone treatment. In breast tissue, inhibition of sulfatase activity and stimulation of sulfotransferase activity leads to a reduced local estrogenic activity of both endogenous and exogenous estrogenic metabolites[4,5]. Tibolone and its metabolites do not inhibit or stimulate the enzyme aromatase[3]. In the endometrium, estrogenic stimulation is prevented by the local formation of the Δ-4 isomer, a metabolite with progestagenic and androgenic activity[6]. The local formation of the Δ-4 isomer in the endometrium is very important because the peripheral circulating levels of the Δ-4 isomer are low and, due to the short half-life of the Δ-4 isomer, levels are undetectable after a few hours[7].

The tissue-selective effects of tibolone are mediated by means of regulating pre-receptor events in contrast to selective estrogen receptor modulators (SERMs) that accomplish their tissue selectivity by means of modulating the ER. Tibolone is the first in a new class of compounds called 'selective tissue estrogenic activity regulators' (STEARs)[8].

## THE EFFECTS OF TIBOLONE ON BREAST

The observational UK Million Women Study (MWS) reported for the first time an increased breast cancer risk for tibolone (relative risk (RR), 1.45; 95% confidence interval (CI), 1.25–1.67) similar to estrogens only (RR, 1.30; 95% CI, 1.21–1.40), but substantially less compared to combined estrogen and progesterone products (RR, 2.00; 95% CI, 1.88–2.12)[9]. These results are surprising and at odds with the preclinical and clinical data about the effects of tibolone on breast, which will be briefly discussed further on. The data are also not biologically plausible, taking into account the specific mechanism of action of tibolone on breast tissue (see the editorial by Speroff[10] for more details).

## PRECLINICAL *IN VIVO* DATA

In the DMBA rat breast cancer model, tibolone exerts protective effects similar to tamoxifen[1] and in cynomolgus monkeys, tibolone did not increase breast proliferation, as measured by the proliferation marker Ki67. This in contrast to estrogens only and, even more notably, estrogens combined with progestins[11].

## CLINICAL DATA

A number of studies have demonstrated that the incidence of breast pain is clearly less in tibolone treated patients compared to continuous combined estrogen-progestin therapy (CCEPT)[12]. Also, the well-known increase in mammographic density seen with CCEPT is practically absent with tibolone[12,13]. The proliferation marker Ki67 in postmenopausal women on tibolone also reflects an absence of breast stimulation[13,14].

## EPIDEMIOLOGICAL DATA

The MWS has recruited over 1 million women in the UK between 50 and 64 years of age via the national breast screening centers. Data about the type and duration of HT use were collected at baseline and the average follow-up period for breast cancer detection was 2.6 years and for death due to breast cancer 4.1 years. The results suggest that all types of hormone therapy are associated with a statistically significantly increased risk of breast cancer (Table 1).

The magnitude of the risk was substantially greater for estrogen plus progestins than for estrogens alone and tibolone ($p < 0.0001$).

The relative risks observed in the MWS are higher than most other published data on estrogen plus progestin therapy (EPT) and estrogen-only therapy (ET)[15]. As such, the MWS is an outlier in the magnitude of the increase in risk of breast cancer found with ET, EPT and tibolone (see below). A possible explanation for this is that the study recruited participants from breast cancer screening centers (a population know to be self-selected and to have a higher baseline risk for breast cancer). For a detailed discussion about the MWS, see the contribution of Shapiro in this volume.

To date, one other epidemiological study has investigated the relation between tibolone and breast cancer. This is a case-control study using the UK GPRD database[16]. This study did not find an increased risk of breast cancer for tibolone and the data from that study on ET and EPT are similar to those of the previously published data (Table 2).

Recently, the National Institutes of Health have announced the discontinuation of the randomized placebo-controlled estrogen-only arm of the WHI study. One of the most important findings of this study was that no increase in breast cancer risk has been observed in women taking estrogen only for about 7 years. This further supports the impression that the relative risks in the MWS are overestimated. The British Menopause Society mentioned, in their position statement[17] about the discontinued estrogen-only arm, 'Estrogen alone does not increase breast cancer risk according to this WHI study, and hence, since the Million Women Study found that tibolone had the same risk for breast cancer as unopposed estrogen, it is probable that tibolone also does not increase breast cancer risk'.

An additional factor that might contribute to the unexpected increase in breast cancer risk for

**Table 1** The Million Women Study: hormone therapy and breast cancer risk

| | *Relative risk* | *95% confidence interval* |
|---|---|---|
| Estrogen + progestin | 2.00 | 1.88–2.12 |
| Estrogens only | 1.30 | 1.21–1.40 |
| Tibolone | 1.45 | 1.25–1.68 |

**Table 2** The UK GPRD Study: hormone therapy and breast cancer risk

| | *Million Women Study* | *Allen et al.*[16] |
|---|---|---|
| Observation period | 1996–2001 | 1992–1998 |
| Breast cancers | 7140 | 7192 |
| *Relative risk (95% confidence interval)* | | |
| Estrogen + progestin | 2.00 (1.88–2.12) | 1.21 (1.12–1.30)* |
| Estrogen only | 1.30 (1.21–1.40) | 0.97 (0.86–1.08) |
| Tibolone | 1.45 (1.25–1.68) | 1.02 (0.78–1.33) |

*The Allen data refer to the use of sequential estrogen + progestin therapy only because the later introduction of continuous combined estrogen + progestin therapy in the UK market occurred later in the observation period. This resulted in a too limited number of cases of women treated with continuous combined estrogen + progestin therapy

tibolone in the MWS is selective prescribing of tibolone to women at greater risk for breast cancer, as suggested in editorials about the MWS by Speroff[9] and Olsson[18]. In fact, if this phenomenon indeed exists, then most likely all observational trials would show an inflated relative risk for breast cancer with tibolone.

## PREFERENTIAL PRESCRIBING OF TIBOLONE: QUALITATIVE RESEARCH

In 2000, qualitative research was initiated to investigate whether preferential prescribing of tibolone occurred in European countries. The study was conducted in five European countries by means of indepth face-to-face interviews. In total, 50 gynecologists or gynecological oncologists were interviewed from five different countries, each treating an average of 79 menopausal patients per month. The results presented in Table 3 make it evident that there was preferential prescribing of tibolone in patients at risk for breast cancer, by a factor of 3–4.

## PREFERENTIAL PRESCRIBING OF TIBOLONE: A UK DATABASE STUDY

Quantitative research about preferential prescribing was conducted by Velthuis and colleagues in the Mediplus database, which is a primary-care UK database[19]. In this study, the risk factors associated with breast cancer were compared in women who were prescribed either tibolone (Livial) or EPT. The results show that women most recently prescribed Livial have more frequently than expected a history of breast diseases (about 20%) and a history of breast cancer (about three times).

**Table 3** Selective prescribing of tibolone

| | *All patients (mean)* | *Only patients at risk for breast cancer (mean)* |
|---|---|---|
| Netherlands | 25% | 90% |
| UK | 20% | 64% |
| Germany | 17% | 80% |
| Austria | 17% | 94% |
| Switzerland | 13% | 61% |

## CLINICAL TRIAL DATA

The above-mentioned data indicate that preferential prescribing of tibolone to patients with an increased risk for breast cancer occurs. This has consequences for the outcome of observational trials, as they will all tend to overestimate the risk for breast cancer with tibolone. Only large, randomized trials of sufficient duration will reveal the relation between tibolone treatment and the risk for breast cancer. An estimate can be achieved from Organon's own clinical trial database. This database does not yet have sufficient numbers of breast cancer events to produce a reliable estimate, but at this time available data do not suggest an increased risk (Table 4).

Data from landmark clinical trials, such as the ongoing placebo-controlled, randomized LIFT trial (bone fracture rate trial; 4538 subjects enrolled; 5-year study) will most likely provide enough data to achieve a reliable estimate of the relative risk.

The ongoing LIBERATE trial is seeking to enroll at least 2600 women with a history of breast cancer. This randomized, double-blind, placebo-controlled trial investigates the effects of tibolone treatment on the disease-free interval (breast cancer recurrence) in this specific target population. The main analysis is planned 4 years after randomizing the 1st subject. At present (April 1, 2004), more than 1900 subjects have been recruited.

**Table 4** Organon's clinical trial database: breast cancer incidence and relative risk during tibolone treatment

| | *Tibolone* | *Placebo* | *Relative risk (95% confidence interval)* |
|---|---|---|---|
| Number of subjects | 3412 | 1229 | |
| Exposure (woman-years) | 3716 | 1815 | 0.61 (0.22–1.78) |
| Breast cancer incidence | 2.69 | 4.41 | |

## CONCLUSION

Preferential prescribing of tibolone to patients with increased risk for breast cancer has been demonstrated in both quantitative as well as qualitative research. This phenomenon may bias observational studies like the Million Women Study and may lead to overestimated relative risks in those studies. A case-control study with similar numbers of breast cancer patients as in the Million Women Study did not reveal an increased risk and neither did randomized, clinical trials. Large tibolone trials are ongoing and will establish the relation between (long-term) tibolone treatment and the risk for breast cancer.

# References


1. Kloosterboer HJ. Tibolone: a steroid with a tissue-selective mode of action. *J Steroid Biochem Mol Biol* 2001;76:231-8
2. De Gooyer ME, Deckers GH, Schoonen WGEJ, Verheul HAM, Kloosterboer HJ. Receptor profiling and endocrine interactions of tibolone. *Steroids* 2003;68:21-30
3. De Gooyer ME, Oppers-Tiemissen HM, Leysen D, Verheul HAM, Kloosterboer HJ. Tibolone is not converted by human aromatase to 7α-methyl-17α-ethynylestradiol (7α-MEE): analysis with sensitive bio-assays for estrogens and androgens and with LC-MSMS. *Steroids* 2003;68:235-43
4. De Gooyer ME, Overklift GT, Kleyn V, *et al.* Tibolone: a compound with tissue specific inhibitory effects on sulfatase. *Mol Cell Endocrinol* 2001; 183:55-62
5. Chetrite GS, Pasqualini JR. The selective estrogen enzyme modulator (SEEM) in breast cancer. *J Steroid Biochem Mol Biol* 2001;76:95-104
6. Tang B, Markiewicz L, Kloosterboer HJ, Gurpide E. Human endometrial 3β-hydroxysteroid dehydrogenase/isomerase can locally reduce intrinsic estrogenic/progestagenic activity ratios of a steroidal drug (Org OD 14). *J Steroid Biochem Mol Biol* 1993; 45:345-51
7. Vos RM, Krebbers S, Verhoeven C, Delbressine L. *In vivo* human metabolism of tibolone. *Drug Metab Dispos* 2002;30:106-12
8. Smith CL, O'Malley BW. Coregulator function: a key to understanding tissue specificity of selective receptor modulators. *Endocr Rev* 2004;25:45-71
9. Million Women Study Collaborators. Breast cancer and hormone replacement therapy in the Million Women Study. *Lancet* 2003;362:419-27
10. Speroff L. The Million Women Study and breast cancer. *Maturitas* 2003;46:1-6
11. Cline JM, Register TC, Clarkson TB. Effects of tibolone and hormone replacement therapy on the breast of cynomolgus monkeys. *Menopause* 2002; 9:422-9
12. Lundström E, Christow A, Kersemaekers W, *et al.* Effects of tibolone and a continuous combined hormone replacement therapy on mammographic breast density. *Am J Obstet Gynecol* 2002; 186:717-22
13. Valdivia I, Campodónico I, Tapia A, Capetillo M, Espinoza A, Lavín P. Effects of tibolone and continuous combined hormone therapy on mammographic breast density and breast histochemical markers in postmenopausal women. *Fertil Steril* 2004;81:617-23
14. Conner P, Christow A, Kersemaekers W, *et al.* A comparative study of breast cell proliferation during hormone replacement therapy: effects of tibolone and continuous combined estrogen-progestogen treatment. *Climacteric* 2004;7:50-9
15. Gambacciani M, Genazzani AR. The study with a million women (and hopefully fewer mistakes). *Gynecol Endocrinol* 2003;17:359-62
16. Allen DS, de Vries CS, Farmer RDT. Pharmaceutical content and regimen of hormone replacement therapy and risk of breast cancer. *Pharmacoepidemiology Drug Safety* 2002;11(Suppl 1):296
17. Stevenson J, Rees M. Termination of the oestrogen alone arm of the Women's Health Initiative 2004. http://www.the-bms.org/news.htm
18. Olsson H. What we can learn from the Million Women Study. *Maturitas* 2003;46:87-9
19. Velthuis-te Wierik EJM, Hendricks PT, Boerstoel-Streefland M. Clinical background of women prescribed tibolone or combined estrogen + progestogen therapies: a UK Mediplus® study. *Climacteric* 2004;7:197-209

# Specific products for individual therapy 17

*R. Schürmann and T. Faustmann*

## INTRODUCTION

The results of the Women's Health Initiative (WHI) study on hormone replacement therapy (HRT) contribute to a growing body of information on the prevention and control of major medical diseases that affect postmenopausal women. Since the trial examined only the daily combination of 0.626 mg of conjugated equine estrogens (CEE) plus 2.5 mg of medroxyprogesterone acetate (MPA) (Prempro®), the observed risk profile may not apply to lower doses or other types of hormones. Further study limitations (e.g. high number of drop-outs, unblinding, population selection, duration of treatment) must be taken into consideration when interpreting the study results. In addition, the study did not include the most beneficial effects of HRT, for instance relief of menopausal symptoms, in its overall benefit and risk evaluation. This is important because symptom relief is the primary motivation for women to start therapy. Therefore, the results of the WHI intervention trial are not sufficient to provide an all-encompassing assessment of the harm and benefit for HRT in the typical user population, neither for CEE/MPA nor for HRT in general.

### Schering's approach to future HRT

HRT is the most effective treatment for menopausal symptoms and the need for therapy of menopausal symptoms remains undisputed. The results of the WHI HRT study do not justify a general limitation of the use of continuous combined HRT products. An individual risk profile is essential for every woman contemplating hormone therapy and use of hormone therapy should be consistent with individual treatment goals.

Based on results of recent studies, trends towards *lower-dose* hormone therapy and *other administration routes* (patches, intrauterine systems) should be considered. Compounds with *additional benefits* are needed to offer individual therapeutic options. Highly differentiated products with unique potentials are expected to be available in the near future.

## LOWERING THE DOSE

Lowering the estrogen dose may minimize side-effects, while still providing a significant effect on menopausal symptoms and bone protection. Minimizing treatment side-effects may improve adherence to treatment schedules.

The efficacy and tolerability of very low-dose estrogen therapies for preventing postmenopausal bone loss are currently being assessed - and it seems possible that levels lower than those previously believed to be effective are in fact effective. A recently published placebo-controlled study assessed the effects of 3 years of treatment with a low dose of 0.25 mg/day of micronized 17β-estradiol on bone mineral density (BMD) in healthy older postmenopausal women. The results showed significant increases in BMD at all measured sites compared with controls. A meaningful difference in the incidence of side-effects, such as breast tenderness and changes in endometrial thickness, was not found between the verum and placebo groups[1]. However, is appears that this is still not the minimal effective estrogen dose. Cummings and colleagues[2] and Ettinger and colleagues[3] reported that postmenopausal women have an increased risk of hip and vertebral fracture with very low serum estradiol levels (levels below 5 pg/ml). In line with these observations, the concept of ultra-low-dose estrogen therapy was developed.

Menostar® is a *transdermal* delivery system containing estradiol in an acrylate adhesive matrix in a patch that is only 3.25 $cm^2$ large. Transdermal delivery is maintained over 7 days, delivering 14 μg estradiol daily - half the lowest dose available today. The therapeutic goal is to increase low endogenous estradiol to levels of at least 10 pg/ml.

## Results of an ultra-low-dose study

A multicenter, double-blind, randomized, placebo-controlled phase III study was performed to evaluate the efficacy and safety of this ultra-low-dose estradiol patch in the prevention of osteoporosis. A total of 417 postmenopausal women aged 60 years and older with intact uteri were included in the study. The primary efficacy variable was the percentage change of lumbar spine BMD from baseline to 2 years. The primary safety variable was the incidence of endometrial hyperplasia or cancer after 2 treatment years. All subjects took daily supplements of 800 mg calcium and 400 IU vitamin D in addition to the study treatment.

*Efficacy*

The ultra-low-dose estradiol patch was clinically and statistically superior to placebo in the prevention of osteoporosis in postmenopausal women over a 24-month period. In this group, the mean percentage increase (from baseline) of the lumbar spine BMD - the primary measure of efficacy - was statistically significantly increased ($p < 0.001$) after 24 months. The mean percentage increase in the total hip BMD - the secondary measure of efficacy - was also increased for the verum group after 24 months. The patients treated with ultra-low-dose estradiol also had significantly ($p < 0.001$) greater mean percentage increases in BMD of the lumbar spine and total hip, compared with placebo subjects, after 12 months (Table 1).

*Safety*

After 12 months, hyperplasia was not diagnosed in either treatment group. After 24 months, there was one (0.5%) ultra-low-dose estradiol patient with atypical endometrial hyperplasia. Endometrial cancer was not diagnosed at any time throughout the study in either treatment group. Overall, the endometrial biopsy data demonstrated endometrial safety for 24 months of unopposed treatment with estradiol. However, until more data are available, clinical surveillance is important during this therapy. Menostar® was well tolerated. Typical estrogen-related side-effects (such as vaginal bleeding, breast tenderness) were comparable to those with placebo.

*Summary*

In contrast to standard doses of estrogen used for HRT, treatment with Menostar® targets blood levels below 15 pg/ml and provides prevention of postmenopausal osteoporosis without simultaneous stimulation of the endometrium. Therefore, the ultra-low-dose estradiol patch is intended for unopposed estrogen in women with or without an intact uterus. Once approved, it will

**Table 1** Mean percentage change in bone mineral density from baseline in lumbar spine and total hip

| | *Lumbar spine* | | | *Total hip* | | |
|---|---|---|---|---|---|---|
| *Endpoint* | *Ultra-low estradiol* ($N = 208$) | *Placebo* ($N = 209$) | *p Value* | *Ultra-low estradiol* ($N = 208$) | *Placebo* ($N = 209$) | *p Value* |
| 12 months | $n = 189$<br>2.29 | $n = 186$<br>0.51 | < 0.001 | $n = 189$<br>0.90 | $n = 184$<br>–0.22 | < 0.001 |
| 24 months | $n = 189$<br>2.99 | $n = 186$<br>0.54 | < 0.001 | $n = 189$<br>0.84 | $n = 185$<br>–0.71 | < 0.001 |

$n$ = number of subjects with data available; $N$ = total number of subjects

be the only estrogen product without the need for a concomitant progestogen for women with an uterus. Menostar® represents a new treatment paradigm for prevention of postmenopausal osteoporosis based on an ultra-low estradiol dose.

## LOCAL ACTION

The Mirena® levonorgestrel intrauterine system (LNG-IUS) releases 20 µg/day levonorgestrel into the uterine cavity at a relatively constant rate for 5 years. In addition to contraception, the LNG-IUS can be used for therapeutic indications, such as the treatment of idiopathic menorrhagia. The perimenopause is characterized by increased occurrence of dysfunctional uterine bleeding. The LNG-IUS can be used, together with an estrogen of choice, for the treatment of climacteric symptoms that begin in the perimenopause.

Effectiveness in endometrial protection is supported by the lack of any endometrial hyperplasia in the re-evaluation of 1891 endometrial samples taken during the clinical studies of LNG-IUS use in combination with estrogen therapy[4].

The Mirena® concept has been further improved with the intention that it is more suitable for women with advanced uterine atrophy. The menopausal levonorgestrel system (MLS) was developed as a 3-year progestogen intrauterine treatment for postmenopausal women on estrogen replacement therapy. MLS releases approximately 10 µg of levonorgestrel *in vitro*. The rationale for the development of the MLS was to provide an even lower local dose of levonorgestrel than Mirena® to counteract the estrogen-induced stimulation of the endometrium. Because of the high *local* concentration of levonorgestrel, unscheduled bleeding and spotting, as well as effects attributable to systemic progestogens, are further reduced. The small size of the MLS makes insertion easier compared to Mirena® for postmenopausal women who have an involuted uterus and narrowed cervical canal. At 1 year after insertion, the amenorrhea rates for women using MLS and Mirena® in conjunction with estrogen therapy are 76% and 91%, respectively. Endometrial hyperplasia is effectively prevented in women using the MLS combined with estrogen therapy after up to 3 years of follow-up[5].

*Summary*

Mirena® and MLS are excellent options for effective local endometrial progestogenic effects while minimizing systemic side-effects. Selecting the estrogen component, based on the lowest effective dose and preferred application mode, allows for high flexibility when tailoring hormone therapy to an individual woman's needs.

## DIFFERENTIATED PROGESTOGEN

Angeliq® is a new low-dose (1 mg 17β-estradiol) product, which contains drospirenone, a novel progestogen with aldosterone receptor antagonist activity and antiandrogenic activity.

Progestogen should be added to estrogen therapy for all postmenopausal women with an intact uterus to prevent the elevated risk of estrogen-induced endometrial hyperplasia and adenocarcinoma[6]. By changing the progestogen type, route, or regimen, clinicians can individualize therapy to minimize side-effects. Natural progesterone has low oral bioavailability, unfavorable metabolism and a short plasma half-life, and so it has been necessary to synthesize suitable alternatives in order to develop effective hormonal replacement therapies. While certain progestogens used in continuous combined HRT preparations may counteract the positive effects of estradiol, aldosterone antagonists (e.g. spironolactone and eplerenone) have cardiovascular benefits based on their mode of action. Some of the possible cardiovascular benefits associated with aldosterone antagonism include:

(1) Increased sodium excretion and prevention of edema and weight gain[7-9];

(2) Improved diastolic function[10];

(3) Decreased systolic and diastolic blood pressure[11-13].

Ideally, synthetic progestogens should demonstrate the same hormonal properties as progesterone itself, i.e. a combination of progestogenic, antialdosterone and antiandrogenic properties.

The only currently available progestogen which closely matches the pharmacological profile of endogenous progesterone is drospirenone[14]. The antimineralocorticoid effect of 3 mg drospirenone is equivalent to approximately 20–25 mg of spironolactone. This antialdosterone activity has not been found for any other synthetic progestogen. Clinical studies with Angeliq® also evaluated cardiovascular effects known to be due to aldosterone receptor antagonism.

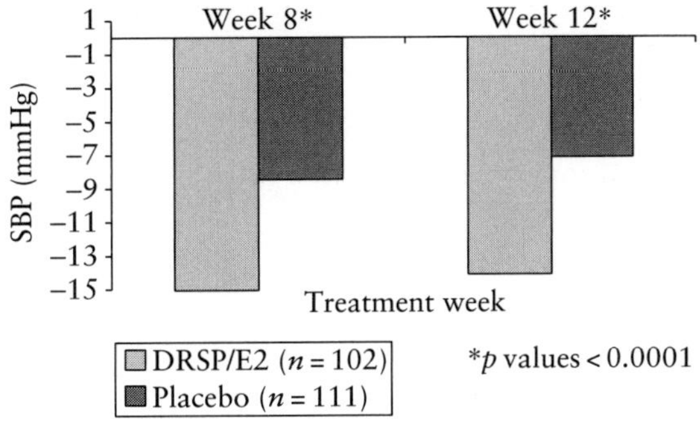


**Figure 1** Effects of 3 mg drospirenone/1 mg 17β-estradiol (DRSP/E2) on blood pressure in women with stage I hypertension: change from baseline in systolic blood pressure (SBP). *n*, number of subjects with data available

## Blood pressure effects of drospirenone/estradiol in women with stage I hypertension

A multicenter, double-blind, randomized, placebo-controlled phase III study was performed to evaluate the effect of a continuous combined HRT preparation containing 3 mg drospirenone and 1 mg 17β-estradiol (DRSP/E2) on blood pressure in postmenopausal women with stage I hypertension.

Changes in systolic blood pressure were measured as the primary efficacy parameter. Secondary efficacy parameters were changes in diastolic blood pressure, mean blood pressure and, using ambulatory blood pressure monitoring (ABPM) over a 24-h period (performed at baseline and week 12 in a subgroup of 43 patients), changes in mean systolic and diastolic 24-h blood pressure. A total of 213 mildly hypertensive postmenopausal women, aged 45–80 years were randomized and treated for 12 weeks.

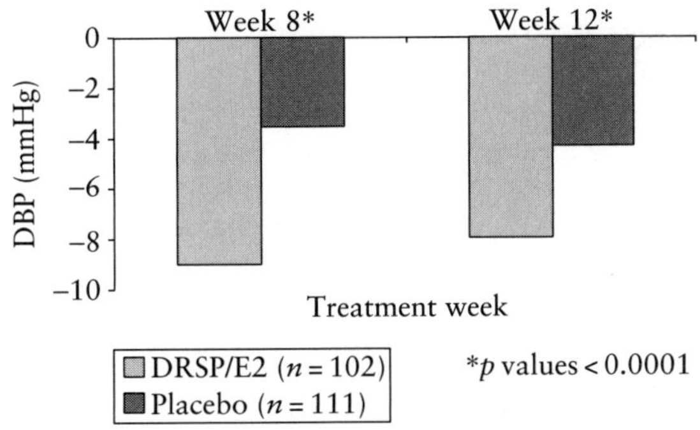


**Figure 2** Effects of 3 mg drospirenone/1 mg 17β-estradiol (DRSP/E2) on blood pressure in women with stage I hypertension: change from baseline in diastolic blood pressure (DBP). *n*, number of subjects with data available

*Results*

The DRSP/E2 group exhibited statistically significantly greater reductions (from baseline) in systolic and diastolic blood pressures at the week 8 and week 12 end-points, compared with the placebo group (Figures 1 and 2). At week 12 in the ABPM subgroup, reductions in mean systolic blood pressure values measured over a 24-h period as well as during the daytime were statistically significant in the DRSP/E2 group compared with the placebo group (Figure 3). The mean difference in reduction from baseline in daytime diastolic blood pressure between the two groups was statistically significant at week 12. In both groups, the mean systolic blood pressure decreased from baseline values of about 145 mmHg already in week 2. The reduction was consistently more pronounced in the DRSP/E2 group. After discontinuation of medication, the blood pressures in both groups were similar (Figure 4). For the mean diastolic blood pressure, similar data were recorded, however on a lower level.

*Summary*

In summary, consistent statistically and clinically significant reductions in systolic and diastolic

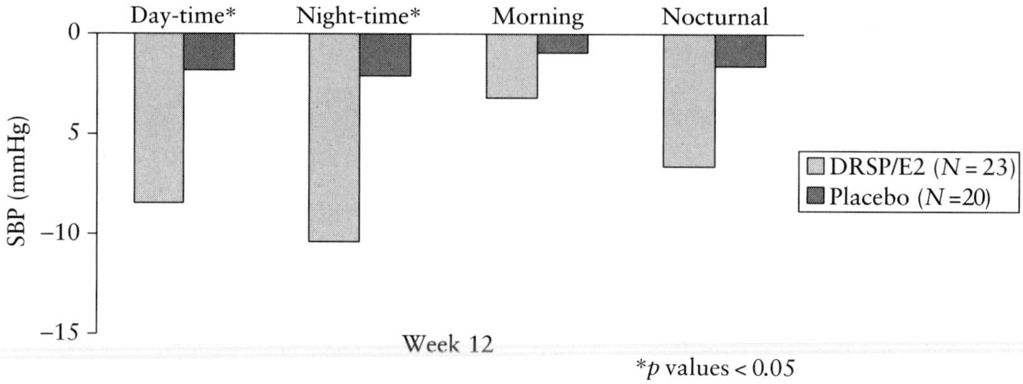


Day-time, 06:00–22:00; Night-time, 22:00–06.00; Morning, 04:00–08:00

**Figure 3** Effects of 3 mg drospirenone/1 mg 17β-estradiol (DRSP/E2) on blood pressure in women with stage I hypertension: ambulatory systolic blood pressure measurement (SBP). *N*, total number of subjects

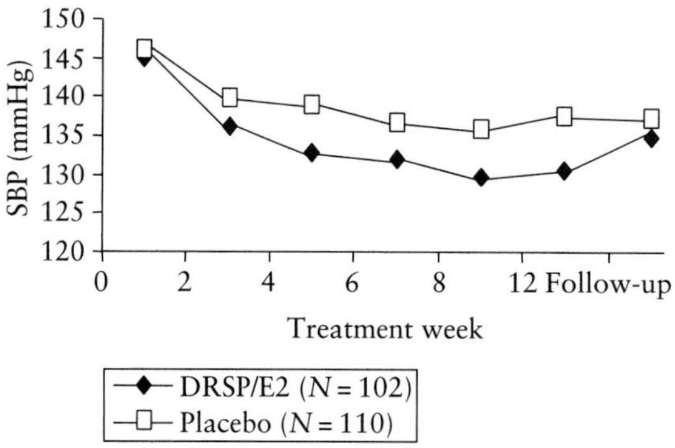


**Figure 4** Effects of 3 mg drospirenone/1 mg 17β-estradiol (DRSP/E2) in women with stage I hypertension: mean systolic blood pressure (SBP)

blood pressure with DRSP/E2 compared to placebo were demonstrated. This HRT preparation effectively lowers blood pressure in mildly hypertensive postmenopausal women.

*Why are the blood pressure results of the Angeliq® studies important?*

There is a high prevalence of hypertension in industrialized countries (30–40%). In the USA, the prevalence of hypertension in women between the ages of 50 and 79 years ranges from 36% in Caucasian women to 59% in African-American women[15]. The American Heart Association reported that about 17 000 women in the USA died from hypertension and 267 000 women were discharged from hospital with hypertension in 1999 alone[16]. Hypertension is a major risk factor for cardiovascular disease, which is still the leading cause of death in European and North American societies[17]. Elevated blood pressure is the most important and the most prevalent modifiable risk factor for stroke[18]. A blood pressure reduction of 10–12 mmHg systolic and 5–6 mmHg diastolic can lead to a 38% decline in stroke incidence and 19% reduction of coronary heart disease events[19].

The blood pressure-lowering effect of Angeliq® is a beneficial treatment effect, especially in mildly hypertensive women. When combined with drospirenone, the well-known favorable effects of estradiol are not attenuated.

## CONCLUSIONS

There is an unequivocal need for therapies that safely and effectively address climacteric symptoms and prevent osteoporosis as a significant medical problem. Acknowledging the recent trends in view of the recent studies, lower-dose hormone therapy (e.g. Menostar®) and other administrations routes (Mirena®) should be considered. Compounds with additional benefits (e.g. the new progestogen drospirenone) will offer individual therapeutic options.

# References


1. Prestwood KM, Kenny AM, Kleppinger A, *et al.* Ultralow-dose micronized 17beta-estradiol and bone density and bone metabolism in older women: a randomized controlled trial. *J Am Med Assoc* 2003;90:1042–8
2. Cummings SR, Browner WS, Bauer D, *et al.* Endogenous hormones and the risk of hip and vertebral fractures among older women. *N Engl J Med* 1998;339:733–8
3. Ettinger B, Pressman A, Sklarin P, *et al.* Associations between low levels of serum estradiol, bone density, and fractures among elderly women: the study of osteoporotic fractures. *J Clin Endocrinol Metab* 1998;83:2239–43
4. Villikka K. Mirena protection from endometrial hyperplasia during estrogen replacement therapy. *Schering Oy Expert report* 1.4.2003
5. Raudaskoski T, Tapanainen J, Tomas E, *et al.* Intrauterine 10 μg and 20 μg levonorgestrel systems in postmenopausal women receiving oral oestrogen replacement therapy: clinical, endometrial and metabolic response. *Br J Obstet Gynaecol* 2002;109:136–44
6. The North American Menopause Society. Role of progestogen in hormone therapy for postmenopausal women: Position statement of The North American Menopause Society. *Menopause* 2003;10:113–32
7. Cody RJ. Sodium and water retention on congestive heart failure – the pivotal role of the kidney. *Am J Hypertens* 1988;1:395S–401S
8. Horisberger JD, Rossier BC. Aldosterone regulation of gene transcription leading to control of ion transport. *Hypertension* 1992;19:221–7
9. Whorwood CB, Ricketts ML, Stewart PM. Regulation of sodium-potassium adenosine triphosphate subunit gene expression by corticosteroids and 11 beta-hydroxysteroid dehydrogenase activity. *Endocrinology* 1994;135:901–10
10. Tsutamoto T, Wada A, Maeda K, *et al.* Spironolactone inhibits the transcardiac extraction of aldosterone in patients with congestive heart failure. *J Am Coll Cardiol* 2000;36:838–44
11. Sato A, Suzuki Y, Saruta T. Effects of spironolactone and angiotensin-converting enzyme inhibitor on left ventricular hypertrophy in patients with essential hypertension. *Hypertens Res* 1999;22:17–22
12. Zannad F. Vascular and cardiac actions of aldosterone and spironolactone. *Z Kardiol* 1991;80 (Suppl 7):103–5
13. Plouin PF, Battaglia C, Alhenc-Gelas F, *et al.* Are angiotensin converting enzyme inhibition and aldosterone antagonism equivalent in hypertensive patients over fifty? *Am J Hypertens* 1991; 4:356–62
14. Fuhrmann U, Krattenmacher R, Slater EP, *et al.* The novel progestin drospirenone and its natural counterpart progesterone: biochemical profile and antiandrogenic potential. *Contraception* 1996;54: 243–51
15. Wasserheil-Smoller S, Anderson G, Psaty BM, *et al.* Hypertension and its treatment in postmenopausal women: baseline data from the women's health initiative. *Hypertension* 2000;36: 780–9
16. American Heart Association. *2002 Heart and Stroke Statistical Update*. Dallas, Texas: American Heart Association, 2001
17. Thom TJ. International mortality from heart disease: rates and trends. *Int J Epidemiol* 1989;18 (Suppl 1):520–9
18. Collins R, Peto R, MacMahon S, *et al.* Blood pressure, stroke, and coronary heart disease. 2. Short-term reductions in blood pressure: overview of randomised drug trials in their epidemiological context. *Lancet* 1990;335:827–39
19. MacMahon S. Blood pressure and the prevention of stroke. *J Hypertens Suppl* 1996;14:S39–46

# Are all HRT preparations the same? 18

*E. Lang and V. Rakov*

## INTRODUCTION

The findings from the Heart and Estrogen/progestin Replacement Study (HERS)[1] and from the Women's Health Initiative (WHI) study[2] have resulted in a revision of the benefit and risk profile of hormone treatment in postmenopausal women. These studies alerted physicians and patients not only to the use of hormone replacement therapy (HRT) for cardiovascular prevention, but questioned the cardiovascular safety of HRT in general. At the same time, these investigations, partially due to the press and mass media reaction, dwarfed the other studies with controversial results and significantly restricted the view on the benefit and risk profile of HRT.

In this paper, we do not intend to criticize the HERS and the WHI study; the strengths and weaknesses of these studies have already been analyzed by many leading HRT experts. Our starting position is the statement issued at the National Institutes for Health (NIH) meeting in October 2002: '*Equine estrogens may have different pharmacodynamic properties from other estrogens; medroxyprogesterone acetate is not a component of any other combination hormone product, and therefore it is not possible to extrapolate the dose and toxicity findings from the WHI*'[3]. Indeed, only one HRT combination has been investigated in both clinical trials: 0.625 mg conjugated equine estrogens (CEE) and 2.5 mg medroxyprogesterone acetate (MPA). Other HRT combinations, for instance containing estradiol (E2) + norethisterone acetate (NETA), differ from CEE/MPA in their chemical composition and pharmacological and clinical profiles. Low-dose combinations like 1 mg E2 and 0.5 mg NETA also possess a different estrogenic potency because of a lower dose of estrogen compared to 0.625 mg CEE. The differentiation of E2 and NETA compared to CEE and MPA with regard to their pharmacokinetic and pharmacodynamic profiles is the focus of this paper.

## MATTER OF DIFFERENT SUBSTANCES

### Conjugated equine estrogens versus 17β-estradiol

Conjugated equine estrogens, derived from pregnant mares' urine, are comprised of a mixture of estrogens and possibly more than 200 other chemical components, including progestins and androgens[4-8]. To date, ten of the estrogen components of Premarin have been documented in the literature (Figure 1). The United States Pharmacopeia (USP) provides standards for five of the ten identified estrogen components of Premarin (Table 1)[9], which are believed to comprise less than 50% of the total steroidal content of Premarin[10].

In estradiol-containing combinations, 17β-estradiol is the only one estrogen component that is chemically and biologically identical to the endogenous human hormone.

Comparison of the pharmacokinetics of the estrogens in preparations containing 17β-estradiol and CEE is difficult because of the variety of CEE components. The pharmacokinetic parameters for E2 are easy to obtain and they are reported in every package insert for the HRT products with E2. The package insert for Premarin/Prempro includes pharmacokinetic information for estrone and equilin, but not for their significantly more potent metabolites, 17β-estradiol and 17β-dihydroequilin[4].

There are investigations demonstrating that it is impossible to assess quantitatively the expected conversion of the estrogen precursors like estrone

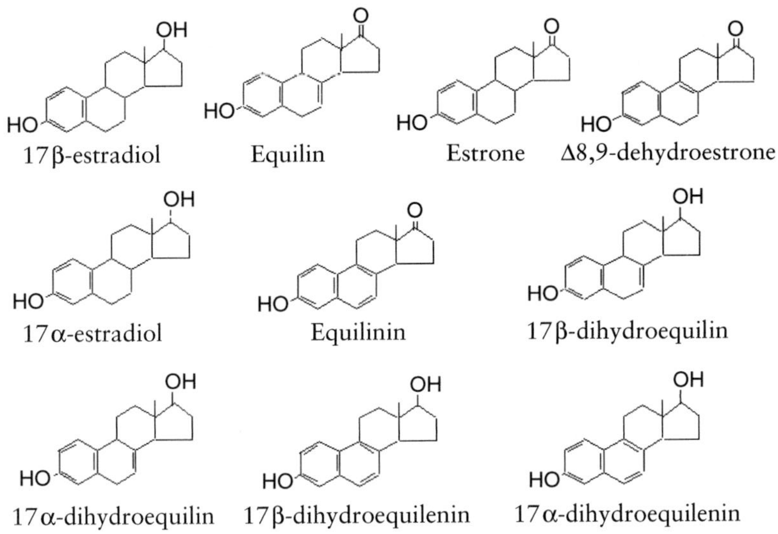


**Figure 1** Documented estrogen components of Premarin

**Table 1** United States Pharmacopeia monograph for conjugated estrogens

| *Estrogen* | *% of labelled content* |
|---|---|
| Estrone | 52.5–61.5* |
| Equilin | ≤ 30 |
| 17α-dihydroequilin | 13.5–19.5 |
| 17α-estradiol | 2.5–9.5 |
| 17β-dihydroequilin | ≤ 4.0 |

*Total of estrone + equilin to be 79.5–88% of label claim

or equilin into their hormonally active metabolites. For example, tablet concentrations of estrone are more than twice those of equilin, but serum levels of 17β-dihydroequilin (active metabolite of equilin) are 1.6 times as high as those of 17β-estradiol (active metabolite of estrone)[5]. Also, the detectable serum concentration of the dehydroestrone sulfate (DHES) metabolite, 17β-Δ8,9-dehydroestradiol, is significantly higher (one-half that of 17β-estradiol) than expected from the tablet content of DHES[5], and the 'diols' are known to be the most potent form of estrogens *in vivo*.

In addition to the substantial differences in the pharmacokinetic profile between E2 and CEE, one can state that estrogens do not exert their effects in a uniform manner with respect to different target tissues. The differential effects may be due to variable pharmacokinetics and tissue metabolism, or tissue-specific transcription factors as well.

Recent work investigating the mechanism of gene activation by estrogens and antiestrogens, particularly in non-reproductive tissue, suggests that estrogen receptors in combination with different estrogens may be able to regulate more than one hormone responsive element on the DNA[11]. This can explain why one estrogen can be more active than another in a specific tissue or organ. The FDA Memorandum also refers to the results of clinical studies which suggest that CEE may also have different effects on cardiovascular risk parameters, such as lipoprotein levels, peroxidation, and vasodilatation[5]. The results of recent clinical studies have shown that the clinical consequences of such differences are still not known and that favorable changes of surrogate parameters do not necessarily mean the improvement of cardiovascular safety.

## Medroxyprogesterone acetate versus norethisterone acetate

MPA (a 17α-hydroxyprogesterone derivative) and NETA (a 19-nortestosterone derivative) differ in their chemical structure, as shown in Figure 2. This difference may account for their different

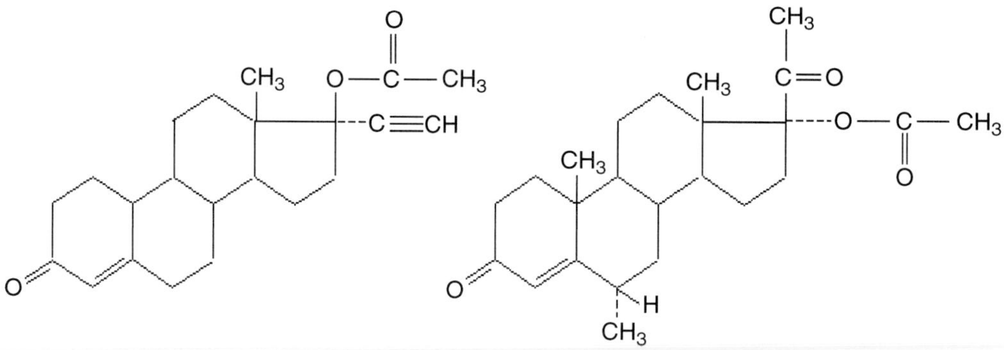

Norethisterone acetate (NETA) Medroxyprogesterone acetate (MPA)

**Figure 2** Structure of norethisterone acetate and medroxyprogesterone acetate

**Table 2** Spectrum of progestin effects*

| *Progestin* | *Antiestrogenic* | *Estrogenic* | *Androgenic* | *Antiandrogenic* | *Glucocorticoid* | *Anitmineralocorticoid* |
|---|---|---|---|---|---|---|
| Progesterone | + | – | – | (+) | (+) | + |
| Medroxyprogesterone acetate | + | – | (+) | – | + | – |
| Norethisterone | + | (+) | + | – | – | – |

*As demonstrated in preclinical studies; +, effect observed; (+), weak effect observed; –, no effect observed

affinities for steroid receptors and therefore for their different pharmacokinetic and pharmacodynamic profiles.

NETA and MPA exhibit different pharmacokinetic profiles. When given in combination with E2 or CEE, the half-life of MPA is more than three times longer than the half-life of NETA. It can be speculated that the half-life can influence the biological activity of the different progestins, potentially leading to differences in clinical effects.

As shown in Table 2, all progestins exhibit antiestrogenic effects, but differ in their affinities for other steroid receptors[12]. For example, comparing MPA and NETA, MPA demonstrates some glucocorticoid effects while NETA does not. In a clinical setting, glucocorticoid activity could play a role in expression of thrombin receptors and therefore in the pathophysiology of thrombosis[13].

The partial effects of the progestin component have been implicated in the safety and effectiveness of different estrogen–progestin combination therapies. Differences in receptor-binding activity can influence the pharmacodynamic profile of the preparations containing MPA or NETA. For example, the androgenic activity of NETA may be the reason for the observed additional anabolic effect of NETA on bone mass in patients treated with E2 and NETA[14]. Because of its partial glucocorticoid activity, MPA may be associated with adverse vascular effects in patients treated with CEE and MPA[1,2].

The interaction of different steroids with the various receptors may be relevant with regard to their effects on the cardiovascular system. Studies with cynomolgus monkeys, rabbits, and with human coronary artery smooth muscle cells have demonstrated distinctions between NETA and MPA regarding their respective vascular effects[15–20].

In a study in cynomolgus macaques with diet-induced atherosclerotic plaques, MPA reversed the positive effect of CEE on plaque size (Figure 3)[15]. In ovariectomized cholesterol-fed rabbits, treatment with NETA reduced aortic cholesterol content (Figure 4)[16]. In a direct comparison in

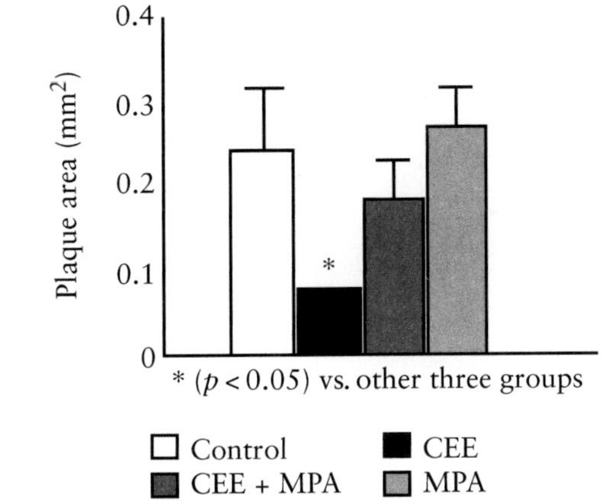


**Figure 3** Reversal of conjugated equine estrogens (CEE) reduction in diet-induced plaque formation by medroxyprogesterone acetate (MPA) in cynomolgus macaques

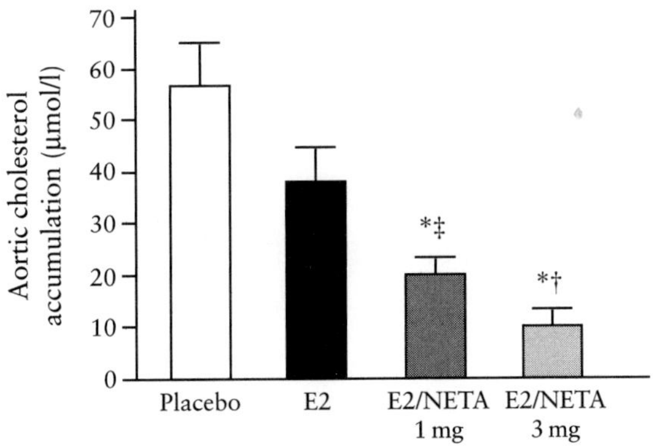


* Significantly different ($p = 0.001$) from placebo
‡ Significantly different ($p < 0.01$) from E2
† Significantly different ($p = 0.001$) from E2

**Figure 4** Reduction by norethisterone acetate (NETA) of cholesterol accumulation in the proximal thoracic aorta of ovariectomized cholesterol-fed rabbits. E2, 17β-estradiol

rabbits, MPA treatment resulted in significantly higher vascular reactivity than did treatment with NETA (Figure 5)[19].

The higher vascular reactivity has also been demonstrated in monkeys treated with CEE + MPA compared to those that were treated with ethinylestradiol and NETA (Figure 6)[20].

Summarizing, one can note the following results from the preclinical studies with MPA and NETA:

(1) In monkeys, MPA reversed the positive effect of CEE treatment on plaque size;

(2) In rabbits, NETA showed an additive effect to E2 in reducing aortic cholesterol content compared to placebo and E2 alone;

(3) In rabbits and in monkeys, NETA was associated with less vascular reactivity than MPA;

(4) In *in vitro* and *in vivo* experiments, NETA did not stimulate thrombin receptor production in smooth muscle cells and blood cells. MPA did stimulate thrombin receptor production in these studies.

It is possible that the observed differences in cardiovascular effects between MPA and NETA in these experimental and animal studies may be partly attributed to MPA's glucocorticoid activity.

## MATTER OF DOSE

As has already been mentioned, it is difficult to compare the doses of preparations containing CEE and E2 based on pharmacokinetic parameters, because the information about the active metabolites of CEE is scarce. There are some clinical studies, mostly investigating the influence of HRT on bone mineral density, which showed an average E2 concentration in patients treated with 0.625 mg CEE or different E2 dosages. In these studies, reported E2 levels with 1 mg E2 treatment were approximately 25–40 pg/ml compared to 40–109 pg/ml with 0.625 mg CEE treatment (Table 3)[21–23]. Reginster and colleagues[21] reported E2 levels observed after 6 months of treatment with 0.625 mg CEE that were approximately four times the level observed for subjects treated with 1 mg E2. Palacios and colleagues[22] reported serum E2 levels of approximately 40 pg/ml after 1 and 2 years of treatment with 0.625 mg CEE; similar E2 levels were reported by Delmas and colleagues[23] for 2 years of treatment with 1 mg E2. Serum E2 levels reflect the total estrogen potency of preparations containing E2. In studies with CEE, only one of the active or

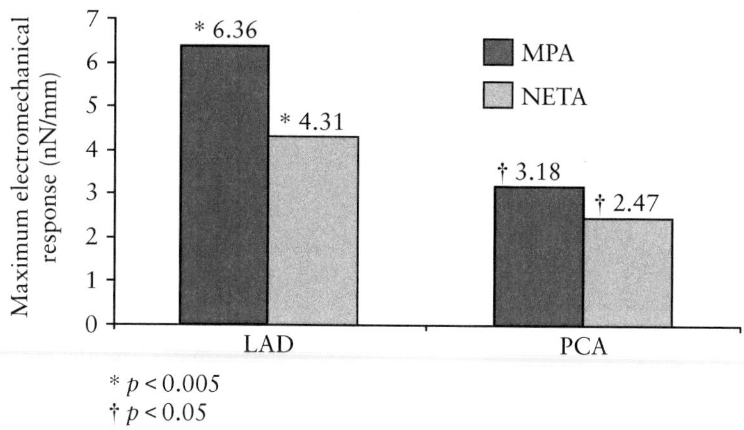


**Figure 5** Effect of medroxyprogesterone acetate (MPA) and norethisterone acetate (NETA) on electromechanical response in rabbit arteries. LAD, anterior descending coronary artery; PCA, posterior cerebral artery

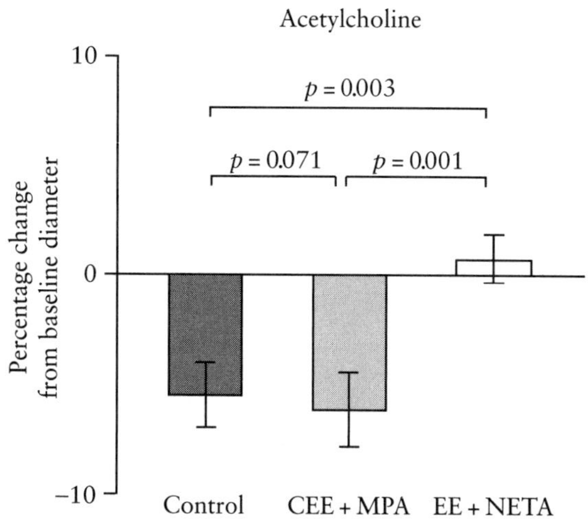


**Figure 6** Percentage of change from baseline in diameters of arteries as reaction to acetylcholine in Cynomolgus macaques. CEE, conjugated equine estrogens; MPA, medroxyprogesterone acetate; EE, ethinylestradiol

potentially active estrogen components of the CEE can be measured.

The interpretation of serum E2 levels in CEE-treated subjects is confounded by the known cross-reactivity of the different estrogen components of CEE for the E2 assay. Nevertheless, the total estrogenic potency of CEE is likely to be greater than that reflected by serum E2 levels, because of the added potency of the other estrogen components.

The comparison of the different dosages of CEE and E2 based on the clinical effects, like hot flushes, is also problematic because even relatively low doses of estrogens have a high impact on vasomotor complaints[24,25]. The measurement of specific biological parameters such as follicle stimulating hormone (FSH) and sex hormone binding globulin (SHBG) allows a more quantitative assessment of the biological effects of estrogens, compared to assessment of the effects on subjective symptoms such as hot flushes. In a study reported by Archer and colleagues, 12 weeks of treatment with 0.625 mg CEE reduced serum FSH levels by 50.3 mIU/ml compared to 34.6 mIU/ml after treatment with 1 mg E2, indicating a higher hypothalamic/pituitary effect of CEE as compared to E2[26]. As assessed by its effect on serum binding globulins, the potency of 0.625 mg CEE appears to be greater than that of 1 mg E2. 1 mg E2 is rather comparable with 0.3 mg CEE in its effect on hepatic metabolism as a quantifiable parameter for estrogenic potency (Table 4)[27].

The reduction of estrogen dose could be a crucial issue for the balanced efficacy and safety profile. This is confirmed in some recently published clinical studies and epidemiological investigations.

**Table 3** Serum estradiol (E2) levels observed in studies in prevention of postmenopausal bone loss

| *Study* | *Duration* (months) | *Daily estrogen treatment(s)* | *Estradiol serum level** (pg/ml) |
|---|---|---|---|
| Reginster[21] | 6 | 1 mg E2 valerate ($n$ = 14) | 25.3 |
| | | 2 mg E2 valerate ($n$ = 18) | 105.1 |
| | | 0.625 mg CEE ($n$ = 35) | 109.2 |
| Palacios[22] | 24 | 0.625 mg CEE ($n$ = 20) | 41.8 ± 3.9 (12 months) |
| | | | 39.6 ± 4.6 (24 months) |
| Delmas[23] | 24 | 1 mg E2/0.25 mg NETA ($n$ = 44) | 39 |
| | | 1 mg E2/0.5 mg NETA ($n$ = 46) | 41 |

*Serum levels of additional estrogens not reported for CEE treatments; CEE, conjugated equine estrogens; NETA, norethisterone acetate

**Table 4** Effect of different estrogens and doses on serum binding globulins

| *Estrogen* | *SHBG* | *CBG* | *Renin substrate* |
|---|---|---|---|
| E2 oral 1 mg | +60% | – | +85% |
| E2 oral 2 mg | +120% | +20% | +180% |
| CEE 0.3 mg | +50% | – | +50% |
| CEE 0.625 mg | +80% | +20% | +100% |
| CEE 1.25 mg | +120% | +50% | +250% |

SHBG, sex hormone binding globulin; CBG, corticosteroid binding globulin; E2, 17β-estradiol; CEE, conjugated equine estrogens

## DIFFERENT STUDIES, DIFFERENT OUTCOMES

Epidemiological data on dose relationship indicate that the reduction of estrogen dose may lead to the reduction of adverse events. Jick and colleagues[28] demonstrated the lowering of thromboembolic events in patients treated with 0.3 mg CEE compared to those treated with 0.625 mg or 1.25 mg CEE, with relative risks of 2.1, 3.3 and 6.9, respectively.

The recent evaluation from the Nurses' Health Study[29] clearly showed a significantly decreased risk of stroke in patients treated with 0.3 mg CEE (relative risk (RR), 0.54; 95% confidence interval (CI) 0.28–0.6), whereas the risk for women who received 0.625 mg or 1.25 mg CEE was increased (RR, 1.35; CI, 1.08–1.68 and RR, 1.63; CI, 1.18–2.26, respectively).

The results of controlled clinical studies suggest that E2 and NETA may have different effects on the cardiovascular safety parameters and clinical outcomes.

### The EPAT Study

The Estrogen and Prevention of Atherosclerosis Trial (EPAT) assessed the effects of unopposed 1 mg E2 and placebo on the progression of subclinical atherosclerosis by measuring carotid intima media thickness in postmenopausal women without pre-existing cardiovascular disease but with low density lipoprotein (LDL) cholesterol levels above 130 mg/dl[30]. Patients with LDL cholesterol levels above 160 mg/ml also received statin therapy. Progression of atherosclerosis was slowed in patients receiving unopposed E2 compared to patients receiving placebo. Additionally, E2 did not negatively affect the success of statin therapy.

### The ESPRIT Study

In the Estrogen Therapy for Prevention of Reinfarction in Postmenopausal Women (ESPRIT) study, 2 mg estradiol valerate was compared to placebo for the prevention of re-infarction in 1017 postmenopausal women aged 50–69 years who had survived a first myocardial infarction[31]. Evaluation of the results after 24 months of treatment showed a neutral effect of the treatment with estradiol. The frequency of re-infarction or cardiac death did not differ between the estradiol and placebo groups (RR, 0.99; CI, 0.7–1.41). A non-significant reduction in all-cause mortality in the estradiol group was also observed (RR, 0.79; CI,

0.5–1.27). The lowest risk of any death (RR, 0.56; CI, 0.23–1.33) and of cardiac death (RR, 0.33; CI, 0.11–1.01) was observed in estradiol-treated patients 3 months post-recruitment.

## The WHISP Pilot Study

The Women's Hormone Intervention Secondary Prevention (WHISP) pilot study assessed the safety of combined 1 mg E2 + 0.5 mg NETA and placebo in postmenopausal women with acute coronary syndrome[32]. The primary objective of the study was the assessment of the effect on cardiovascular surrogate parameters. Clinical outcomes, such as death and myocardial infarction, were assessed as secondary parameters. As shown in Table 5, there were no significant differences in clinical outcomes after 3 months of treatment, although there were significantly more coronary angiograms performed in the placebo group than in the 1 mg E2/0.5 mg NETA group. The results of this study did not suggest the presence of any increased risk with regard to cardiovascular safety associated with a low-dose HRT in this patient population.

**Table 5** Clinical outcomes reported in the WHISP study (3 months)

| *Clinical outcome* | *1 mg E2/0.5 mg NETA* ($n$ = 47) | *Placebo* ($n$ = 48) |
|---|---|---|
| Death, MI, stroke | 2 (4%) | 3 (6%) |
| Death, MI, stroke, CVD admissions | 8 (17%) | 12 (25%) |
| Gynecological events | 1 (2%) | 0 |
| Pulmonary embolism | 1 (2%) | 1 (2%) |

MI, myocardial infarction; CVD, cardiovascular disease; E2, 17β-estradiol; NETA, norethisterone acetate

## The Danish Osteoporosis Prevention Study

The Danish Osteoporosis Prevention Study (DOPS) was designed to study primary prevention of fractures in postmenopausal women receiving hormone treatment for a total follow-up period of 20 years. Data on serious adverse events such as cardiovascular and cerebrovascular incidents were also collected. A total of 723 women received either 2 mg E2 + 1 mg NETA as a sequential combination or 2 mg E2 unopposed; 1293 women received no treatment. The results from 5 years of follow-up were reported by Mosekilde and colleagues[33]. Four cases of cardiovascular events were reported in the treated group compared to seven cases in the non-treated group. There were no reports of venous thromboembolism in the study.

## CONCLUSIONS

It is beyond controversy that different hormonal substances possess different pharmacokinetic and pharmacodynamic profiles, different receptor affinities, and different effects on reproductive and non-reproductive organs (e.g. cardiovascular system). Despite the limitation of interpreting results from experimental studies for human beings, these results are of value and may even be an explanation of different outcomes in clinical studies with hormonal preparations containing different substances in different dosages.

Obviously, dose of hormones significantly influences not only the efficacy but also the safety profile of HRT and this should be one of the focuses of the future investigations and of the elaboration of the guidance for hormonal treatment.

Taking into consideration the presented differences between different HRT preparations, the results from the HERS and the WHI study should be interpreted cautiously and their extrapolation to the HRT in general is not justified. Even the authors of the study mentioned almost in each publication of the study results: '*The results (of WHI) do not apply to low doses of these products, to other formulations of estrogens and progestins, or to estrogens and progestins administered through the transdermal route.*'

# References


1. Hulley S, Grady D, Bush T, *et al.* Randomized trial of estrogen plus progestin for secondary prevention of coronary heart disease in postmenopausal women. *J Am Med Assoc* 1998;280:605–13
2. Writing Group for the Women's Health Initiative Investigators. Risk and benefits of estrogen plus progestin in healthy postmenopausal women. *J Am Med Assoc* 2002;288:321–33
3. Woodcock J. Bridging what is known and what is not known, FDA perspective and response. NIH meeting, October 2002
4. Prempro package insert
5. FDA Memorandum, Approvability of a Synthetic Generic Version of Premarin, 1997, 1–41
6. Dey M. The new science of hormone replacement therapy. *J Br Menopause Soc* 1999;S2:4–5
7. Lippert TH, Seeger H, Mueck AO. Clinical and pharmacological characteristics of the conjugated equine estrogens. *Arzneimitteltherapie* 1999;17:362–4
8. Lippert TH, Seeger H, Mueck AO. Pharmacology and toxicology of different estrogens. *Gynecol Endocrinol* 2001;15:26–33
9. USP 24 (The United States Pharmacopeia)/NF 19 (The National Formulary)/ Conjugated estrogens. United States Pharmacopeial Convention, Inc., Rockville, MD, effective 1 January 2000:681
10. Lippert TH, Seeger H, Mueck AO. Estrogens and the cardiovascular system: role of estradiol metabolites in hormone replacement therapy. *Climacteric* 1998;1:296–301
11. Yang NN, Venugopalan M, Hardikor S, Glasebrook A. Identification of an estrogen response element activated by metabolites of 17β-estradiol and raloxifene. *Science* 1996;273:1222–5
12. Kuhl H. In *Klimakterium, Postmenopause und Hormonsubstitution*. Germany: UNI-MED Verlag AG, 1999:169
13. Herkert O, Kuhl H, Sandow J, *et al.* Sex steroids used in hormonal treatment increase vascular procoagulant activity by inducing thrombin receptor (PAR-1) expression. Role of the glucocorticoid receptor. *Circulation* 2001;104:2826–31
14. Juel Riis B, Lehmann H-J, Christiansen C. Norethisterone acetate in combination with estrogen: effects on the skeleton and other organs. A review. *Am J Obstet Gynecol* 2001;187:1101–16
15. Adams MR, Register TC, Golden DL, *et al.* Medroxyprogesterone acetate antagonizes inhibitory effects of conjugated equine estrogens on coronary artery atherosclerosis. *Arterios Throm Vasc Biol* 1997;17:217–21
16. Alexandersen P, Haarbo J, Sandholt I, *et al.* Norethindrone acetate enhances the antiatherogenic effect of 17β-estradiol: a secondary prevention study of aortic atherosclerosis in ovariectomized cholesterol-fed rabbits. *Arterios Throm Vasc Biol* 1998;18:902–7
17. Clarkson TB, Anthony MS, Klein KP. Hormone replacement therapy and coronary artery atherosclerosis: the monkey model. *Br J Obstet Gynaecol* 1996;103(Suppl 1):53–8
18. Seeger H, Wallwiener D, Mueck AO. Effect of medroxyprogesterone acetate and norethisterone on serum-stimulated and estradiol-inhibited proliferation of human coronary artery smooth muscle cells. *Menopause* 2001;8:5–9
19. Pedersen NG, Pedersen S, Dalsgaard T, *et al.* Endothelin-1 induced vasoconstriction variates with the progestogen used for pre-treatment. Presented at the *XVI FIGO World Congress of Gynecology and Obstetrics*, 3–8 September 2000, Washington, DC
20. Suparto IH, Williams JK, Ckine JM, *et al.* Contrasting effects of two hormone replacement therapies on the cardiovascular and mammary gland outcomes in surgical postmenopausal monkeys. *Am J Obstet Gynecol* 2003;188:1132–9
21. Reginster YV, Sarlet N, Deroisy R, Albert A, Gaspard U, Franchimont P. Minimal levels of serum estradiol prevent postmenopausal bone loss. *Calcif Tissue Int* 1992;51:340–3
22. Palacios S, Menendez C, Jurado AR, Vargas JC. Effects of percutaneous oestradiol versus oral oestrogens on bone density. *Maturitas* 1995;20: 209–13
23. Delmas PD, Confavreux E, Garnero P, *et al.* A combination of low doses of 17β-estradiol and norethisterone acetate prevents bone loss and normalizes bone turnover in postmenopausal women. *Osteoporos Int* 2000;11:177–87
24. Notelovitz M, Lenihan JP, McDermott M, *et al.* Initial 17β-estradiol dose for treating vasomotor symptoms. *Obstet Gynecol* 2000;95:726–31
25. Utian WH, Shoupe D, Bachmann G, *et al.* Relief of vasomotor symptoms and vaginal atrophy with lower doses of conjugated equine estrogens and medroxyprogesterone acetate. *Fertil Steril* 2001;75: 1065–79
26. Archer DF, Fisher LA, Rich D, *et al.* Estrace vs Premarin for treatment of menopausal symptoms: dosage comparison study. *Adv Ther* 1992; 9:21–31
27. Kuhl H. Adverse effects of estrogen treatment: natural versus synthetic estrogens. Sex steroids and the cardiovascular system. *The Proceeding of the 1st Interdisciplinary Workshop*, Tuebingen, Germany, October 1996. Carnforth, UK: Parthenon Publishing, 1998:201–10

28. Jick H, Derby LE, Myers MW, *et al.* Risk of hospital admission for idiopathic venous thromboembolism among users of postmenopausal oestrogens. *Lancet* 1996;348:981–3
29. Grodstein F, Manson JE, Colditz GA, *et al.* A prospective, observational study of postmenopausal hormone therapy and primary prevention of cardiovascular disease. *Ann Intern Med* 2000; 133:933–41
30. Hodis HN, Mack WJ, Lobo RA, *et al.* Estrogen in the prevention of atherosclerosis : a randomized, double blind, placebo-controlled trial. *Ann Intern Med* 2001;135:939–53
31. The ESPRIT team. Estrogen therapy for prevention of reinfarction in postmenopausal women: a randomized placebo controlled trial. *Lancet* 2002; 360:2001
32. Collins P, Flather M, Lees B, *et al.* The Women's Hormone Intervention Secondary Prevention (WHISP) pilot study. Presented at *10th World Congress on the Menopause*, 2002, Berlin, Germany
33. Mosekilde L, Beck-Nielsen H, Sorensen O. Hormonal replacement therapy reduces forearm fracture incidence in recent postmenopausal women – results of the Danish Osteoporosis Prevention Study. *Maturitas* 2000;36:181–93

# Breast cancer risk: differences between hormone preparations?

19

*H. Kuhl*

## INTRODUCTION

The premature termination of the Women's Health Initiative (WHI) trial after an average follow-up of 5.2 years was based on the organizers' decision that the risks pretendedly exceeded health benefits[1]. Subsequently published sub-analyses revealed, however, that the most important adverse effects, the increases in the risks of coronary heart disease and breast cancer, were due to flaws in the study design and selection bias.

The dramatic increase in the incidence and severity of coronary heart disease after menopause is due to the accelerated development of atherosclerosis associated with the long-term estrogen deficiency. There is little doubt that primary prevention of coronary heart disease with estrogens is only possible when no severe lesions of the arterial endothelium exist. A detailed analysis of the WHI study confirmed the suspicion that the increase in coronary heart disease events during the first year of treatment with 0.625 mg conjugated estrogens and 2.5 mg medroxyprogesterone acetate (CEE/MPA) was due to the long-term estrogen deficiency and high atherosclerosis risk of those women in whom the menopause occurred at least 20 years ago. In women with an estrogen deficiency of less than 10 years, which is also a very long period, the relative risk was 0.89[2]. Therefore, the WHI study investigated the secondary prevention rather than the primary prevention of coronary heart disease.

## HRT AND BREAST CANCER RISK

A more important flaw is the 26% increase in breast cancer risk reported by the WHI authors that became obvious in the sub-analysis published 1 year later[3]. It is generally accepted that the risk of breast cancer is, among other factors, determined by the total duration of exposure to endogenous or exogenous estrogens. The increase in the incidence of breast cancer observed in postmenopausal women during long-term hormone replacement therapy (HRT) is one of the most important issues which largely influences the acceptance of hormone treatment by the public. Many observational studies carried out in the past revealed quite inconsistent results which were summarized and re-analyzed in 1997 in the Collaborative Study[4]. This reanalysis revealed a 35% increase in the relative risk of breast cancer for women who had used HRT for 5 years or longer (average 11 years). It also showed that, 5 or more years after discontinuation of treatment, the relative risk returned to 0.90 in women who had been treated for 5–9 years[4]. This suggested that the increase in breast cancer diagnoses during HRT is not due to the induction of new breast cancers, but to an acceleration of growth of already existing occult tumors. It has been shown, in an autopsy study, that, in 39% of the women aged between 40 and 50 years, small foci of breast cancer are present, mostly in the form of ductal carcinoma *in situ*[5].

The increase in breast cancer risk during 5.2 years of treatment with CEE/MPA, as observed in the WHI study, referred only to those women who had already been treated with hormones prior to the initiation of the WHI study (Table 1)[4]. In women not pretreated before the WHI study, the risk was not elevated (hazard ratio 1.09). The higher breast cancer risk in the pretreated women could be interpreted as a long-term effect of an early mutagenic/carcinogenic effect of prior HRT, but the time course of breast cancer diagnoses during the WHI study did not differ between the women with HRT prior to the study and those without previous hormone treatment. There was, however, a significant difference in the placebo group of the WHI study between women with and without prior hormone therapy (Table 1)[4]. In women who had received hormones prior to the WHI study, the rate of breast cancer diagnoses was profoundly lower during placebo treatment as compared to never-users, who can be regarded as the true controls[4]. It can be suggested that, during the hormone treatment prior to the WHI study, the growth of occult tumors had been considerably accelerated, resulting in earlier diagnoses. The lack of these diagnoses in the placebo group of the WHI study was causative for the higher breast cancer risk, i.e. the result was due to a selection bias, and there was no reason to stop the WHI study prematurely.

## DIFFERENCE BETWEEN ESTROGEN-ONLY AND ESTROGEN/PROGESTIN COMBINATIONS

In contrast to the WHI study arm with CEE/MPA, the arm with CEE only did not reveal an increase in breast cancer risk after 6.8 years of treatment. This indicated that the additional progestin enhances the proliferative effect of estrogens on breast tumors. In fact, most of the recent studies demonstrated that current or ever-use for 5 or more years of estrogen/progestin combinations was associated with a higher breast cancer risk than with estrogens only (Table 2)[6-12]. This is indirectly confirmed by the finding that, in young women with anovulation, the relative risk of breast cancer is reduced by 60% as compared to women with normal cycles[13].

**Table 1** Time course of the incidence of invasive breast cancer (number per 1000 women per year) in women treated with either placebo or conjugated equine estrogens/medroxyprogesterone acetate (CEE/MPA) with or without hormone therapy (HRT) prior to the initiation of the WHI study[4]

| *Treatment group* | *n* | *Year 1* | *Year 2* | *Year 3* | *Year 4* | *Year 5* | *Year 6+* |
|---|---|---|---|---|---|---|---|
| CEE/MPA without prior HRT | 6277 | 1.1 | 2.4 | 3.1 | 5.8 | 5.4 | 6.9 |
| Placebo without prior HRT | 6020 | 2.3 | 3.7 | 3.3 | 4.0 | 3.4 | 5.6 |
| CEE/MPA with prior HRT | 2225 | 2.3 | 5.0 | 4.6 | 4.2 | 8.2 | 3.9 |
| Placebo with prior HRT | 2079 | 2.4 | 4.9 | 1.5 | 2.0 | 2.3 | 1.7 |

**Table 2** Risk of breast cancer during replacement therapy with estrogens only (ERT) or estrogen/progestin combinations (HRT)

| | | *Relative risk* | |
|---|---|---|---|
| *Study* | *Treatment* | *ERT* | *HRT* |
| WHI | current 5.2 years | 0.77 | 1.24* (cc) |
| MWS | current 2.6 years | 1.30* | 2.00* |
| Weiss *et al.*, 2002 | current ≥ 5 years | 0.81 | 1,54* (cc) |
| Kirsh & Kreiger, 2002 | ever ≥ 10 years | 1.74 | 3.48* (cc + seq) |
| Porch *et al.*, 2002 | current ≥ 5 years | 0.99 | 1.76* (cc + seq) |
| Daling *et al.*, 2002 | ever > 5 years lobular | 1.30 | 2.50* (cc) |
| Li *et al.*, 2003 | ever lobular | 1.30 | 2.50* (cc + seq) |
| Chen *et al.*, 2002 | current lobular | 1.98* | 3.91* (cc + seq) |
| Magnusson *et al.*, 1999 | ever | 1.94* | 1.63* (cc + seq) |

*, Significant; cc, continuous combined therapy; seq, sequential therapy

## DIFFERENCES BETWEEN ESTROGENS?

Concerning the question whether or not there are differences between the various formulations with respect to the risk of breast cancer, no sufficient epidemiological data are available. Neither the Collaborative Study nor the Million Women Study found significant differences between the various types and doses of estrogens (Table 3)[4,14]. This might be explained by the hypothesis that the maximal effect of estrogens on tumor growth is possibly reached at relatively low concentrations. Investigations on breast cancer risk and serum levels of estradiol in postmenopausal women revealed a significant association showing a five-fold higher risk at serum concentration of more than 11.5 pg/ml as compared to levels below 8.6 pg/ml[15].

**Table 3** Relative risk of breast cancer in users of various estrogen preparations as found in the Million Women Study[14]

| *Hormone preparation* | *Relative risk* | *Confidence interval* |
|---|---|---|
| Estrogen only | 1.30 | 1.22–1.38 |
| ≤ 0.625 mg CEE | 1.25 | 1.11–1.41 |
| ≥ 0.625 mg CEE | 1.36 | 1.14–1.61 |
| < 1 mg (ethinyl)estradiol | 1.25 | 1.12–1.40 |
| > 1 mg (ethinyl)estradiol | 1.19 | 0.89–1.58 |
| Oral estrogens | 1.32 | 1.21–1.45 |
| Transdermal estrogens | 1.24 | 1.11–1.39 |
| Estrogen implants | 1.65 | 1.26–2.16 |

CEE, conjugated equine estrogens

## DIFFERENCES BETWEEN PROGESTINS?

There are only few data on the relative breast cancer risk in women treated with different HRT preparations. In contrast to the WHI study and nearly all case-control studies including the Million women study, a Swedish case-control study found the highest relative risk (1.94) with estrogen-only preparations, while that with estrogen/progestin combinations was lower (1.63) (Table 2). Among the various types of progestins, formulations containing estrogens combined with nortestosterone derivatives were found to have a higher relative risk that those with progesterone derivatives. The overlapping confidence intervals indicated, however, no significant differences[12].

In the Million Women Study, the relative risk calculated for estrogen-only was 1.30, while, for estrogens combined with norethisterone, MPA or norgestrel/levonorgestrel, it was similar, between 1.53 and 1.97[14]. Using tibolone, the elevated breast cancer risk was in a similar range, 1.45 (Table 4)[14].

## MECHANISMS INVOLVED IN THE DEVELOPMENT OF BREAST CANCER

In face of the high burden of the human organism with carcinogens taken up daily with the normal diet which originate from boiled, grilled or baked proteins, carbohydrates, and fat, but which are also naturally contained in plants and fruit[16,17], the weak mutagenic effect of estrogens or estrogen metabolites is negligible. On the other hand, a protective effect of progestins, which was claimed on the basis of *in vitro* results, has been refuted by the epidemiological reality. Still today, it is argued

**Table 4** Relative risk of breast cancer in users of various hormone therapy preparations, as found in the Million Women Study[14]

| *Hormone therapy* | *Relative risk* | *Confidence interval* |
|---|---|---|
| Estrogen-only | 1.30 | 1.22–1.38 |
| Tibolone | 1.45 | 1.25–1.67 |
| Estrogen + medroxyprogesterone acetate | 1.60 | 1.33–1.93 |
| Estrogen + norethisterone | 1.53 | 1.35–1.75 |
| Estrogen + norgestrel/levonorgestrel | 1.97 | 1.74–2.33 |

that certain steroids may act as protective by local suppression of estrogen-stimulated growth of tumor cells via inhibition of enzymes like sulfatases or aromatase, even though very low estrogen concentrations are obviously associated with an increased breast cancer risk[15,18]. Estrogens and, even more markedly, estrogen/progestin combinations promote the development of breast carcinoma by an acceleration of growth. This may be caused by direct or indirect stimulation of growth. There is no doubt that stroma cells have a profound stimulatory effect on the growth of tumor cells mediated by paracrine actions of cytokines and growth factors[19-21]. This might explain the finding that, in postmenopausal monkeys, treatment with CEE/MPA increases proliferation of breast epithelium considerably more than CEE only, although both estrogen receptors and progesterone receptors were profoundly suppressed[22]. Another aspect is the influence of estrogens and progestins on the vascularization and blood flow which are essential for the development of cancer.

## EFFECT OF SEX STEROIDS ON THE PROLIFERATION OF BREAST EPITHELIUM AND TUMORS

The present epidemiological, animal-experimental and clinical knowledge suggests that it is the acceleration of growth of tumor cells by estrogens and progestins which promotes the development of breast cancers. This is indirectly confirmed by the return of increased breast cancer risk to baseline or below 5 years after discontinuation of long-term treatment with HRT[4]. Investigations with tissue samples of invasive breast cancers demonstrated that the mitosis rate during the luteal phase is double that in the follicular phase. This concerns not only the estrogen receptor/progesterone receptor-positive cases, but also, to a lesser degree, the receptor-negative cases[23]. This pattern agrees with that in healthy breast tissue; in premenopausal women, normal mammary epithelium also shows the maximal mitosis rate in the luteal phase and the lowest proliferation rate in the follicular phase[24].

Clinical studies with postmenopausal women treated continuously with hormones revealed a slight increase in the proliferation rate of breast epithelium with CEE only and a markedly higher rate with CEE/MPA, which was comparable with that during the luteal phase in premenopausal women[25]. Similar results were observed with ovariectomized monkeys which showed a higher proliferation rate with CEE/MPA than with CEE only[22,26]. Contrary to this, in postmenopausal women who were treated with tibolone or combinations of estrogens and norethisterone or levonorgestrel, no increased proliferation was observed[27]. In the monkey model, a combination of ethinylestradiol and norethisterone acetate did not increase the proliferation of mammary epithelium, in contrast to CEE/MPA[28]. It is not clear whether the lack of stimulation of epithelial proliferation is due to the androgenic activity of norethisterone or levonorgestrel. In ovariectomized monkeys treated with sex steroid-containing implants, physiological levels of testosterone reduced estrogen-induced proliferation of breast epithelium[29]. On the other hand, not only a combination of 2 mg estradiol and 1 mg norethisterone, but also a combination of 2 mg estradiol valerate and 2 mg dienogest, which shows antiandrogenic properties, did not stimulate breast cell proliferation in postmenopausal women[30].

## TIBOLONE AND BREAST CANCER

The results of the Million Women Study suggest that tibolone increases the risk of breast cancer to a similar extent as estrogen/progestin combinations (Table 4)[14]. This appears plausible, as tibolone is a prodrug that, after oral administration, is rapidly converted in the liver to various hormonally active metabolites. These are the weak progestin 7α-methyl-norethisterone (delta-4-isomer) which has a strong androgenic activity comparable to that of testosterone, the potent estrogen 7α-methyl-ethinylestradiol, and two 3-hydroxy-metabolites of tibolone with weak estrogenic properties[31,32].

In animal experiments, the estrogenic metabolite 7α-methyl-ethinylestradiol has been found to be as potent as ethinylestradiol[33], and the time course of its serum concentration is comparable with that of ethinylestradiol after intake of a low-dose oral contraceptive (Figure 1)[34].

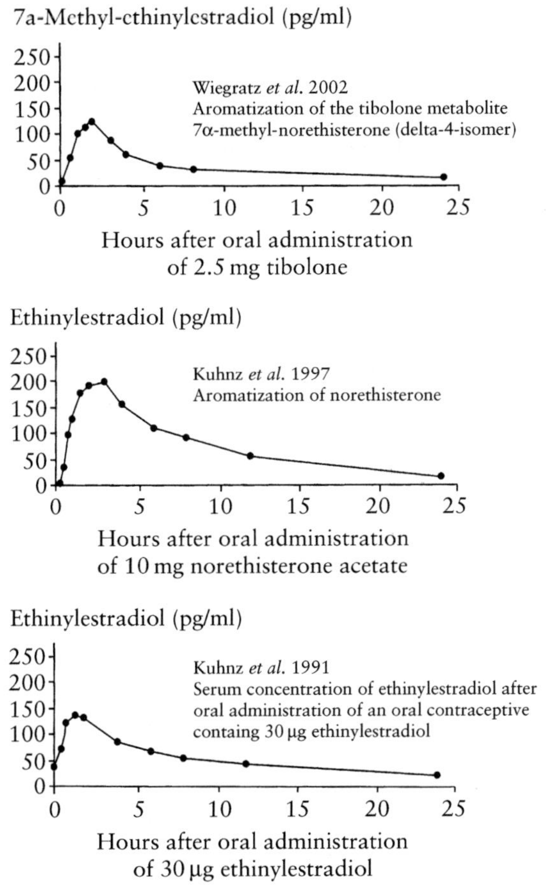


**Figure 1** Time course of the serum concentrations of 7α-methyl-ethinylestradiol after oral administration of 2.5 mg tibolone, and of ethinylestradiol after intake of 10 mg norethisterone acetate or an oral contraceptive containing 30 μg ethinylestradiol[31,34,35]

It has been claimed that, due to the lack of aromatase activity in the adult liver, the conversion of tibolone to 7α-methyl-ethinylestradiol must be an artifact. This can be easily refuted, as it has been demonstrated that, in postmenopausal women, norethisterone is also rapidly aromatized to ethinylestradiol (Figure 1)[35,36]. Moreover, *in vitro* investigations with primary human hepatocytes or homogenates of normal adult human liver samples clearly demonstrated a marked conversion of tritium-labelled norethisterone to ethinylestradiol (Table 5)[37,38]. As there are differences between the capacity of hepatic tissue regarding the aromatization of nortestosterone derivatives like norethisterone or tibolone and the endogenous substrates testosterone and androstenedione, differential enzyme systems have been suggested as being responsible for endogenous androgens (i.e. aromatase) and the synthetic nortestosterone derivatives[38].

**Table 5** Aromatization of norethisterone in adult human liver tissue. Tritium-labelled norethisterone was incubated for 2 h at 37°C with homogenates of healthy liver, cirrhotic liver, and liver cancer. After extraction and isolation by means of column chromatography and thin layer chromatography, the tritium-labelled ethinylestradiol (EE) originating from norethisterone was co-crystallized with ethinylestradiol to constant radioactivity, which was measured[36] (ethinylestradiol: 100 fmol = 30 pg)

| *Liver tissue* | *Formation of EE* (fmol/100 mg protein) |
|---|---|
| Male, 48 years, cirrhosis | 157 |
| Male, 54 years, cancer | 24 |
| Male, 54 years, healthy | 169 |
| Female, 48 years, cancer | 54 |
| Female, 40 years, cirrhosis | 1121 |
| Female, 69 years, cirrhosis | 699 |
| Female, 48 years, cancer | 414 |
| Male, 38 years, healthy | 302 |
| Male, 51 years, healthy | 604 |

Tibolone, which in women shows strong androgenic effects on various metabolic parameters, caused only a slight increase in epithelial tissue in the breast of ovariectomized monkeys. Histopathological investigations revealed only minor degrees of mammary lobuloalveolar hyperplasia (Table 6)[26].

## EFFECTS OF SEX STEROIDS ON VASCULARIZATION AND BLOOD FLOW

Vascularization and blood supply play an essential role in the development and growth of tumors. In malignant tumors, the angiogenesis is regulated by different mechanisms involving angiogenic factors produced by the tumor like VEGF (vascular endothelial growth factor) and MMP (matrix-metalloproteinases), as well as antiangiogenic factors like angiostatin. Hypoxia of tumors may promote mechanisms leading to the spread of metastases. The stimulation of vascularization and

**Table 6** Histopathologic findings in ovariectomized monkeys treated for 2 years with conjugated estrogens (CEE) with or without additional medroxyprogesterone acetate (MPA), or with tibolone[26]

| *Histopathological finding* | *Control* | *CEE* | *CEE + MPA* | *Tibolone* |
|---|---|---|---|---|
| Atrophy | 11 | 1 | 1 | 7 |
| Lobuloalveolar hyperplasia | 19 | 27 | 28 | 24 |
| minimal hyperplasia | 17 | 4 | 2 | 12 |
| mild hyperplasia | 2 | 10 | 8 | 9 |
| moderate hyperplasia | 0 | 13 | 18 | 3 |
| Focal ductal hyperplasia | 0 | 2 | 1 | 0 |

blood flow by estrogens and progestins may theoretically increase the growth of occult tumors, but simultaneously decrease the risk of the formation of metastases. Vice versa, the reduction in blood flow might result in a decrease of tumor growth. In most arteries, for example the coronary artery or the thoracic aorta, 17β-estradiol exerts vasodilatory effects, while, in the pulmonary and mesenteric vessels, it may act as a vasoconstrictor.

Long-term treatment of fertile women with daily 8–10 mg norethisterone or norethisterone prodrugs (e.g. lynestrenol) reduced the risk of breast cancer by 50%, while progesterone derivatives or 19-norprogesterone derivatives did not[39]. Although the number of cases was relatively small, the effect was striking. The underlying mechanism is unknown, but the effect might be associated with the reduction in blood flow in the breast observed in patients with mastalgia during treatment of women with daily 5–10 mg norethisterone acetate[40].

It is well known that, in ovulatory women, blood flow in the breast is highest in the luteal phase, reaching a maximum on day 27, followed by a rapid premenstrual fall. This agrees with the maximal mitosis rate of mammary epithelium in the luteal phase. Another interesting relationship exists between the reduced risk of breast cancer in multiparous women and the decrease in breast vascularity. In nulliparous women, breast vascularity increases continuously throughout reproductive life[41]. It rises strongly during every pregnancy, but decreases rapidly after birth. Within the following postpartal year, it increases, but remains lower than in nulliparous women. Therefore, the more births a woman has had, the lower is the vascularity of her breast[41]. It is well known that the risk of breast cancer correlates inversely with the number of births.

Randomized, prospective trials and observational studies showed a significant 40% reduction in the risk of colorectal cancer and lung/bronchial cancer in women treated with HRT[1,42,43]. This is of importance when comparing the death rates because of the various cancers recorded in 2000. In Germany, the mortality was 24/100 000 women for breast cancer, 17/100 000 women for colon cancer, and 10/100 000 women for lung/ bronchial cancer[44]. The decrease in the risk of colon cancer and lung/bronchial cancer during HRT might be associated with a reduced blood flow in these tissues, as no estrogen and progesterone receptors have been found in colon tumors[45]. In contrast to coronary, uterine and other arteries, estradiol may potentiate the effect of vasoconstrictors in pulmonary and mesenterial arteries and decrease blood flow[46–48]. The rapid and lasting improvement of recurrent intestinal bleeding during treatment with oral contraceptives is, however, also dependent on the presence of a progestin, as the use of estrogen-only was ineffective[49]. Whether the glucocorticoid activity of certain progestins plays a role in the development of tumors remains to be clarified.

It has been shown that the tissue factor is involved in the regulation of angiogenic properties of tumor cells by enhancing production of VEGF by the tumor cells[50]. On the other hand, progestins with relatively weak glucocorticoid activity may upregulate the expression of the thrombin receptor (PAR-1 receptor) in the vessel wall and enhance the thrombin-induced production of tissue factor[51]. This has been demonstrated with MPA, 3-keto-desogestrel and gestodene at low concentrations, but not with norethisterone or levonorgestrel[51].

## CONCLUSIONS

Recent epidemiological studies have revealed that the effect of estrogen-only therapy on breast cancer risk is relatively low, while the use of estrogen/progestin combinations causes a marked rise in the relative risk. The increased risk observed in the WHI study is probably an artifact, because it was found only in those women who have been pretreated with hormones before initiation of the WHI study, which led to a very low breast cancer rate in the placebo group. The presence of a progestin seems to be essential for the development of breast cancer, while the estrogen component plays only a minor role. No differences between the various types, doses and routes of administration of estrogens are discernible. In premenopausal women, the mitosis rate in normal breast epithelium as well as in breast cancers is highest during the luteal phase. Both in postmenopausal women and in the monkey model, estrogen/progestin combinations stimulate the proliferation of normal mammary epithelium to a higher degree than estrogens only, whereby combinations of estrogens with MPA seem to be more effective than those with nortestosterone derivatives. Physiological levels of testosterone reduce estrogen-stimulated proliferation of mammary epithelium, but a role of the androgenic activity of progestins regarding breast cancer risk is questionable. Tibolone, which is a prodrug that is rapidly converted to a progestin with strong androgenic activity and to a potent estrogen, increases breast cancer risk in a similar way to estrogen/progestin combinations. There is possibly an association between breast cancer risk and the effect of estrogens and progestins on vascularity and blood flow. On the other hand, progestins with glucocorticoid activity stimulate the expression of tissue factor, which upregulates VEGF production and angiogenesis.

# References


1. Writing Group for the Women's Health Initiative Investigators. Risks and benefits of estrogen plus progestin in healthy postmenopausal women. *J Am Med Assoc* 2002;288:321–33
2. Manson JAE, Hsia J, Johnson KC, *et al.* Estrogen plus progestin and the risk of coronary heart disease. *N Engl J Med* 2003;349:523–34
3. Chlebowski RT, Hendrix SL, Langer RD, *et al.* Influence of estrogen plus progestin on breast cancer and mammography in healthy postmenopausal women. *J Am Med Assoc* 2003;289:3243–53
4. Collaborative Group on Hormonal Factors in Breast Cancer. Breast cancer and hormonal replacement therapy: collaborative reanalysis of data from 51 epidemiological studies of 52,705 women with breast cancer and 108,411 women without breast cancer. *Lancet* 1997;350:1047–59
5. Black WC, Welch HG. Advances in diagnostic imaging and overestimations of disease prevalence and the benefits of therapy. *N Engl J Med* 1993;328:1237–43
6. Weiss LK, Burkman RT, Cushing-Haugen KL, *et al.* Hormone replacement therapy regimens and breast cancer risk. *Obstet Gynecol* 2002;100:1148–58
7. Kirsh V, Kreiger N. Estrogen and estrogen-progestin replacement therapy and risk of postmenopausal breast cancer in Canada. *Cancer Causes Control* 2002;13:583–90
8. Porch JV, Lee IM, Cook NR, *et al.* Estrogen-progestin replacement therapy and breast cancer risk: the Women' Health Study (United States). *Cancer Causes Control* 2002;13:847–54
9. Daling JR, Malone KE, Doody DR, *et al.* Relation of regimens of combined hormone replacement therapy to lobular, ductal, and other histologic types of breast carcinoma. *Cancer* 2002;95:2455–64
10. Li CI, Malone KE, Porter PL, *et al.* Relationship between long durations and different regimens of hormone therapy and risk of breast cancer. *J Am Med Assoc* 2003;289:3254–63
11. Chen CL, Weiss NS, Newcomb P, *et al.* Hormone replacement therapy in relation to breast cancer. *J Am Med Assoc* 2002;287:734–41
12. Magnusson C, Baron JA, Correia N, *et al.* Breast-cancer risk following long-term oestrogen- and

oestrogen-progestin-replacement therapy. *Int J Cancer* 1999;81:339–44
13. Garland M, Hunter DJ, Colditz GA, *et al.* Menstrual cycle characteristics and history of ovulatory infertility in relation to breast cancer risk in a large cohort of US women. *Am J Epidemiol* 1998;147:636–43
14. Million Women Study Collaborators. Breast cancer and hormone-replacement therapy in the Million Women Study. *Lancet* 2003;362:419–27
15. Thomas HV, Key TJ, Allen DS, *et al.* A prospective study of endogenous serum hormone concentrations and breast cancer risk in postmenopausal women on the island of Guernsey. *Br J Cancer* 1997;76:401–5
16. Ames BN, Magaw R, Swirsky Gold L. Ranking possible carcinogenic hazards. *Science* 1987;236: 271–80
17. Sugimura T, Sato S. Mutagens-carcinogens in foods. *Cancer Res* 1983;43(Suppl):2415–21s
18. Cauley JA, Lucas FL, Kuller LH, *et al.* Elevated serum estradiol and testosterone concentrations are associated with a high risk for breast cancer. *Ann Intern Med* 1999;130:270–7
19. Woodward TL, Xie JW, Haslam SZ. The role of mammary stroma in modulating the proliferative response to ovarian hormones in the normal mammary gland. *J Mammary Gland Biol Neoplasia* 1998;3:117–31
20. Reed MJ, Purohit A. Breast cancer and the role of cytokines in regulating estrogen synthesis: an emerging hypothesis. *Endocr Rev* 1997;18: 701–15
21. Lange CA, Richer JK, Shen T, Horwitz KB. Convergence of progesterone and epidermal growth factor signaling in breast cancer. *J Biol Chem* 1998;273: 31308–16
22. Cline JM, Soderqvist G, von Schoultz E, *et al.* Effects of hormone replacement therapy on the mammary gland of surgically postmenopausal cynomolgus macaques. *Am J Obstet Gynecol* 1996; 174:93–100
23. Menard S, Casalini P, Agresti R, *et al.* Proliferation of breast carcinoma during menstrual phases. *Lancet* 1998;352:148–9
24. Potten CS, Watson RJ, Williams GT, *et al.* The effect of age and menstrual cycle upon proliferative activity of the normal human breast. *Br J Cancer* 1988;58:163–70
25. Hofseth LJ, Raafat AM, Osuch JR, *et al.* Hormone replacement therapy with estrogen or estrogen plus medroxyprogesterone acetate is associated with increased epithelial proliferation in the normal postmenopausal breast. *J Clin Endocrinol Metab* 1999;84:4559–65
26. Cline JM, Register TC, Clarkson TB. Effects of tibolone and hormone replacement therapy on the breast of cynomolgus monkeys. *Menopause* 2002; 9:422–9
27. Hargreaves DF, Knox F, Swindell R, *et al.* Epithelial proliferation and hormone receptor status in the normal postmenopausal breast and the effects of hormone replacement therapy. *Br J Cancer* 1998; 78:945–9
28. Suparto IH, Koudy Williams J, Cline JM, *et al.* Contrasting effects of two hormone replacement therapies on the cardiovascular and mammary gland outcomes in surgically postmenopausal monkeys. *Am J Obstet Gynecol* 2003;188:1132–40
29. Dimitrakakis C, Zhou J, Wang J, *et al.* A physiologic role for testosterone in limiting estrogenic stimulation of the breast. *Menopause* 2003;10:292–8
30. Conner P, Söderqvist G, Skoog L, *et al.* Breast cell proliferation in postmenopausal women during HRT evaluated through fine needle aspiration cytology. *Breast Cancer Res Treat* 2003;78:159–65
31. Wiegratz I, Sänger N, Kuhl H. Formation of 7alpha-methyl-ethinylestradiol during treatment with tibolone. *Menopause* 2002;9:293–5
32. Schoonen WGEJ, Deckers GH, de Gooijer ME, *et al.* Hormonal properties of norethisterone, 7alpha-methyl-norethisterone and their derivatives. *J Steroid Biochem Mol Biol* 2000;74:213–22
33. Bodine PVN, Harris HA, Lyttle CR, *et al.* Estrogenic effects of 7α-methyl-17α-ethinylestradiol: a newly discovered tibolone metabolite. *Steroids* 2002;67:681–6
34. Kuhnz W, Sostarek D, Gansau C, *et al.* Single and multiple administration of a new triphasic oral contraceptive to women: pharmacokinetrics of ethinylestradiol and free and total testosterone levels in serum. *Am J Obstet Gynecol* 1995;165: 596–602
35. Kuhnz W, Heuner A, Hümpel M, *et al.* *In vivo* conversion of norethisterone and norethisterone acetate to ethinyl estradiol in postmenopausal women. *Contraception* 1997;56:379–85
36. Klehr-Bathmann I, Kuhl H. Formation of ethinylestradiol in postmenopausal women during continuous treatment with a combination of estradiol, estriol and norethisterone acetate. *Maturitas* 1995; 21:245–50
37. Yamamoto T, Yoshiji S, Yasuda J, *et al.* Aromatization of norethisterone to ethinylestradiol in human adult liver. *Endocrinol Jpn* 1986;33:527–31
38. Yamamoto T, Kitawaki J, Shiroshita K, *et al.* The confirmation of norethisterone aromatisation in primary human hepatocytes by the vitafiber-II cell culture system. *Acta Obstet Gynaecol Jpn* 1988; 40:87–9
39. Plu-Bureau G, Le MG, Sitruk-Ware R, *et al.* Progestogen use and decreased risk of breast cancer in a cohort study of premenopausal women with benign breast disease. *Br J Cancer* 1994;70:270–7
40. Madjar H, Vetter M, Prömpeler H, *et al.* Doppler measurement of breast vascularity in women under pharmacologic treatment of benign breast disease. *J Reprod Med* 1993;38:935–40

41. Simpson HW, McArdle CS, George WD, *et al.* Pregnancy postponement and childlessness leads to chronic hypervascularity of the breasts and cancer risk. *Br J Cancer* 2002;87:1246–52
42. Kreuzer M, Gerken M, Heinrich J, *et al.* Hormonal factors and risk of lung cancer among women? *Int J Epidemiol* 2003;32:263–71
43. Olsson H, Bladstrom A, Ingvar C. Are smoking-associated cancers prevented or postponed in women using hormone replacement therapy? *Obstet Gynecol* 2003;102:565–70
44. Jemal A, Thomas A, Murray T, *et al.* Cancer statistics, 2002. *CA Cancer J Clin* 2002;52:23–47
45. Slattery ML, Samowitz WS, Holden JA. Estrogen and progesterone receptors in colon tumors. *Am J Clin Pathol* 2000;113:364–8
46. Farhat MY, Ramwell PW. Estradiol potentiates the vasopressor response of the isolated perfused rat lung to the thromboxane mimic U-46619. *J Pharmacol Exp Ther* 1992;261:686–91
47. Farhat MY, Abi-Younes S, Dingaan B, *et al.* Estradiol increases cyclic adenosine monophosphate in rat pulmonary vascular smooth muscle cells by a nongenomic mechanism. *J Pharmacol Exp Ther* 1996;276:652–7
48. Vargas R, Delaney M, Farhat MY, *et al.* Effect of estradiol 17β on pressor response of rat mesenteric bed to norepinephrine, K+, and U-46619. *J Cardiovasc Pharmacol* 1995;25:200–6
49. Barkin JS, Ross BS. Medical therapy for chronic gastrointestinal bleeding of obscure origin. *Am J Gastroenterol* 1998;93:1250–4
50. Zhang Y, Deng Y, Luther T, *et al.* Tissue factor controls the balance of angiogenic and anti-angiogenic properties of tumor cells in mice. *J Clin Invest* 1994;94:1320–7
51. Herkert O, Kuhl H, Sandow J, *et al.* Sex steroids used in hormonal treatment increase vascular procoagulant activity by inducing thrombion receptor (PAR-1) expression: role of the glucocorticoid receptor. *Circulation* 2001;104:2826–31

# Observational studies and randomized controlled trials of hormone therapy: effect of stage of menopause on outcomes

20

*R. A. Lobo*

## INTRODUCTION

Important hormonal and pathophysiological changes occur in women, beginning around the time of the menopausal transition. A recent consensus meeting[1] outlined various stages that occur around the time of the final menstrual period (FMP), which defines the onset of menopause (Figure 1). The menopausal transition (previously known as the perimenopause) precedes the FMP and is followed by 'early' and 'late' postmenopausal stages. We know from prospective studies[2–4] that estradiol levels decline gradually during the perimenopause and then decrease abruptly to low levels (below the premenopausal range) beginning 6 months before the FMP. The falling levels of estradiol continue until a nadir is reached beginning about 4 years after the FMP. This 4-year stage after the FMP, which is referred to as 'early' (Figure 1), is when many pathophysiological changes begin to occur. These changes include accelerated bone loss[5], an exaggerated increase in cholesterol[6] and the greatest prevalence of postmenopausal symptoms, such as the hot flush[7]. This stage, therefore, constitutes a 'window of opportunity' for the use of hormonal therapy (HT) in postmenopausal women, if it is indicated because of symptoms. It is hypothesized that HT at this 'early' stage after menopause may be protective for coronary vessels, the integrity of bone and possibly for the preservation of neuronal systems as well. It is now clear that

Final menstrual period (FMP)

| *Stages:* | −5 | −4 | −3 | −2 | −1 | 0 | +1 | +2 |
|---|---|---|---|---|---|---|---|---|
| *Terminology:* | Reproductive | | | Menopausal transition | | | Postmenopause | |
| | Early | Peak | Late | Early | Late* | | Early* | Late |
| | | | | Perimenopause | | | | |
| *Duration of stage:* | variable | | | variable | | ⓐ 1 yr | ⓑ 4 years | until demise |
| *Menstrual cycles:* | variable to regular | regular | | variable cycle length (*>7 days different from normal*) | ≥2 skipped cycles and an interval of amenorrhea (*≥60 days*) | *Amen × 12 mos* | none | |
| *Endocrine:* | normal FSH | | ↑ FSH | ↑ FSH | | | ↑ FSH | |

**stages most likely to be characterized by vasomotor symptoms* ↑ *= elevated*

**Figure 1** Stages/nomenclature of normal reproductive aging in women. Reproduced from the Recommendations of Stages of Reproductive Aging Workshop (STRAW), Park City, Utah, USA, July 2001

initiation of HT at a later stage imparts some cardiovascular risk (rather than being protective) and may not be beneficial for cognitive activity, as will be discussed below.

## OBSERVATIONAL STUDIES AND RANDOMIZED CONTROLLED TRIALS

Use of hormonal therapy has been studied for over 50 years. Only in the last 20 years have the results from several prospective cohorts been reported. During this time period, we have also seen many small prospective randomized trials (RCTs) of short duration, providing us with information on the effects of various HT regimens on biochemical and surrogate end-points (cardiovascular risk factors, blood flow, bone mass, etc.). In the last 5 years, we have seen results from a few large randomized controlled trials where hard end-points have been analyzed (myocardial infarction, breast cancer, hip fractures). The largest of these, the HT trial of the Women's Health Initiative (WHI), which was terminated after an average of 5.2 years of therapy[8], will provide the basis of comparisons with observational studies. A detailed description or an analysis of this trial is beyond the scope of this review.

Table 1 provides a comparison of results from several reports from the Nurses' Health Study (NHS), which is representative of most observational data, and the more recently published data from WHI. There is good agreement in the results for all the listed end-points except for coronary heart disease (CHD) and risk of Alzheimer's disease. While observational studies have shown a protective effect of HT on CHD and the development of Alzheimer's (or slowing of its onset)[9], in WHI, HT was reported to cause early coronary harm with an increase in the rate of non-fatal myocardial infarction[10] and to have no effect (or a worsening) in cognitive function[11]. In all the other illnesses listed, the benefits and risks of HT are similar between the observational studies and WHI.

A hypothesis, which seeks to explain these differences, has been put forward[12] and will be expanded upon here. In that the characteristics of the women in the NHS and WHI were quite different (use of HT during the menopausal transition and early menopause in the NHS, and in older women with more risk factors in the WHI), the timing of initiation of HT is 'menopause- and age-sensitive' for the effect of HT on CHD and Alzheimer's risk. Table 2 depicts some of these differences in the two studies. In WHI, the mean age of women was 63 years and, even though a third of the women were between ages 50 and 59 years, very few (17%) were within 5 years of menopause and only 12.5% had significant hot flush symptoms[13]. In the Alzheimer's risk (cognitive decline) sub-study[11], all the women enrolled were over 65 years, which is in sharp contrast with the younger, generally healthier cohort in the NHS[9,14].

**Table 1** Comparison of results from the Nurses' Health Study, an observational study, and from the Women's Health Initiative, a randomized controlled trial

| | *Agree* |
|---|---|
| Osteoporosis | yes |
| Breast cancer | yes |
| Colon cancer | yes |
| Uterine cancer | yes |
| Venous thromboembolism and pulmonary embolism | yes |
| Stroke (dose) | yes |
| Coronary heart disease* | no |
| Alzheimer's disease* | no |

*Hypothesis: age/menopause-sensitive

**Table 2** Baseline characteristics of the populations of women in the Nurses' Health Study (NHS) and the Women's Health Initiative (WHI). Rates of hypertension and diabetes were similar

| *Characteristic* | *WHI* | *NHS* |
|---|---|---|
| Age range at study onset (years) | 50–79 | 30–55 |
| Smokers (past and present) | 49.9% | 6.9% |
| Mean body mass index (kg/m$^2$) | 28.5* | 25.1 |
| Using aspirin | 19.1% | 43.9% |

*34.1% had a body mass index ≥ 30 kg/m$^2$
Data from *J Am Med Assoc* 2002;28:321–33; *Ann Intern Med* 2000;133:933–41; *N Engl J Med* 1996;335:453–61

## OLDER WOMEN AND CORONARY HEART DISEASE (SECONDARY PREVENTION RCTS)

Older women and particularly those with known CHD do not benefit from HT and increase their risk of harm in the first 1-2 years when initiating HT. Table 3 lists those RCTs which were designed to show a benefit of HT in secondary prevention of CHD[15-21]. Lack of benefit and the occurrences of early harm are listed. Various regimens were used: oral conjugated equine estrogens/ medroxyprogesterone (CEE/MPA), transdermal estradiol with norethindrone, and oral estradiol. In this table, WHI[8,10] is listed as being both a primary and secondary prevention trial because of the large age span of the women in the study. Several lines of evidence point to the fact that, once significant coronary atherosclerosis exists, estrogen does not exert beneficial and potentially protective effects (as has been shown in young healthy women) and increases the likelihood of early harm after initiation of therapy. A subanalysis of NHS, looking only at those women with CHD[22], is also consistent with this in that a trend towards early harm (although not statistically significant) was witnessed. Based on these data, it appears clear that HT should not be prescribed to older women with CHD with the expectation that it will be beneficial for CHD.

In WHI, women ≥ 65 years who initiated HT had a decline in cognitive activity[11]. Although the observational data are extremely consistent in showing a protective effect on Alzheimer's risk[9], one recent observational study[14] provides evidence that older individuals initiating estrogen in the sixth and seventh decades may have a worsening of cognitive function, while those who initiated estrogen early and continued the treatment for many years had a benefit.

## CORONARY HEART DISEASE IN YOUNGER WOMEN

An attempt to pool data from several trials was reported by Hemminki and McPherson[23,24]. In 22 trials encompassing 4124 women, the effect of various forms of HT was assessed for CHD. This was a very heterogeneous group of studies of variable duration (3 months for hot flushes to 3 years for assessment of bone mass). Although no early harm was reported, the odds ratio for CHD was 1.39 (95% confidence interval (CI), 0.38-3.95), leading the authors to conclude that HT is not protective for CHD. While this conclusion may be correct, the short length of these trials in younger, healthier women does not lend itself to provide this interpretation.

## EARLY HARM IN YOUNG AND OLDER WOMEN

In the WHI, the overall CHD risk was not significant (hazard ratio (HR), 1.24; CI, 1.0-1.54)[10], but the data did show significantly more CHD events in year 1 (HR, 1:81; CI, 1.09-3.01), with a decreasing trend thereafter ($p = 0.02$). In the 50-59-year age group, we do not know the age of menopause but data were provided to show that the overall hazard ratio in women less than 10 years from menopause was 0.89 (CI, 0.5-1.5), compared to

**Table 3** Randomized controlled trials designed to show a benefit of hormone therapy in secondary prevention of coronary heart disease

| *Trial* | *Mean age* (years) | *Relative risk* | *95% confidence interval* | *Early harm* |
|---|---|---|---|---|
| HERS | 67 | 0.99 | 0.81-1.22 | yes |
| Papworth | 66 | 1.29 | 0.84-1.95 | ns |
| ESPRIT | 63 | 1.99 | 0.70-1.41 | ns |
| CARS | 65 | 1.2 | 1.1-2.0 | yes |
| WHI* | 63 | 1.24 | 1.0-1.54 | yes |
| Angiographic trials: ERA, WAVE, WELL HART | 66 | no benefit | | not powered |

*Both primary and secondary; ns, not significant

1.71 (CI, 1.2–2.7) in women who entered the trial more than 20 years from menopause. This is consistent with the hypothesis brought forth.

In the 50–59-year-old age group, even though the overall HR was 1.27 (CI, 0.7–2.1), and was not significantly increased, there remains concern for the possibility of early harm in younger women initiating HT. It is my view that the women in the 50–59-year-old age group in the WHI (menopausal age unknown) are not representative of symptomatic or even asymptomatic younger women at the onset of menopause. A combination of greater age from the time of menopause and the existence of other risk factors is likely to have influenced this risk assessment.

The total number of CHD events in the approximately 2800 women aged 50–59 years in the WHI was 37 vs. 27 in those who were receiving placebo. Although data for events in each year were not provided, I have calculated that there were 9.2 events in 1 year for the HT group vs. 5 in the placebo arm. This translates into a CHD event rate of 3.2/1000 with HT and 1.9/1000 with placebo, which is consistent with the 2/1000 from various databases[24].

The year-1 event rate of over 3/1000 in the 50–59-year age group in the WHI is not representative of healthy women in the early menopause who initiate HT for symptomatic relief, or those who enter prospective trials to assess the efficacy of HT. Evidence for this is provided below.

A compilation of data from 7000 women from four large clinical trials in young healthy women (mean age 53 years) was conducted and presented elsewhere[25]. Data for years 1 and 2 in these women were calculated to assess the incidence of early harm in this population, which was about three times the size of the 50–59-year-old age group in WHI. The four trials were homogeneous in that these protocols assessing HT had consistent inclusion and exclusion criteria, as is required for randomized trials with HT. The observed rate in these trials for CHD was 0.17/1000 vs. 3.2/1000 in the WHI, as stated above. An analysis of just two of these trials, which include published data using only CEE and MPA (the same HT products in the WHI) has recently been published[26]. Here, there were zero events in over 4000 women, 2500 of whom were using continuous combined CEE/MPA. Recent data were also analyzed for the year-1 effects of estradiol and drospirenone in 1142 women, aged 56 years. Although this is a smaller group than the studies cited above, there were no CHD occurrences of early harm (0/1000 recorded in this trial). These data suggest that young healthy women near to the onset of menopause do not experience early harm, as was reported by the WHI investigators. Further, it is conceivable that, during the early postmenopausal phase, the 'window of opportunity' for treatment provides some cardioprotection by inhibiting atherosclerosis, as was demonstrated in the observational trials.

HT initiated early, before coronary atherosclerosis progresses significantly, results in the possible inhibition of atherosclerosis and therefore cardioprotection (Figure 2). HT initiated later (as a secondary prevention trial) is too late to affect atherosclerosis and may induce early harm because of plaque instability and up-regulation of tissue factors such as MMP-9[27], which eventually causes plaque rupture and thrombosis. Clearly, whether she has had a coronary event or not, a woman in her sixties with risk factors would be expected to have coronary vessels which have advanced atherosclerosis, and HT initiated at this time should be appropriately considered to be a 'secondary' prevention trial, which we now know shows no coronary benefit and may induce early harm. Standard HT should not be used in this scenario.

No reliable data are available assessing the occurrence of early harm when using lower than standard doses of HT. It is possible that the risk equation presented above might be different when using lower-dose therapy or perhaps by different routes of administration. In terms of potential benefit, there are data from the NHS showing an equivalent coronary benefit with doses of CEE of 0.625 and 0.3 mg, and a reduction in the incidence of stroke with the lower dose[27].

## CONCLUSION

The early time period after menopause provides a 'window of opportunity' for hormone therapy

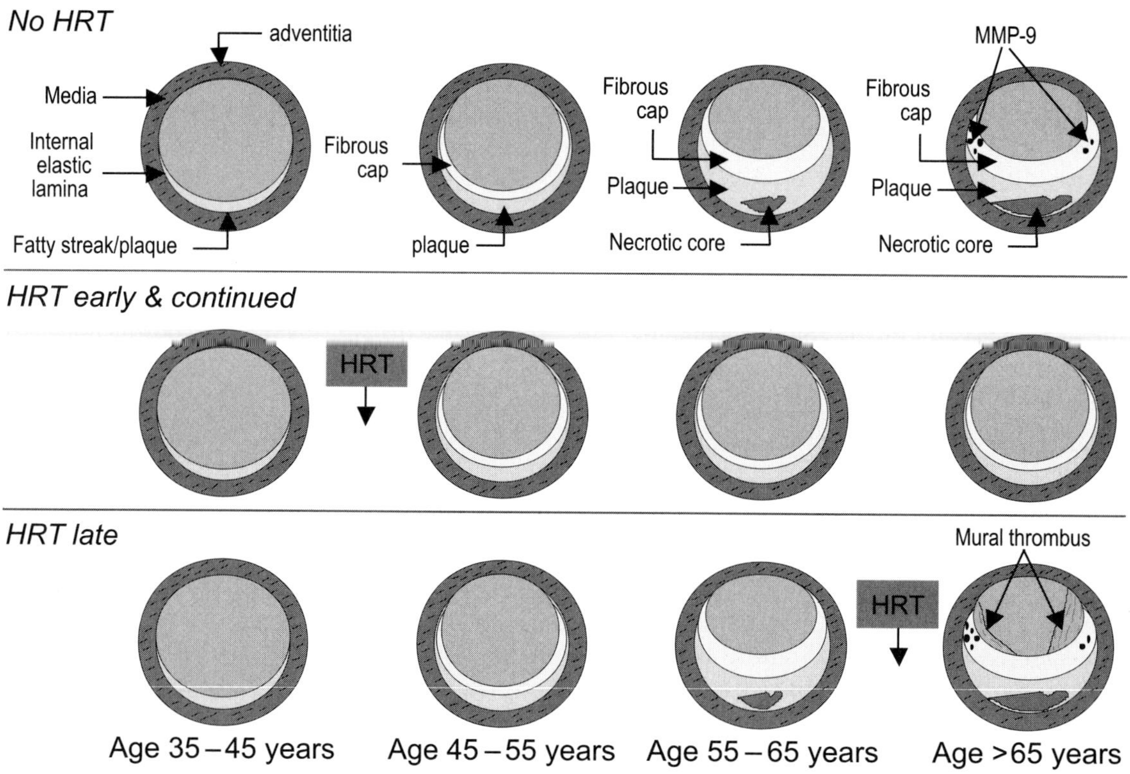


**Figure 2** Hypothetical sequence of early and late initiation of hormone replacement therapy (HRT); with early initiation potentially attenuating atherosclerosis development and late initiation potentially causing harm

if treatment is warranted based on menopausal symptoms and/or an increased risk of osteoporosis. However, not all women should begin hormone therapy and it remains an individual decision. The potential benefit of hormone therapy in young healthy women at the onset of menopause is not represented by the results of the recent randomized controlled trials.

# References


1. Soules MR, Sherman S, Parrott E, *et al.* Executive summary: Stages of Reproductive Aging Workshop (STRAW). *Fertil Steril* 2001;76:874–8
2. Burger HG, Dudley EC, Hopper JL, *et al.* The endocrinology of the menopausal transition: a cross-sectional study of a population-based sample. *J Clin Endocrinol Metab* 1995;80:3537–45
3. Rannevik G, Jeppsson S, Johnell O, Bjerre B, Laurell-Borulf Y Svanberg L. A longitudinal study of the perimenopausal transition: altered profiles of steroid and pituitary hormones, SHBG and bone mineral density. *Maturitas* 1995;21:103–13
4. Randolph JF, Sowers M, Gold EB, *et al.* Reproductive hormones in the early menopausal transition: relationship to ethnicity, body size and menopausal status. *J Clin Endocrinol Metab* 2003;88: 1516–22
5. Slemenda C, Hui SL, Longcope C, Johnston CC. Sex steroids and bone mass: a study of changes about the time of menopause. *J Clin Invest* 1987; 80:1261–9

6. Kannel WB, Hjortland MC, McNamara PM, Gordon T. Menopause and the risk of cardiovascular disease. The Framingham Study. *Ann Intern Med* 1976;85:447–52
7. Oldenhave A, Jaszmann LJ, Haspels AA, Everaerd WT. Impact of climacteric on well-being. A survey based on 5213 women 39 to 60 years old. *Am J Obstet Gynecol* 1993;168:772–80
8. Writing Group for the Women's Health Initiative Investigators. Risks and benefits of estrogen plus progestin in healthy postmenopausal women: Principal results from the Women's Health Initiative randomized controlled trial. *J Am Med Assoc* 2002;288:321–33
9. Le Blanc ES, Janowsky J, Chan BK, Nelson HD. Hormone replacement therapy and cognition: systematic review and meta-analysis. *J Am Med Assoc* 2001;285:1489–99
10. Manson JE, Hsia J, Johnson KC, Rossouw JE, Assaf AR, Lasser NL. Estrogen plus progestin and the risk of coronary heart disease. *N Engl J Med* 2003;349:523–34
11. Shumaker SA, Legault C, Rapp SR, *et al.* Estrogen plus progestin and the incidence of dementia and mild cognitive impairment in postmenopausal women: the Women's Health Initiative Memory Study: a randomized controlled trial. *J Am Med Assoc* 2003;289:2651–62
12. Mikkola TS, Clarkson TB. Estrogen replacement therapy, atherosclerosis, and vascular function. *Cardiovasc Res* 2002;53:605–19
13. Hays J, Ockene JK, Brunner RL, *et al.* Effects of estrogen plus progestin on health-related quality of life. *N Engl J Med* 2003; 348:1839–54
14. Zandi PP, Carlson MC, Plassman B, *et al.* Hormone replacement therapy and incidence of Alzheimer disease in older women: the Cache County Study. *J Am Med Assoc* 2002;288:2123–9
15. Hulley S, Grady D, Bush T, *et al.* Randomized trial of estrogen plus progestin for secondary prevention of coronary heart disease in postmenopausal women. Heart and Estrogen/progestin Replacement Study (HERS) Research Group. *J Am Med Assoc* 1998; 280:605–13
16. Clarke SC, Kelleher J, Lloyd-Jones H, Slack M, Schofiel PM. A study of hormone replacement therapy in postmenopausal women with ischaemic heart disease: the Papworth HRT atherosclerosis study. *Br J Obstet Gynaecol* 2002;109:1056–62
17. Cherry N, Gilmour K, Hannaford P, *et al.* Oestrogen therapy for prevention of reinfarction in postmenopausal women: a randomized placebo controlled trial. *Lancet* 2002; 360:2001–8
18. Alexander KP, Newby LK, Hellkamp AS, *et al.* Initiation of hormone replacement therapy after acute myocardial infarction is associated with more cardiac events during follow-up. *J Am Coll Cardiol* 2001;38:1–7
19. Herrington DM, Reboussin DM, Brosnihan KB, *et al.* Effects of estrogen replacement on the progression of coronary artery atherosclerosis. *N Engl J Med* 2000;343:522–9
20. Waters DD, Alderman El, Hsia J, et al. Effects of hormone replacement therapy and antioxidant vitamin supplements on coronary atherosclerosis in postmenopausal women: a randomized controlled trial. *J Am Med Assoc* 2002;288:2432–40
21. Hodis HN, Mack WJ, Azen SP, *et al.* For the Women's Estrogen-Progestin Lipid Lowering Hormone Atherosclerosis Regression Trial Research Group. *N Engl J Med* 2003;349:535–46
22. Grodstein F, Manson JE, Stampfer MJ. Postmenopausal hormone use and secondary prevention of coronary events in the Nurses' Health Study. A prospective, observational study. *Ann Intern Med* 2001;135:1–8
23. Hemminki E, McPherson K. Impact of perimenopausal therapy on cardiovascular events and cancer: pooled data from clinical trials. *Br Med J* 1997;315:149–53
24. Hemminki R, McPherson K. Value of drug-licensing documents in studying the effect of postmenopausal hormone therapy on cardiovascular disease. *Lancet* 2000;355:566–9
25. Lobo RA, Pickar JH. Evaluation of cardiovascular-event rates with hormone replacement therapy in healthy postmenopausal women. *Obstet Gynecol* 2003;101:95S
26. Lobo RA. Evaluation of cardiovascular event rates with hormone therapy in healthy, early postmenopausal women: results from two large clinical trials. *Arch Intern Med* 2004; in press
27. Zanger D, Yang BK, Ardans J, *et al.* Divergent effects of hormone therapy on serum markers of inflammation in postmenopausal women with coronary artery disease on appropriate medical management. *J Am Coll Cardiol* 2000;36:1797–802

# How representative are the results of the WHI for daily clinical decisions about hormone therapy in other regions of the world?

21

*M. H. Birkhäuser*

## THE WOMEN'S HEALTH INITIATIVE: BASICS

The Women's Health Initiative (WHI) was designed as a large, National Institutes of Health-sponsored, randomized, multicenter study. A total of 27 000 women were included, aged 50–79 years, with a mean age of about 63 years. The recruitment lasted from 1993 to 1998. The hormone replacement therapy subgroup consisted of a combined estrogen–progestin arm (HRT arm) and an estrogen-alone arm in hysterectomized women (ERT arm). The aim of the trial was to evaluate the risk–benefit analysis of the long-term results of an administration of ERT and HRT for the prevention of diseases. The primary benefit was coronary heart disease and non-lethal myocardial infarction or death by coronary heart disease; the primary risk was invasive breast cancer. A global index was chosen to evaluate the sum of all risks and benefits. The end of the study was planned for 2005.

However, the HRT arm[1] was stopped in 2002 by the Data and Safety Monitoring Board because the sum of the risks exceeded the sum of the benefits (predetermined limits reached). The mean follow-up of the combined HRT arm was 5.2 years. In the HRT arm, the treatment consisted in the combined administration of conjugated equine estrogens (CEE; 0.625 mg/day) + medroxyprogesterone acetate (MPA; 2.5 mg/day) ($n = 8506$) or placebo ($n = 8102$). The total drop-out rate was 42% in the HRT arm and 38% in the placebo arm. The ERT arm was stopped in February 2004[2]. The mean follow-up of the estrogen-alone arm was 6.8 years. In the ERT arm, the treatment consisted in the administration of CEE (0.625 mg/day) alone ($n = 5310$) or placebo ($n = 5429$). The characteristics of the participants in both arms are presented on Tables 1 and 2.

The age at recruitment was unusually high: the mean ages of the women in the WHI were 63.2 years (HRT arm) and 63.6 years (ERT arm) at inclusion, bringing the mean ages at termination of the study up to 68 and 70 years, respectively.

Looking at the health situation at baseline, it was surprising to find values of the body mass index ranging from overweight to obesity, an unusual high incidence of arterial hypertension at inclusion, particularly in the ERT arm, and a high percentage of participants using aspirin or statins at inclusion. All these findings point to the presence of cardiovascular risk factors in about half of the study population. These women cannot be called 'healthy'.

## HYPOTHESIS

There were several serious biases, rendering difficult the comparison with women in other regions of the world at initiation of HRT/ERT. The study design is typical for a trial for secondary and not primary cardiovascular prevention:

(1) The population studied in the WHI does not correspond to the postmenopausal women treated by HRT/ERT in Europe and in other regions of the world, considering its age, its body masss index and its pre-existing cardiovascular risk factors, such as the high incidence of arterial hypertension at inclusion.

(2) The WHI was designed for the study of cardiovascular prevention in elderly women. The

**Table 1** Baseline characteristics: combined arm

| *Characteristics* | *HRT* ($n = 8506$) | *Placebo* ($n = 8102$) |
|---|---|---|
| Age at screening (years)* | 63.2 (7.1) | 63.3 (7.1) |
| Prior hormone use (%) | 26.1 | 25.6 |
| Body mass index (kg/m$^2$)* | 28.5 (5.8) | 28.5 (5.9) |
| Never smokers (%) | 49.6 | 50.0 |
| Diabetes (%) | 4.4 | 4.4 |
| Elevated cholesterol levels needing treatment (%) | 12.5 | 12.9 |
| Hypertension (%) | 35.7 | 36.4 |
| Statin use at baseline (%) | 6.9 | 6.8 |
| Aspirin use at baseline (%) | 19.1 | 20.1 |
| Family history of breast cancer (%) | 16.0 | 15.3 |
| History of myocardial infarction (%)† | 1.6 | 1.9 |
| History of CABG/PTCA (%)† | 1.1 | 1.5‡ |

*Values are means (standard deviation); †overall incidence of prior cardiovascular disease, 7.7%; ‡$p = 0.04$ vs. hormone replacement therapy (HRT); CABG/PTCA, coronary artery bypass graft/percutaneous transluminal coronary angioplasty

**Table 2** Baseline characteristics: conjugated equine estrogens-only arm

| *Characteristics* | *ERT* ($n = 5310$) | *Placebo* ($n = 5429$) |
|---|---|---|
| Age at screening (years)* | 63.6 (7.3) | 63.6 (7.3) |
| Prior hormone use (%) | 47.8 | 48.9 |
| Body mass index (kg/m$^2$)* | 30.1 (6.1) | 30.1 (6.2) |
| Never smokers (%) | 51.9 | 50.4 |
| Diabetes (%) | 7.7 | 7.6 |
| Elevated cholesterol levels needing treatment (%) | 14.5 | 15.9 |
| Hypertension (%) | 48.0 | 47.4 |
| Statin use at baseline (%) | 7.4 | 7.9 |
| Aspirin use at baseline (%) | 19.4 | 19.7 |
| Family history of breast cancer (%) | 18.0 | 17.1 |
| History of myocardial infarction (%)† | 3.1/5.1 | 3.2/5.7 |
| History of CABG/PTCA (%)† | 2.3 | 2.1‡ |

*Values are means (standard deviation); †overall incidence of prior cardiovascular disease, 7.7%; ‡$p = 0.04$ vs. estrogen replacement therapy (ERT); CABG/PTCA, coronary artery bypass graft/percutaneous transluminal coronary angioplasty

women recruited for the WHI were essentially free of climacteric symptoms, whereas, in clinical routine, HRT/ERT is prescribed to women in their menopausal transition primarily to treat climacteric symptoms. The WHI used exclusively a per oral combination of CEE and MPA.

(3) The risk-benefit balance based on the population selected for the WHI was therefore not representative for other regions and countries. The results of the WHI cannot be applied to other routes of administration and other progestins.

## POINTS TO SUPPORT THIS HYPOTHESIS

### Age at initiation of therapy

The mean ages of the women included in the WHI were 63.2 years (HRT) and 63.6 years (ERT). In the HRT arm, 33.4% of the volunteers were between 50 and 59 years, 45.3% between 60 and 69 years and 21.3% between 70 and 79 years old. The age distribution in the ERT arm was similar[2]. As a consequence, about two-thirds of all women included in the WHI were between the ages of 60 and 80 years when HRT/ERT was started. In contrast, the population starting HRT or ERT around menopause in Bern (Switzerland) is much younger: 97% of all women starting HRT are aged between 45 and 59 years.

## Cardiovascular risk factors

As defined by the World Health Organization, the body mass index for underweight is < 18.5 kg/m$^2$, for normal weight from 18.5 to 24.9 kg/m$^2$, for overweight from 25 to 29.9 kg/m$^2$, and for obesity ≥ 30 kg/m$^2$. In the WHI, the mean body mass indices were 28.5 (HRT arm) and 30.1 kg/m$^2$ (ERT arm), corresponding to the definitions of overweight and obesity, respectively. In contrast, the mean body mass index of European women at the age of recruitment for HRT/ERT is clearly lower (Table 3), showing that European women are less exposed to this important risk factor.

Arterial hypertension is present in the HRT arm at baseline in 35.7% and in the ERT arm in 48.0% of the participants, compared to a much lower incidence in Switzerland: only 13.6% of our women beginning HRT/ERT suffer from arterial hypertension. Furthermore, in the WHI, the combined use of statins and aspirin at baseline is 26% in the HRT and 26.8% in the ERT arm, pointing again to the presence of cardiovascular risk factors at baseline in a high percentage of all volunteers.

**Table 3** Body mass index: comparison between women in Switzerland* and the USA (WHI[1])

| *Mean body mass index* (kg/m$^2$) | *Percentage of women* | |
|---|---|---|
| | *Switzerland** | *WHI* |
| < 25 (normal or low) | 56.2 | 30.6 |
| 25–29 (overweight) | 29.1 (A1) | 35.2 (B1) |
| ≥ 30 (obese) | 11.4 (A2) | 34.1 (B2) |
| | A1 + A2 = 40.5 | B1 + B2 = 69.4 |

*Women aged 50–64 years, Bundesamt für Statistik, 2003

## Reason to prescribe HRT: its impact on the results found

In the WHI, the reason to start HRT/ERT was cardiovascular prevention, whereas, in Europe and other regions of the world, the main indication for HRT is the presence of climacteric symptoms and of a decreased quality of life as a consequence of estrogen deficiency. Because, in the WHI, about only 10% of all women had climacteric symptoms, the WHI was not able to show a significant improvement of quality of life in women receiving HRT or ERT. In contrast, a Swedish observational study published by Wiklund and colleagues[3], carried out in symptomatic women, has shown a significant improvement of quality of life in women receiving a hormonal substitution. This apparent contradiction is not due to the different design of the two studies (observational study versus randomized controlled trial), but to the different selection of the women studied, as has been illustrated by another randomized controlled trial, the Heart and Estrogen/progestin Replacement Study (HERS). In the HERS, it was found that improvement of depressive symptoms and mental health depends on the presence or absence of hot flushes prior to the start of HRT[4].

During the period of recruitment for the WHI, in the USA too, in daily medicine HRT/ERT was prescribed mostly because of hot flushes[5]. In 46%, the reason for the prescription of HRT was the presence of climacteric symptoms, in 31% prevention of osteoporosis and in only 15% the prevention of cardiovascular diseases. Therefore, the WHI is not representative for the current indications of hormonal treatment in the USA during the 1990s. The WHI has been designed to study a minor, but at that time promising potential indication for HRT, and not to evaluate the risk-benefit balance of the main indication for HRT, namely climacteric symptoms.

## The WHI is not designed to study primary prevention of cardiovascular diseases

The 2763 participants of the HERS[6] with established coronary disease had a mean age of 66.7 years, the WHI participants mean ages of 63.2 (HRT arm) and 63.6 (ERT arm) years, respectively.

Women starting HRT/ERT for climacteric symptoms are in their menopausal transition or immediately postmenopausal. Therefore, the WHI population is about 12 years older than women starting HRT in our daily practice, and only 3 years younger than the HERS participants. The baseline characteristics of the women recruited for the WHI reveal the presence of cardiovascular risk factors in the majority of the participants at inclusion (see above) and we may suppose that a high percentage already had atherosclerotic lesions of their coronary arteries, a fact that is much less probable in younger women starting HRT/ERT immediately after cessation of their endogenous estrogen production. Therefore, it must be admitted that the WHI was not designed to study primary prevention *sensu strictiori*. This is confirmed by the subanalysis of the WHI data by Manson and colleagues[7]. The hazard ratio of 0.89 in women having a distance from menopause of less than 10 years is much lower than the increased cardiovascular risk published earlier[1] for the total cohort. Unfortunately, the WHI population was strongly underpowered and therefore unable to show a cardioprotective effect in women starting HRT/ERT during the menopausal transition[8]. However, the risk found in the WHI subgroup of younger women resembles much more the results of the Nurses' Health Study[9–11] and the Estrogen in the Prevention of Atherosclerosis Trial (EPAT)[12], and is compatible with the experimental data in monkeys published by the group of Clarkson and colleagues[13,14]; all these studies point to a cardioprotective effect in females starting HRT/ERT immediately after menopause.

## The role of the progestin used

Gerhard and colleagues have shown that progesterone does not neutralize the endothelium-dependent vasodilatation of the brachial artery induced by estradiol therapy in postmenopausal women[15]. In monkeys, progesterone did not neutralize the protective effect given by 17β-estradiol[13]. Therefore, natural progesterone has no negative effect on the arterial wall. In contrast, the experimental data for the combination of CEE with MPA are contradictory[16–19]. The WHI supports the hypothesis that MPA might neutralize the favorable effect of estrogens alone. In contrast to the opinion prevailing in the USA, clinicians in other regions do not agree that a progestin class effect can be deduced from this observation. The earlier data obtained in monkey experiments do not support such a class effect. Adams and colleagues have shown that the combination of estradiol + progesterone[12] does not exert the same negative effect on the arterial wall as does the combination of CEE and MPA[17]: MPA but not progesterone neutralizes the benefit given by estrogens. Although later results obtained by the same group do not support these findings for MPA[18,19], the current experimental[12–19] and clinical[1,2] data do not exclude that some progestins might attenuate the cardiovascular benefits of estrogens. In the WHI, there were clinically important differences between the use of unopposed CEE[2] and the combined administration of CEE and MPA[1,7]. In particular, CEE alone did not result in an increase of the cardiovascular risk and of the risk of breast cancer.

Furthermore, some progestins might have a negative effect on the central nervous system, antagonizing the positive effect of estrogens. Sherwin[20] compared the effect on a depression score of CEE (0.625 mg and 1.25 mg/day) + placebo versus CEE (0.625 mg and 1.25 mg/day) + MPA (5 mg/day). She found that MPA counteracted the positive effect of CEE on the depression score.

## Route of administration

Oral and non-oral routes of administration of HRT/ERT may have different effects and side-effects. This is best illustrated by the different influences on the thromboembolic risk induced by oral and transdermal estrogen administration. Scarabin and colleagues[21] compared, in a multicenter, hospital-based, case–control study in postmenopausal women, the effect on the thromboembolic risk of oral ERT with the risk of transdermal ERT. The adjusted matched odds ratio was 3.9 (95% confidence interval (CI), 2.0–7.6) for oral and 1.0 (CI, 0.5–1.7) for transdermal estradiol. The authors suggest that oral but not transdermal ERT is associated with the risk of venous thromboembolism in postmenopausal women, and that transdermal ERT might be safer than oral ERT in respect to the thrombotic risk. It is, therefore, hazardous to conclude from the WHI that non-oral HRT/ERT follows automatically the same risk-benefit pattern as oral HRT/ERT.

## CONCLUSIONS

(1) The WHI is an excellent study for women in their later postmenopause, possessing, at least in part, several cardiovascular risk factors. The WHI is a study beyond others. It has to be taken for its real value and not promoted as a myth. The WHI was not designed to study the effect of HRT and ERT on symptomatic peri- and immediately postmenopausal women. Therefore, the results of the WHI and HERS cannot be applied to women with early (40–50 years) or premature (< 40 years) menopause.

(2) Taking the characteristics of the population studied, the WHI resembles more a trial of secondary than of primary cardiovascular prevention. Whereas the results of its combined arm (CEE and MPA) are in frank contradiction with earlier data from solid observational studies, such as the Nurses' Health Study, its CEE-only arm shows no increase of the cardiovascular risk. There is no increase either in the combined arm in the subgroup of the younger women (50–59 years) participating in the study. In younger women, HRT/ERT should not be prescribed only for primary cardiovascular prevention. However, estrogens may have a beneficial effect on the cardiovascular system by inducing a risk reduction if HRT is started during the menopausal transition or immediately after menopause ('true' primary prevention). By design, the WHI population was underpowered and therefore unable to show cardioprotection of women starting hormone treatment during the menopausal transition. Thus, we have to rely on observational studies showing cardioprotection in peri- and early postmenopausal women. In elderly women, HRT is contraindicated for secondary cardiovascular prevention. Randomized controlled trials are urgently needed to test cardioprotection in women starting treatment during the menopausal transition.

(3) It is likely that, for some preventive effects of HRT/ERT, there is a 'window of opportunity'. If ERT/HRT is started during the menopausal transition or immediately after menopause, a cardioprotective effect is possible; if HRT/ERT is started later, the effects might be negative. Therefore, the metabolic effect of HRT/ERT seems to depend on menopausal age.

(4) In the USA, the results of the WHI led to the conclusion that there is a class effect for progestins. This conclusion is not generally accepted outside of the USA because the different progestins have different affinities, different properties and different metabolic effects. The results obtained with MPA cannot be simply transferred to other progestins used frequently outside the USA. Based on the WHI data, the importance of the role and the type of the progestin used have been underestimated. We need studies investigating the metabolic effects of other progestins than MPA.

(5) The route of administration of the estrogen and the progestin components might influence the risk-benefit balance. Therefore, transdermal HRT/ERT might have other metabolic consequences than oral HRT/ERT[21]. We need studies comparing oral and non-oral administration of 17β-estradiol.

(6) Therefore, the conclusions of the WHI should not be applied uncritically to women from other regions and other countries, living in other conditions, taking HRT/ERT for other indications, starting it at a different age and using different compounds[22].

# References


1. Writing Group for the Women's Health Initiative Investigators. Risks and benefits of estrogen plus progestin in healthy postmenopausal women: principal results from the Women's Health Initiative randomized controlled trial. *J Am Med Assoc* 2002:288:321–3
2. The Women's Health Initiative Steering Committee. Effects of conjugated equine estrogen in postmenopausal women with hysterectomy. The Women's Health Initiative randomized controlled trial. *J Am Med Assoc* 2004;291:1701–12
3. Wiklund I, Karlberg J, Mattsson LA. Quality of life of postmenopausal women on a regimen of transdermal estradiol therapy: a double-blind placebo-controlled study. *Am J Obstet Gynecol* 1993;168:824–30
4. Hlatky MA, Boothroyd D, Vittinghoff E, Sharp P, Whooley MA, for the HERS Research Group. Quality-of-life and depressive symptoms in postmenopausal women after receiving hormone therapy. Results from the HERS Trial. *J Am Med Assoc* 2002;287:591–7
5. Newton KM, LaCroix AZ, Leveille SG, Rutter C, Keenan NL, Anderson LA. Women's beliefs and decisions about hormone replacement therapy. *J Womens Health* 1997;6:459–65
6. Hulley S, Grady D, Bush T, *et al.* for the HERS Research Group: Randomized trial for estrogen plus progestin for secondary prevention of coronary heart disease in postmenopausal women. *J Am Med Assoc* 1998;280:605–13
7. Manson JE, Hsia J, Johnson KC, Rossouw JE, *et al.* for the Women's Health Initiative Investigators. Estrogen plus progestin and the risk of coronary heart disease. *N Engl J Med* 2003;349:523–34
8. Naftolin F, Taylor HS, Karas R. Early initiation of hormone therapy and clinical cardioprotection: the Women's Health Initiative (WHI) could not have detected cardioprotective effects of starting hormone therapy during the menopausal transition. *Fertil Steril* 2004;81:1498–501
9. Grodstein F, Manson JE, Colditz GA, Willett WC, Speizer FE, Stampfer MJ. A prospective, observational study of postmenopausal hormone therapy and primary prevention of cardiovascular disease. *Ann Intern Med* 2000;133:933–41
10. Grodstein F, Stampfer MJ, Manson JE, *et al.* Postmenopausal estrogen and progestin use and the risk of cardiovascular disease. *N Engl J Med* 1996;335:453–61
11. Grodstein F, Stampfer MS, Colditz GA, *et al.* Postmenopausal hormone therapy and mortality. *N Engl J Med* 1997;336:1769–75
12. Hodis HN, Mack WJ, Lobo RA, *et al.* for Estrogen in the Prevention of Atherosclerosis Trial Research Group. Estrogen in the prevention of atherosclerosis: a randomised, double-blind, placebo-controlled trial. *Ann Intern Med* 2001;135:939–53
13. Adams MR, Kaplan JR, Manuck SB, *et al.* Inhibition of coronary artery atherosclerosis by 17-beta estradiol in ovariectomized monkeys. Lack of an effect of added progesterone. *Arteriosclerosis* 1990; 10:1051–7
14. Williams JK, Anthony MS, Honoré EK, *et al.* Regression of atherosclerosis in female monkeys. *Arterioscler Thromb Vasc Biol* 1995;15:827–36
15. Gerhard M, Walsh BW, Tawakol A, *et al.* Estradiol therapy combined with progesterone and endothelium-dependent vasodilation in postmenopausal women. *Circulation* 1998;98:1158–63
16. Adams MR, Register TC, Golden DL, Wagner JD, Williams JK. MPA antagonizes inhibitory effects of CEE on coronary artery atherosclerosis. *Arterioscler Thromb Vasc Biol* 1997;17:217–21
17. Register TC, Adams MR, Golden DL, Clarkson TB. Conjugated equine estrogens alone, but not in combination with medroxyprogesterone acetate, inhibit aortic connective tissue remodeling after plasma lipid lowering in female monkeys. *Arterioscler Thromb Vasc Biol* 1998;18:1164–71
18. Clarkson TB, Appt SE. MPA and postmenopausal coronary artery atherosclerosis revisited. *Steroids* 2003;68:941–51
19. Mikkola TS, Clarkson TB. Estrogen replacement therapy, atherosclerosis, and vascular function. *Cardiovasc Res* 2002;15:605–19
20. Sherwin BB. The impact of different doses of estrogen and progestin on mood and sexual behavior in postmenopausal women. *J Clin Endocrinol Metab* 1991;72:336–43
21. Scarabin P-Y, Oger E, Plu-Bureau G, for the EStrogen and THromboEmbolism Risk (ESTHER) Study Group. Differential association of oral and transdermal oestrogen-replacement therapy with venous thromboembolism risk. *Lancet* 2003;362: 428–32
22. Guidelines for the hormone treatment of women in the menopausal transition and beyond. Position Statement by the Executive Committee of the International Menopause Society. http://www.imsociety.org

# Effects of HRT on the risks of breast cancer and cardiovascular disease: the validity of the epidemiological evidence

22

*S. Shapiro*

## INTRODUCTION

In the annals of female hormone use, hormone replacement therapy (HRT), either in its original incarnation as one or another of the unopposed estrogens, or in its reincarnation as one or another of the estrogen plus progestin combinations, has undergone more swings and roundabouts in terms of claimed benefit versus risk than any other therapy of which I can think. It is generally agreed that HRT has beneficial effects on menopausal symptoms and related conditions such as atrophic vaginitis and, perhaps, cystitis. But for other outcomes, verdicts, especially concerning long-duration HRT, have sometimes been favorable, sometimes null, and sometimes unfavorable, depending on when they were reached, and who reached them. I am most familiar with what took place in the United States, and a brief and deliberately oversimplified chronology helps to illustrate some of the shifts in fashion.

In the United States, in the 1950s and early 1960s, unopposed estrogens could do no wrong. Initially, these products, principally conjugated estrogens, were aggressively promoted by the manufacturers with the promise of prolonged if not eternal youth (unconfirmed), beauty (unconfirmed), and sexuality (partly confirmed). Unopposed estrogens were then found to cause endometrial cancer, with dose- and duration-related increases in the risk (overwhelmingly confirmed). Subsequently, they were found to reduce the risk of osteoporosis (confirmed). Then, they were found to reduce the risk of coronary heart disease (CHD) (thought for a good long time by some investigators, but not by others, to be confirmed), but at the same time to increase the risk of venous thromboembolism (confirmed). Then, they were found to reduce the risk of large bowel cancer (confirmed). Current unopposed estrogen use (but not past use) was thought possibly to increase the risk of breast cancer ever so slightly, a suspicion that had been present at a low level *ab initio*, but one which grew with the passage of time, despite somewhat conflicting evidence. More strident claims were made for a cardioprotective effect, not only of unopposed estrogen therapy but of combined HRT as well (and with the added advantage that the latter therapy appeared not at the same time to increase the risk of endometrial cancer). Then, suspicions of a link with breast cancer grew stronger, with combined therapy thought possibly to increase the risk more than did unopposed estrogen, but still only a little bit more (and, on this matter, confirmation or non-confirmation was in the eye of the beholder, principally because the data were scanty).

Against this background, until recently, the predominant view was that, despite the nagging possibility of an increased risk of breast cancer, the anticipated benefits of long-term HRT (especially a reduced incidence of CHD) were likely in the aggregate to outweigh the risks. Consumption of unopposed estrogens among hysterectomized women, and of combined HRT among non-hysterectomized women, reached all-time highs, and stayed there – until July, 2002.

Since that date, the use of HRT, combined therapy in particular, has plummeted. Based on findings published by the Women's Health Initiative (WHI)[1], it is now claimed that there is clear-cut evidence that combined HRT indeed increases the risk of breast cancer; that it does not decrease, but instead increases, the risk of CHD; and that it also increases the risk of stroke, and of pulmonary embolism. Still further, the WHI investigators claim that the joint effects of these adverse outcomes have been shown quantitatively to outweigh the benefits of decreased risks of osteoporosis and large bowel cancer.

More specifically with regard to breast cancer risk, it is further claimed that the findings from two additional studies, an earlier meta-analysis (The Collaborative Re-analysis[2]) which incorporated almost all of the world's epidemiological studies conducted up to that time, and a study published soon after the WHI study, The Million Women Study (MWS)[3] have documented the same associations. When considered in conjunction with the findings from the WHI, it is claimed that the three studies have definitively established that HRT, and especially combined therapy, increases the risk of breast cancer.

Here I show that the three studies have not ruled out the possibility that they shared similar biases and confounders, and that these are plausible alternatives to causality as explanations for the reported increases in the risk of breast cancer and of cardiovascular disease. For illustrative purposes, in the short space allotted to me, I concentrate on one single bias, detection bias. References are made to other biases in passing. The three studies are considered in chronological order.

## THE COLLABORATIVE RE-ANALYSIS

In a meta-analysis of data derived from 51 studies (the great majority of them case-control studies) in 21 countries, 17 949 postmenopausal cases of breast cancer and 35 916 controls were compared[2]. Among women last exposed to HRT 5 years or more previously, there was no association with breast cancer risk. For women who last used HRT less than 5 years previously, the confounder-adjusted odds ratios (relative risks) for durations of use of < 1, 1–4, 5–9, 10–14, and ≥ 15 years were 0.99, 1.08, 1.31, 1.24, and 1.56, respectively (trend test, $p = 0.003$) (Table 1). Among women exposed for ≥ 5 years, the relative risk was 1.35 (95% confidence interval, 1.21–1.49).

Could these results be accounted for by detection bias and, if so, how great would that bias have to be? It is known that breast cancer can sometimes remain 'occult' or 'clinically silent' for many years, but be detected by screening. Indeed, screening mammography is advocated as public health policy because it results in the detection of clinically silent cases earlier and at a less advanced stage than they would otherwise be detected. (For a more detailed consideration of how detection bias might arise, see reference 4.)

**Table 1** Collaborative Reanalysis: relative risks of breast cancer according to duration of HRT use among women exposed to HRT within the previous 5 years

| *Duration of HRT use* (years) | *Relative risk** |
|---|---|
| < 1 | 0.99 |
| 1–4 | 1.08 |
| 5–9 | 1.31 |
| 10–14 | 1.24 |
| ≥ 15 | 1.56 |
| ≥ 5 | 1.35 (95% CI, 1.21–1.49) |

*Trend test: $2p = 0.003$
HRT, hormone replacement therapy; CI, confidence interval

Women receiving HRT would have been under greater medical surveillance than non-recipients because they needed to have their prescriptions filled, and because there would inevitably have been greater anxiety among them, and their medical attendants about possible HRT-induced breast cancer risk. Moreover, consciousness of and concern about a possibly increased risk could have become greater with increasing duration of exposure.

Consider a hypothetical group of 100 postmenopausal women. In Table 2, column 2 gives the distribution of HRT use and never-use in the preceding 5 years according to duration of exposure, as calculated from the control distribution in the data from the Collaborative Re-analysis. In columns 3 and 4, the numbers in each of the duration categories are multiplied by the corresponding relative risks, to yield expected numbers of cases. In column 5, the differences between columns 4 and 3 yield the expected excess numbers of cases in each of the categories, which are then summed to give the total excess.

Based on these data, application of the relative risk estimates reported in the Collaborative Re-analysis data yields a total expected excess of

**Table 2** Collaborative Reanalysis: excess number of cases in a hypothetical population of 100 women exposed to HRT within the previous 5 years

| *Duration of HRT use* (years) | *Number of women* ($n = 100$) | *Relative risk* | *Expected number of cases* | *Excess* |
|---|---|---|---|---|
| Never | 74.5 | 1.00 | 74.50 | 0.00 |
| < 1 | 2.7 | 0.99 | 2.67 | −0.03 |
| 1–4 | 6.4 | 1.06 | 6.78 | 0.38 |
| 5–9 | 4.0 | 1.31 | 5.24 | 1.24 |
| 10–14 | 2.0 | 1.24 | 2.48 | 0.48 |
| ≥ 15 | 1.6 | 1.56 | 2.50 | 0.90 |
| | | | Total excess | 3.01 |
| | | | Excess per year of HRT use | < 0.20 |

HRT, hormone replacement therapy

cases among HRT recipients of about 3% over a span of ≥ 15 years, or an average of < 0.2% per year.

For a difference in incidence among HRT-exposed and non-exposed women of 0.2% a year, or less, it is impossible to distinguish between causation and detection bias as alternative explanations for the Collaborative Re-analysis findings. Still further, the absence of an increased risk ≥ 5 years after stopping HRT is exactly what would be anticipated under the hypothesis of detection bias, since consciousness of and concern about breast cancer risk would become less intense with the passage of time after stopping HRT.

There was also quantitative evidence in the Collaborative Re-analysis to suggest detection bias. Table 3 gives relative risks according to breast cancer stage and duration. In all duration categories extending to ≥ 10 years, the relative risk estimates were higher for localized than for widespread disease - which is what would have been expected, since surveillance would have led to earlier detection.

Some additional salient limitations to the Collaborative Re-analysis data were, first, that, in the case-control studies (which contributed most of the data), information bias could not be ruled out, and was even likely; and, second, that confounding (e.g. by socioeconomic status) was not adequately controlled.

In the face of the strong likelihood of detection bias, as well as other biases, the low-magnitude relative risk estimates observed in the Collaborative Re-analysis do not constitute valid evidence of an increased risk of breast cancer among HRT users[5]. Moreover, the fact that the estimates were statistically significant does not change that assessment: in a meta-analysis, the effect of combining data from a series of studies, the majority of which share the same biases, is simply to set narrower confidence limits around the magnitude of those biases[6].

**Table 3** Collaborative Reanalysis: HRT < 5 years previously. Relative risks of breast cancer according to stage and duration of use

| | *Stage* | |
|---|---|---|
| *Duration* (years) | *Early* | *Late* |
| < 1 | 1.09 | 0.68 |
| 1–4 | 1.32 | 0.90 |
| 5–9 | 1.67 | 1.04 |
| ≥ 10 | 1.42 | 1.25 |

HRT, hormone replacement therapy

## THE WOMEN'S HEALTH INITIATIVE RANDOMIZED CONTROLLED TRIAL

In the WHI, 8506 and 8102 postmenopausal women, respectively, were randomized to estrogen plus progestin, or placebo[1]. Initially, they were followed for an average of 5.2 years, and, in later reports on the risks of CHD[7] and breast cancer[8], the follow-up was extended to 5.6 years. The findings for the two follow-up periods were not materially different, and for convenience the 5.2-year follow-up is considered here. (Elsewhere,

I have published a more detailed critique of the WHI findings[4]).

The hazard ratio for breast cancer was 1.26 (95% confidence interval, 1.00–1.59), and the estimates for CHD, stroke and pulmonary embolism were 1.29 (1.02–1.63), 1.41 (1.07–1.85), and 2.13 (1.39–3.25), respectively (Table 4). The study was stopped for two reasons: an increased risk of breast cancer, and a global index that 'was supportive of overall harm' (page 325). The outcomes that together accounted for the adverse global index were breast cancer, CHD, stroke, and pulmonary embolism. For all other outcomes included in the index, the hazard ratios were below unity.

The findings of an increased breast cancer risk, and of an adverse global index, were considered definitive because they were documented in what was represented to be a randomized, double-blind, controlled trial. However, it was predictable that the study would not remain double-blind because recipients of estrogen plus progestin would commonly and inevitably develop symptoms, such as breakthrough bleeding, and breast enlargement and tenderness, which would make them aware of their treatment status. Hence, it was predictable that there would be a potential for detection bias. As a consequence of the unblinding, it was also predictable that there would be a potential for confounding because of differential non-adherence to the assigned treatments, as well as cross-overs among the treatment groups.

As expected, the study fulfilled the prediction and ceased to be double-blind. By the time the study ended, 44.4% of the estrogen plus progestin recipients, as against 6.8% of the placebo recipients, had become aware of their exposure status, principally because of persistent vaginal bleeding: a relative difference of 6.5-fold, and an absolute difference of 37.6%. There was also major non-adherence to the assigned treatments, amounting to 42% and 38% among the estrogen plus progestin and placebo recipients, respectively, and cross-overs were also common (6% and 11%).

Against that background, consider the possibility of detection bias. How this bias might arise for breast cancer has been considered above, and in greater detail elsewhere[4]. With regard to myocardial infarction, stroke and pulmonary embolism, the women were twice warned, first about 2.5 years after the study commenced, and then again a year later, about possible increased risks in estrogen plus progestin users. Despite the inevitable anxieties that these warnings would first have provoked, and then have accentuated, the women were nevertheless asked to continue with their assigned treatments. In addition, consciousness of myocardial infarction risk was already present before the warnings were issued, since at baseline the women were informed that the objective of the WHI was to determine whether estrogen plus progestin reduces the risk of myocardial infarction.

How might detection bias arise for the cardiovascular outcomes? It is unlikely that severe or classical myocardial infarction, stroke, or pulmonary embolism would differentially have been detected among estrogen plus progestin and placebo recipients. But there could have been differential detection of mild or atypical cases (e.g. myocardial infarction masquerading as 'indigestion'; hemiparesis with recovery in a few

**Table 4** Women's Health Initiative: hazard ratios and differences in incidence rates of breast cancer, coronary heart disease, stroke and pulmonary embolism

| | | | *Incidence* (per $10^4$/year) | | |
|---|---|---|---|---|---|
| | *Hazard ratio* | *95% CI* | *Estrogen plus progestin* | *Placebo* | *Excess* |
| Breast cancer | 1.26 | 1.00–1.59 | 3.8 | 3.0 | 0.8 |
| Coronary heart disease | 1.29 | 1.02–1.63 | 3.7 | 3.0 | 0.7 |
| Stroke | 1.41 | 1.07–1.05 | 2.9 | 2.1 | 0.8 |
| Pulmonary embolism | 2.13 | 1.39–3.25 | 1.6 | 0.8 | 0.8 |

CI, confidence interval

days; pulmonary embolism masquerading as 'influenza' or 'bronchitis').

How great would detection bias have to be to account for the findings for all four outcomes? Table 4 gives average annual incidence rates of breast cancer, CHD, stroke, and pulmonary embolism among the estrogen plus progestin and placebo recipients. Among the estrogen plus progestin recipients, the excess incidence rates for the four outcomes were, respectively, 0.8, 0.7, 0.8, and 0.8 per 1000 exposed women per year.

In the face of the massive and much greater unblinding that occurred among the estrogen plus progestin recipients relative to the placebo recipients, it is entirely plausible that detection bias, alone, could have accounted for the low-magnitude association for breast cancer, which in any case only '. . . almost reached nominal statistical significance' (page 327), to begin with. Given these data, it is once again impossible to distinguish between detection bias and causation as alternative explanations for the findings.

As for the cardiovascular outcomes, in the face of women who were aware that they were assigned to estrogen plus progestin after having been warned, not once, but twice, about an increased risk, it is questionable whether the WHI findings should be considered admissible evidence at all. But if they are considered, detection bias once again cannot be excluded. Other studies have documented an increased risk of pulmonary embolism and venous thromboembolism among HRT users, an association which is consistent with the well-established effects of oral contraceptives among younger women, and it is likely that that relationship is causal. However, it would not be possible to reach that conclusion based on the WHI findings alone. And for myocardial infarction and stroke, it is abundantly clear not only that detection bias could explain the findings, but that bias may well be the most plausible explanation.

An additional defect in the WHI was that the low adherence rates, amounting to 38–42%, combined with common cross-overs from HRT to no treatment, and vice-versa, raised substantial issues of confounding. For example, women who stopped HRT because of a fear of breast cancer might thereafter have examined their breasts more frequently. To deal with that problem, the data were analyzed using intention-to-treat methods. Those methods may be valid as a technique for reducing confounding in relatively short-term trials in which there is little or no unblinding, and in which there are relatively modest non-adherence or cross-over rates. But, in a long-term study with high rates, and in a study in which almost half of the HRT-exposed women become aware of their status, they become meaningless, and they do not eliminate the possibility of major confounding.

How could the WHI findings have been represented as definitive with so little justification? The answer, I suspect, is that this study was thought of as having met the 'gold standard' in epidemiological research, that of a randomized, double-blind, controlled trial. What the investigators appear not to have recognized is that, while the WHI was a controlled trial to begin with, it soon ceased to be one[4,9], and it took on the characteristics of an observational study, with all of the limitations of bias and confounding intrinsic to that methodology.

Once again, as in any other observational study, for the low-magnitude relative risks observed in the WHI, it became impossible to distinguish between bias or confounding, and causation, as alternative explanations for the findings[5]. Contrary to what was claimed, the WHI did not establish that HRT increases the risk of breast cancer, CHD, stroke or pulmonary embolism.

## THE MILLION WOMEN STUDY

In the United Kingdom, all women aged 50–64 years are invited to undergo screening mammographies at 3-year intervals[3]. From May 1996 to March 2001, the MWS sent letters of invitation and questionnaires to women scheduled for routine mammography. A total of 1 084 110 women were recruited and followed for invasive breast cancer incidence and mortality in National Health Service (NHS) Central Registries.

The main analyses were confined to past and present HRT use, as recorded at recruitment (baseline) among 828 923 postmenopausal women. Relative to never-use, among women who had last used HRT more than 1 year before recruitment, there was no evidence of an association with breast cancer, even when such use had lasted as long as 10 or more years. By contrast, among women who were users at recruitment (current users), the relative risk estimates for estrogen alone, estrogen plus progestin, tibolone, and other or unknown HRT exposures were 1.30, 2.00, 1.45, and 1.44, respectively (Table 5); all the associations were statistically significant. The difference between the estimates for estrogen alone versus estrogen plus progestin was also significant ($p < 0.0001$). The relative risks in current users of estrogen, and of estrogen plus progestin, were significantly greater for total durations of use that lasted for ≥ 5 years, relative to shorter-duration use. For fatal breast cancer, the relative risk was 1.22 (95% confidence interval, 1.05–1.41).

Could these results have been accounted for by detection bias? The investigators excluded '. . . women with any cancer *registered before recruitment*' (my emphasis; page 420). Thus, breast cancers identified during the mammography carried out *at the time of recruitment* would have been reported to the cancer registries, and *included*. In addition, in the best of hands, the sensitivity of mammography is only about 70–80%[10] – and among HRT recipients it would be reduced still further because of increased mammographic density[11]. Thus exposed women aware of breast lumps could sometimes have escaped mammographic detection at baseline, and then have been clinically diagnosed as having breast cancer a short time later.

The inclusion of cases diagnosed at baseline would make it likely not only that detection bias was present in the MWS, but that such bias was more pronounced than in either of the other studies reviewed here, for the following reasons.

First, women who attend for screening mammography have been found more commonly to be HRT users[12], and more commonly to have breast lumps which are cases of as yet undiagnosed breast cancer, than non-attenders[13]. Anxiety because of HRT use, or anxiety because of awareness of breast lumps, is a compelling motivation to attend. And the combination of HRT use with awareness of breast lumps would be additive because they constitute two compelling motivations. Moreover, it is likely that anxiety among HRT users would become more marked with increasing duration of use, and it could also be greater among women who use estrogen plus progestin because greater suspicion of breast cancer risk has been focused on that combination than on unopposed estrogen.

Second, the wording of the invitation and questionnaire (available at the study website: http://www.millionwomenstudy.org) would inevitably have added further to any pre-existing anxiety – or among women who were not yet anxious, the invitation would have created it. To quote: 'We have a unique opportunity through the NHS Breast Screening Programme to learn about the way the different types of HRT . . . affect a woman's health, particularly her breasts' (sic) (opening paragraph).

This reasoning is supported by the MWS data. First, among never-users of HRT, the average incidence of breast cancer was 2.8 per 1000 per year (my calculation), while the corresponding incidence in 'developed countries . . . is estimated to be typically 32 in every 1000 between the ages of 50 and 65 years' (page 424), or about 2.1 per 1000 per year. Thus, even among never-users of HRT, the higher incidence in the MWS, as compared with the population at large, indicates that there was indeed a tendency for the selective recruitment of pre-existing cases of breast cancer at baseline.

Second, the MWS investigators carried out a survey in a sample of 1183 women in which they showed that the recruitment of HRT users for mammography was also selective (the rates of HRT use were 32% versus 19% among attenders and non-attenders, respectively)[12]. Thus, the elevated relative risks observed among the women in the MWS could have been accounted for by still greater selective recruitment of women who both used HRT and who were aware of breast lumps.

**Table 5** Million Women Study: relative risk estimates among current users of hormone replacement therapy

| | *Relative risk* | *95% confidence interval* |
|---|---|---|
| Estrogen only | 1.30 | 1.22–1.38 |
| Estrogen plus progestin | 2.00 | 1.91–2.09 |
| Tibolone | 1.45 | 1.25–1.67 |
| Other/unknown | 1.44 | 1.17–1.76 |

**Table 6** Million Women Study: follow-up intervals

| | *Average* (years) |
|---|---|
| *Breast Cancer Registration or diagnosis* | |
| Duration of follow-up | 2.6 |
| Time to diagnosis | 1.2 |
| *Breast cancer death* | |
| Duration of follow-up | 4.1 |
| Time to death | ? |
| Time between diagnosis and death | 1.7 |

Third, in clinical or pathological terms, the findings are inexplicable. Table 6 gives average follow-up intervals. The mean duration of follow-up for the identification of cases of breast cancer was 2.6 years, and the mean time from recruitment to diagnosis was 1.2 years. The mean duration of follow-up for breast cancer mortality was 4.1 years, while the time from recruitment to death was not mentioned. However, since the time between diagnosis and death was 1.7 years, that interval would have been about 2.4 years (4.1–1.7).

It is well established that the majority of breast cancers evolve slowly, over a period of many years. Hence, the short average intervals observed in the MWS, and especially the short interval from recruitment to diagnosis, can only be explained if a substantial proportion of the breast cancers were already present, if as yet undiagnosed, at baseline. Moreover, an average interval of only 1.7 years from diagnosis to death can only be explained if a substantial number of breast cancers had already been present for a considerable length of time before recruitment.

It is also established that the progression of breast cancer, once the tumor enters a phase of active growth, becomes autonomous. Hence, if for the sake of the argument it is assumed that current HRT use does increase the risk, and that the association becomes stronger with long-duration use, it is virtually inconceivable that HRT can cease to have an effect within 1 year of stopping, even when such use has lasted more than 10 years. Indeed, it is difficult to conceive of any explanation for such disparate effects other than detection bias.

Fourth, about 75% of the women invited for screening mammography actually attended, and, of the latter, 71% took part. That is, the participation rate in the MWS was about 53%. With a non-participation rate of 47%, there was ample scope for women to enroll in the MWS, conditional on HRT use, and conditional on having undiagnosed breast lumps - and most conditional of all on the combination of both.

Fifth, the significantly elevated relative risk for tibolone (a compound which blocks the action of estrogen, and which has not been suspected as a possible cause of breast cancer) (Table 5) is added evidence to suggest detection bias.

Could the mortality data have been subject to detection bias? It is well known that death certificates can be unreliable. Consider two hypothetical groups of HRT users and non-users with advanced breast cancer, in all of whom the final event leading to death is bronchopneumonia. Breast cancer, rather than bronchopneumonia, could tend more commonly to have been recorded as the cause of death among the HRT users. Especially for a relative risk estimate as low as 1.26, and a lower 95% confidence limit of 1.05, it is again impossible to rule out detection bias as an explanation.

Not only was there a strong likelihood of detection bias in the MWS, but multiple additional defects were pointed out in correspondence[14]. Among them was failure to properly specify zero time, with the design being 'somewhere in between a prospective cohort and a case-control study' (sic) (page 1330 (Van Leeuwen and Rookus) in reference 14); failure to take into account switches in HRT use over time; failure to record cross-overs in exposure status after recruitment, and, hence, misclassification of current exposure and non-exposure, as well as misclassification of the type of HRT use; and unreliable duration data.

There were also at least 15 errors in the MWS report (I am indebted to Dr Juergen Dinger (Schering AG) for alerting me to these defects). Those errors include discordance between confidence intervals given in the abstract and text; discordance between estimates given in the text and the figures; faulty arithmetic; and incorrect designation of an estrogen product. Occasional errors can sometimes occur in any report, in which case they can subsequently be acknowledged and corrected. However, errors on the scale identified in the MWS report must raise questions about the care with which the study was conducted.

Finally, it again becomes necessary to point out that, in any study that becomes massive enough, virtually any association, no matter how small, and no matter how biased, can become statistically significant[5]. And, once again for the small risk increments observed in the MWS, it is impossible to distinguish between causation and bias as alternative explanations for the findings.

## CONCLUSIONS

It remains to point out that the breast cancer findings among the three studies were discordant. The MWS investigators[3] have claimed that their findings agreed with those of the Collaborative Re-analysis[2]. That claim is incorrect. The Collaborative Re-analysis reported an increased risk among women who were currently using HRT or who had stopped up to 5 years previously; by contrast, in the MWS, the increase was not evident 1 or more years after stopping.

The WHI investigators[1] have claimed that their findings for combined therapy accorded with those of the Collaborative Re-analysis '. . . which reported a 15% increase for...use for less than 5 years and a 53% increase for use for more than 5 years' (page 330). That claim is also incorrect. In the Collaborative Re-analysis, the risk associated with the use of estrogen plus progestin was not analyzed at all: estrogen plus progestin, and progestin alone, were combined and analyzed together in a single category. In addition, an unknown proportion of women in that category had previously used unopposed estrogens. And still further, the increases of 15% and 53% were not statistically significant, and could have been due to chance.

Contrary to what has been widely claimed, the existing epidemiological evidence does not justify the conclusion that HRT, and combined therapy in particular, increases the risk of breast cancer, or that the combined increases in the risk of breast cancer and cardiovascular disease outweigh the benefits. Based on the existing evidence, HRT may or may not be associated with an elevated risk of these outcomes, but, given the low relative risks that have been observed, coupled with multiple methodological limitations in the three studies, it is impossible to distinguish between bias and causation as alternative explanations for the observed associations.

What about future studies, and can epidemiology make any headway in elucidating the hormonal etiology of breast cancer? Since the disease is 100 times more common in women than in men, there is no doubt at all that female hormones do play a crucial role in its etiology. However, we are unlikely to make any progress in understanding that role by repeatedly re-examining the same questions about HRT.

The more relevant question, I suggest, is this: 'Why does HRT not increase the risk of breast cancer 100-fold?' And since it does not, we should direct our attention to the possible role played by female hormones within the breast tissue itself, where the concentration of estrogens and progestins is orders of magnitude greater than in the peripheral blood, whether or not the women are HRT users.

High physiological blood concentrations of estrogens and progestins among breast cancer cases than among non-cases are sometimes invoked as evidence to support the plausibility of HRT as possible cause. But that reasoning ignores the possibility that the high blood concentrations are primarily governed by what is taking place in the breast itself, and that the shifts in blood levels induced by HRT may be without effect, or virtually so. I doubt whether epidemiology can ever resolve the question of whether exogenous female hormones do or do not increase the risk of breast cancer. But collaborative research between pathology and epidemiology, concentrated on what takes place within the breast itself, might help to advance our understanding. Such research may be difficult, but it may be a necessary next step.

# References


1. Writing Group for the Women's Health Initiative investigators. Risks and benefits of estrogen plus progestin in healthy postmenopausal women. Principal results from the Women's Health Initiative randomized controlled trial. *J Am Med Assoc* 2002;288:321–33
2. Collaborative Group on Hormonal Factors in Breast Cancer. Breast cancer and hormone replacement therapy: collaborative reanalysis of data from 51 epidemiological studies of 52 705 women with breast cancer and 108 411 women without breast cancer. *Lancet* 1997;350:1047–59
3. Million Women Study Collaborators. Breast cancer and hormone replacement therapy in the Million Women Study. *Lancet* 2003;362:419–27
4. Shapiro S. Risks of estrogen plus progestin therapy. A sensitivity analysis of findings in the Women's Health Initiative randomized controlled trial. *Climacteric* 2003;68:302–9
5. Shapiro S. Bias in the evaluation of low-magnitude associations: an empirical perspective. *Am J Epidemiol* 2000;151:939–45
6. Shapiro S. Is meta-analysis a valid approach to the evaluation of small effects in observational studies? *J Clin Epidemiol* 1997;50:223–9
7. Manson JE, Hsia J, Johnson KC, *et al.* Estrogen plus progestin and the risk of coronary heart disease. *N Engl J Med* 2003;349:523–4
8. Chlebowski RT, Hendrix SL, Langer RD, *et al.* Influence of estrogen plus progestin on breast cancer and mammography in healthy postmenopausal women. The Women's Health Initiative Randomized Trial. *J Am Med Assoc* 2003;289:3243–53
9. Shapiro S. Looking to the 21st century. Have we learned from our mistakes, or are we doomed to compound them? *Pharmacoepidemiol Drug Safety* 2004;13:257–65
10. Calvin FU, Mello-Thoms C, Kandel HL, Weinstein SP. Course and perception of decision making during mammographic interpretation. *Am J Roentgenol* 2002;179:917–23
11. Greendale GA, Reboussin BA, Sie A, *et al.* Effects of estrogen–progestin on mammographic parenchymal density. *Ann Intern Med* 1999;130:262–9
12. Banks E, Beral V, Cameron R, *et al.* Comparison of various characteristics of women who do and do not attend for breast cancer screening. *Breast Cancer Research* 2001;http://breast-cancer-research.com/content/4/1/R1
13. Morrison AS, Brisson J, Khalid N. Breast cancer incidence and mortality in the Breast Cancer Detection Demonstration Project. *J Natl Cancer Inst* 1988;80:1540–7
14. Garton M, *et al.* Breast cancer and hormone replacement therapy: the Million Women Study (Letter). *Lancet* 2003;362:1328–30

# WHI, HERS and other trials: consequences for clinical practice 23

*H. G. Burger*

## RELEVANT CONCLUSIONS FROM RECENT MAJOR STUDIES OF POSTMENOPAUSAL HORMONE THERAPY

The most important studies of postmenopausal hormone therapy (HT) to have been published in the past 6 years are the Heart and Estrogen/progestin Replacement Study (HERS) I and II[1,2] and the combined continuous hormone therapy arm (CCHT) of the Women's Health Initiative[3], all of which are randomized, controlled trials providing the most dependable evidence available for the populations of women studied. These trials did not involve symptomatic peri- and early postmenopausal women, but generally involved women who were asymptomatic and substantially postmenopausal.

HERS was a trial of CCHT (conjugated equine estrogen 0.625 mg with medroxyprogesterone acetate 2.5 mg daily) in women of average age 67 years, with coronary heart disease (CHD). There was an early increase in cardiovascular events not seen in women on concomitant statin therapy. There was no net benefit for the prevention of recurrent heart disease, and the trial provided clear evidence of an increased risk of venous thromboembolism. Breast cancer risk was not significantly increased in the initial 4 years[1], or during the continued open-label use of HT and placebo for an additional 2.7 years[2].

The Women's Health Initiative CCHT arm[3] was a trial of the same therapy in asymptomatic postmenopausal women of average age 63 years, with the primary end-points of CHD and breast cancer, together with a global index summarizing benefit and risk. Although the majority of participants did not have clinical CHD, two-thirds were overweight or obese, one-third was on treatment for hypertension and half were either past or current smokers. It was therefore highly probable that many had subclinical atherosclerotic vascular disease. Similar to HERS, there was an early increase in CHD events in the hormone-treated group. However, in a subgroup analysis, there was no significant increase in risk in the 36% of participants who were less than 10 years postmenopausal[4].

For women who had not previously used HT, there was no significant increase in breast cancer risk in the 5.2 years of follow-up, prior to early termination of the study. When all women were included in the analysis, including the 26% who had previously been treated with HT, the hazard ratios were 1.24 (95% confidence interval (CI) 1.02–1.50) for total breast cancer, 1.24 (1.01–1.54) for invasive breast cancer, and 1.18 (0.77–1.82) for *in situ* cancer, with a total mean follow-up of 67 months[5]. The absolute increase in breast cancer risk is approximately 1 in 240 for a woman treated for 5 years, i.e. one extra case of breast cancer for 240 women treated for that period of time.

Again, there was a clear increase in risk of venous thromboembolism, and a small increase in the risk of ischemic stroke. There were significant decreases in the risks of fractures, and of colorectal cancer.

Whilst the publication of the Million Women Study[6] received substantial publicity, this was an observational rather than a randomized, controlled trial, which provided additional data on the risk of breast cancer associated with HT. Because data on the use of HT, including its duration, was collected from the subjects only at enrolment, the data in that publication regarding the association between duration of HT use and risk of breast cancer cannot be regarded as strictly reliable.

The above major studies, particularly the randomized, controlled trials, provide an important database to consider implications for current practice. Practical use of hormone therapy is considered for symptomatic peri- and postmenopausal women, and women with significant risk of osteoporotic fracture, while consideration is given to prevention of heart disease and risk reduction for cognitive decline and Alzheimer's dementia.

It is important to reiterate some aspects of the most important trial, the CCHT arm of the WHI:

(1) WHI provides the first randomized, controlled trial of HT (standard-dose oral therapy) for the prevention of chronic disease.

(2) WHI was not conducted in a population of women usually considered for the initiation of HT, and extreme care must be taken in extrapolating its findings to the population conventionally treated, whose absolute risks of major outcomes are lower than in older markedly postmenopausal women.

(3) WHI corroborated much existing data on benefit and risk in an older population, but its findings should not be uncritically applied to the situation of women who have been on long-term HT since menopause and who have not suffered the adverse events found when therapy is commenced at an average age of 63 years, i.e. women who have not suffered a CVD event, stroke, or venous thromboembolism.

(4) The major benefits of WHI which may be reasonably extrapolated are fracture risk reduction and colorectal risk reduction. The major hazards are venous thromboembolism and breast cancer. It is almost certainly inappropriate to extrapolate conclusions regarding cardiovascular disease, stroke or quality of life, in younger perimenopausal women.

(5) The Million Women study essentially corroborated data regarding CCHT but its conclusions regarding other forms of HT await more extensive study in properly designed randomized trials.

## MANAGEMENT OF SYMPTOMATIC PERI- AND POSTMENOPAUSAL WOMEN

Hormone therapy is of proven benefit for the relief of menopausal symptoms, e.g. hot flushes, night sweats, symptoms of urogenital atrophy[7].

Several studies provide evidence that doses of hormones lower than those which have been used conventionally provide comparable symptomatic relief. These include oral preparations containing 1 mg estradiol and 0.5 mg norethisterone, 0.45 mg conjugated equine estrogen and 1.5 mg medroxyprogesterone acetate, and transdermal estradiol delivering 25 μg of estradiol daily[8–10].

There is evidence that the standard-dose combination therapy with estrogen and progestin in uterus-intact women increases the risk of breast cancer after 4–5 years of use (by up to six extra cases per 1000 women over 15 years, treated for the 5 years from age 50 to 55 years)[6].

There is clear evidence for the effect of conventional doses of HT on risk of venous thromboembolism, but there are no reliable data from which the impact of lower-dose combination therapy on risk of breast cancer and venous thromboembolism can be assessed.

In the light of currently available data, lower-dose preparations are appropriately initiated in symptomatic women without specific contraindications to the use of HT. Dose adjustment should be undertaken as necessary and annual reviews of available data and perceptions of benefit and risk, on an individual basis, must be undertaken. It would seem appropriate to attempt treatment withdrawal after 2–4 years, with continuation where symptoms recur and benefit and risk have been discussed fully.

In 20–25% of women, treatment may need to continue for more than 5 years, and efforts should be made to tailor dosage to the minimum necessary for symptom-free maintenance. Although, on general biological principles, and with some evidence from observational studies, reduction of dose should lead to reduction of adverse effects, there are no current data from randomized controlled trials which would allow any reliable conclusions.

## MANAGEMENT OF PERI- AND POSTMENOPAUSAL WOMEN WITH SIGNIFICANT RISKS OF OSTEOPOROSIS AND OSTEOPOROTIC FRACTURE

Significant risks would generally be considered to exist if the likelihood of the occurrence of an osteoporotic fracture is greater than 10% for an individual in the subsequent 10 years. In some countries, for example, Australia, HT is the only reimbursed therapeutic option in osteoporotic women who have not yet suffered a fragility fracture. Low-dose HT is known to have positive effects on bone mineral density, but there are no randomized, controlled trial data except those from standard-dose therapy in a healthy postmenopausal population of US women, where significant risk reduction was demonstrated[3].

On the basis that breast cancer risks emerge only after 4–5 years of standard-dose treatment in older postmenopausal females, it is reasonable to propose that low-dose treatment for 5 years is an appropriate initial strategy for postmenopausal women at significantly increased fracture risk, with extension to 10 years or more for this important indication, if an individualized decision is made between physician and patient. Such women should be considered for lifelong preventative therapy, with a change to a selective estrogen receptor modulator (SERM) or a bisphosphonate after the initial period of HT. Short-term therapy during the early postmenopause does not confer late protection against fracture.

A bone mineral density score of less than –2.5 to –3.0 at age 50 years would provide a reasonable guideline for the initiation of therapy, although fracture risks are influenced by a number of other considerations. It can also be noted that patients with osteoporosis are generally at lower risk of breast cancer.

## RISK REDUCTION FOR CARDIOVASCULAR DISEASE

There is widespread and clear-cut agreement that HT should not be used for reduction of CVD risk in women who have evidence of atherosclerotic vascular disease. There is no place for standard oral HT (and probably not for any form of HT) in women with known vascular disease.

For women without known disease, who are less than about 7 years postmenopausal, the place of preventive therapy is unclear. Known risk factors, such as obesity, sedentary lifestyle, smoking, diabetes, hypertension and hyperlipidemia, should be dealt with by proven approaches. Current opinion would hold that, in general, HT is not indicated even for such primary prevention. However, one category of patient for whom therapeutic decisions are difficult is the patient without known risk factors, but with a family history of CHD (e.g. first myocardial infarct or death in a parent or sibling before age 50). For an individual patient who presents this form of risk and who wishes to minimize it, long-term HT may be a reasonable option, provided that benefit/risk is fully discussed and agreed. Whether HT should be used as an adjunct to other standard measures is unclear from current data.

## RISK REDUCTION FOR COGNITIVE DECLINE AND ALZHEIMER'S DEMENTIA

Randomized, controlled trial evidence for standard oral therapy shows that the treatment of women over 65 years old for this purpose is inappropriate[11]. Observational data suggest that long-term treatment starting around menopause may reduce risks significantly[12]. There are thus no well-based guidelines for making a recommendation in the latter group – but patients with a family history of cognitive decline (Alzheimer's dementia) may wish to use long-term therapy for risk reduction, again following individualized discussion of benefit and risk. This is, however, a highly controversial area and cannot be regarded as a strong recommendation.

## RISK REDUCTION IN COLORECTAL CANCER AND TYPE II DIABETES

Although the WHI demonstrated a clear reduction in colorectal cancer risk from oral CCHT, and HERS demonstrated reduction in risk of developing type II diabetes[13], these have not been regarded as an indication for HT. Recommendations cannot be made, but HT can be considered for those at increased risk.

## OVERALL CONCLUSIONS

Major concerns were expressed by many authorities regarding the widespread use of HT, in the wake of results from WHI, in particular. The appropriateness of extrapolating the entire range of WHI outcomes to symptomatic peri- and early postmenopausal women must be questioned seriously. An increase in CHD and stroke events in the population of women normally targeted for HT seems highly improbable. The trial data should not alter current guidelines regarding optimal HT use for 3-5 years for symptomatic menopausal women and for those at substantially increased osteoporotic fracture risk. The move to initiation and maintenance of therapy with hormone doses lower than those generally prescribed up to the present is to be encouraged.

# References


1. Hulley S, Grady D, Bush T, *et al.* for the Heart and Estrogen/progestin Replacement Study (HERS) Research Group. Randomized trial of estrogen plus progestin for secondary prevention of coronary heart disease in postmenopausal women. *J Am Med Assoc* 1998;280:605–13
2. Grady D, Herrington D, Bittner V, *et al.* for the HERS Research Group. Cardiovascular disease outcomes during 6.8 years of hormone therapy: Heart and Estrogen/progestin Replacement Study follow-up (HERS II). *J Am Med Assoc* 2002;288: 49–57
3. Writing Group for the Women's Health Initiative Investigators. Risks and benefits of estrogen plus progestin in healthy postmenopausal women: principal results from the Women's Health Initiative randomized controlled trial. *J Am Med Assoc* 2002;288:321–33
4. Manson LE, Hsia J, Johnson KC, *et al.* for the Women's Health Initiative Investigators. Estrogen plus progestin and the risk of coronary heart disease. *N Engl J Med* 2003:349:523–53
5. Chlebowski RT, Hendrix SL, Langer RD, *et al.* for the WHI investigators. Influence of estrogen plus progestin on breast cancer and mammography in healthy postmenopausal women: the Women's Health Initiative randomized trial. *J Am Med Assoc* 2003;289:3243–53
6. Million Women Study Collaborators. Breast cancer and hormone-replacement therapy in the Million Women Study. *Lancet* 2003:362:419–27
7. MacLennan A, Lester S, Moore V. Oral estrogen replacement therapy versus placebo for hot flushes: a systematic review. *Climacteric* 2001;4:58–74
8. Gambacciani M, Ciaponi M, Cappagli R, *et al.* Effects of low-dose, continuous combined oestradiol and norethisterone acetate on menopausal quality of life in early postmenopausal women. *Maturitas* 2003;44:157–63
9. Utian WH, Shoupe D, Bachmann G, Pinkerton JV, Pickar JH. Relief of vasomotor symptoms and vaginal atrophy with lower doses of conjugated equine estrogens and medroxyprogesterone acetate. *Fertil Steril* 2001;75:1065–79
10. Brynhildsen J, Hammar M. Low dose transdermal estradiol/norethisterone acetate treatment over 2 years does not cause endometrial proliferation in postmenopausal women. *Menopause* 2002;9:137–44
11. Shumarker SA, Legualt C, Thal L, *et al.* for the WHIMS Investigators. Estrogen plus progestin and the incidence of dementia and mild cognitive impairment in postmenopausal women: the Women's Health Initiative Memory Study: a randomized controlled trial. *J Am Med Assoc* 2003:289:2651–62
12. Zandi PP, Carlson MC, Plassman BL, *et al.* for the Cache County Memory Study Investigators. Hormone replacement therapy and incidence of Alzheimer's disease in older women: the Cache County Study. *J Am Med Assoc* 2002;288:2123–9
13. Kanaya AM, Herrington D, Vittinghoff E, *et al.* Glycemic effects of postmenopausal hormone therapy: the Heart and Estrogen/progestin Replacement Study. A randomized, double-blind, placebo-controlled trial. *Ann Intern Med* 2003;138:1–9

# Do genes determine risk and benefits of hormone therapy?

24

*D. M. Herrington and B. P. McClain*

## INTRODUCTION

Existing data suggested that estrogen replacement therapy should decrease a woman's risk for coronary heart disease[1,2]. Subsequently, the results of the Heart and Estrogen/progestin Study (HERS) were published, showing no effect of 4.1 years of estrogen plus progestin therapy on risk for cardiovascular events in women with established coronary disease[3]. Within the null effect, there was a dramatic and unexpected increase in risk for cardiovascular events in the first year that offset a later benefit after 2 years of treatment. The greatest excess risk occurred during the first 4 months of treatment. The recently announced results of the Women's Health Initiative (WHI) were even more unexpected. In this trial, there was a small but persistently elevated risk for cardiovascular events in largely healthy women randomized to receive hormone therapy (HT)[4].

The proposed positive effects of estrogen on cardiovascular risk were thought to be attributed to improvements in the lipid profile, most notably an increase in high density lipoprotein (HDL) cholesterol. The development of a proinflammatory state has been suggested as a possible mechanism whereby estrogen may exert an early, negative cardiovascular effect. Individual variability of response to estrogen has been suggested and led to a search for genetic influences on the cardiovascular effects of estrogen.

Evidence now suggests that a woman's response to HT with respect to HDL cholesterol and certain inflammatory proteins may vary depending on the presence or absence of one or more common variants of the estrogen receptor-alpha (ER-α) gene. Furthermore, recently published and new preliminary data suggest that postmenopausal women taking hormone replacement and older adult men are at higher risk for clinical or anatomic manifestations of coronary disease if they have the ER-α IVS1-397 C allele or other closely linked variants in the ER-α gene. Ironically, the identical genetic variants associated with increased risk for coronary disease are also associated with greater sensitivity to estrogen with respect to increases in HDL cholesterol. This set of observations suggests that changes in HDL cholesterol induced by exogenous estrogen are less beneficial than previously assumed or that, in individuals with established atherosclerosis, adverse effects of HT, including prothrombotic or proinflammatory effects may outweigh any beneficial effects of increased HDL cholesterol.

## HDL CHOLESTEROL AND CARDIOVASCULAR RISK

Observational studies have consistently reported that elevated HDL cholesterol is a protective factor against coronary heart disease event, independent of low density lipoprotein (LDL) cholesterol[5]. Premature coronary heart disease frequently occurs in patients with low HDL cholesterol or its major apolipoprotein, Apo A-I[6]. Similarly, animal studies suggest a protective effect of HDL cholesterol[7]. The most likely mechanism for a favorable effect of HDL cholesterol is through promotion of reverse cholesterol transport from the vessel wall to the liver for excretion[8]. HDL cholesterol may also supply antioxidants to LDL cholesterol particles, making LDL cholesterol less susceptible to oxidation[9]. Two randomized clinical trials in men with, or at risk, for coronary disease have shown that raising HDL cholesterol with gemfibrozil is associated with a 22–23% reduction in risk for coronary heart disease events[10,11]. Recently, a trial of simvastatin and niacin produced a 42% reduction in LDL cholesterol, a 26% increase in HDL cholesterol, and a 24% reduction in clinical cardiovascular events[12]. In this trial, on-trial HDL2 cholesterol levels were inversely related to angiographic progression of coronary disease ($r = -0.18$; $p = 0.03$).

## ESTROGEN AND HDL CHOLESTEROL

Observational studies[13,14] and randomized clinical trials[15.16] have shown that HT raises HDL cholesterol by augmenting synthesis of apo A-I[17,18]. A man with a disruptive mutation in the ER-α gene demonstrated low levels of HDL cholesterol and apo A-I despite normal estradiol levels. This finding provides indirect evidence that estrogen's effects on HDLcholesterol are ER-α receptor-dependent[19]. Estrogen also decreases hepatic lipase activity[20], reducing the fractional catabolic rate of apo A-I in some[21] but not other[17,18] studies. These effects result in higher numbers of HDL cholesterol particles containing exclusively apo A-I (LpAI). These particles are better cholesterol acceptors *in vitro*[22] and more highly associated with protection of coronary disease in cross-sectional epidemiological studies[23,24]. Thus, there are adequate reasons to assume that estrogen-associated increases in HDL cholesterol might be helpful in slowing atherosclerotic vascular disease. This is further supported by observational studies of estrogen use and risk for coronary heart disease events, which suggest that 25–50% of the apparent benefit of HT can be attributed to its effects on HDL and LDL cholesterol[25,26].

Although evidence suggesting that estrogen-associated changes in HDL cholesterol should be beneficial, both the HERS trial[3] and the ERA trial[27] failed to demonstrate a favorable effect of estrogen replacement on progression of clinical or angiographic coronary disease, even though HDL cholesterol levels were raised by 10–18%. The lack of overall benefit in HERS and ERA may be due to unanticipated adverse effects of estrogen on inflammation or thrombosis[28]. Nevertheless, in the active treatment arm in HERS, women with the highest HDL after 1 year of treatment had significantly fewer coronary heart disease events than those with lower on-trial HDL levels ($p < 0.001$). Thus, genetic or other factors that influence HDL cholesterol response to estrogen may have an important impact on risk for coronary heart disease in certain subgroups, even if the overall effect of HT is null.

## ESTROGEN AND C-REACTIVE PROTEIN

Recently, two large observational studies[29,30] and two clinical trials[31,32] have described significantly elevated levels of C-reactive protein in women taking HT. Women on HT reported 48–260% higher levels of C-reactive protein than women not on therapy, with changes evident in as early as 4 weeks[32]. These recent observations suggest that an estrogen-induced proinflammatory state may diminish the cardioprotective effects of estrogen. An estrogen-associated increase in C-reactive protein is also supported by data from women in labor and early postpartum, showing dramatic increases in C-reactive protein at times when endogenous estrogen levels are elevated[33]. C-reactive protein is an acute-phase reactant that is elevated in subjects with conditions caused by acute and chronic inflammation. In particular, C-reactive protein and the underlying inflammation that it typically reflects have been implicated in the promotion of atherosclerosis and its acute thrombotic implications[34].

## ESTROGEN'S EFFECTS ON E-SELECTIN AND OTHER ADHESION MOLECULES

Estrogen appears to down-regulate various endothelial cell adhesion molecules, potentially contradicting an estrogen-induced proinflammatory effect. During vascular inflammation, endothelial cell adhesion molecules facilitate leukocyte attachment to, and migration across, endothelial cells. Several studies report estrogen inhibition of E-selectin induction, VCAM-1, and ICAM-1 in estrogen receptor-positive endothelial cell lines[35,36], although other studies have demonstrated conflicting reports[37,38].

Recently, additional clinical studies have documented lower serum levels of soluble fragments of E-selectin, VCAM-1 or ICAM-1[29,39] in women receiving estrogen replacement. In observational studies, elevated levels of E-selectin, VCAM-1 or ICAM-1 have been associated with coronary heart disease[40,41], angiographically defined coronary stenoses[42,43], and carotid atherosclerosis[40]. Thus, estrogen-associated reductions in circulating adhesion molecules may reflect an anti-inflammatory effect of estrogen at the level of the endothelium that could account for a cardioprotective effect of estrogen.

## THE ERA TRIAL

The Estrogen Replacement and Atherosclerosis (ERA) trial was a study of 309 postmenopausal women with prior cardiovascular disease randomized to receive either unopposed conjugated equine estrogen 0.625 mg, estrogen plus medroxyprogesterone (MPA) 2.5 mg, or placebo. The mean duration of follow-up was 3.2 years[27]. E-selectin and C-reactive protein levels were recorded at baseline and at 1 year only. Lipid profiles were measured at baseline and at yearly timepoints for the duration of the trial. Two recent studies derived from ERA examined the relationship between genotype at the ER-α gene locus and response to HT. The sequence of particular interest is the first intervening sequence at position-397 (IVS1-397) within the ER-α gene. The effects of HT on HDL cholesterol, C-reactive protein and E-selectin levels were compared among women with the three ER-α IVS1-397 genotypes (C/C, C/T and T/T)[44].

### The IVS1-397 C/C polymorphism and HDL cholesterol

The IVS1-397 C/C genotype was present in 18.9% of the cohort, with C/T and T/T genotypes accounting for 52.3% and 28.8%, respectively. Women receiving either unopposed estrogen or combined estrogen/progestin experienced a significant decrease in LDL cholesterol (9.4% and 16.5%, respectively) and a significant increase in HDL cholesterol (18.8% and 14.2%, respectively)[27]. Subjects not in the active arm (receiving placebo) did not have a significant change in HDL or LDL cholesterol levels. Subjects who had the IVS1-397 C/C polymorphism experienced an augmented increase in HDL cholesterol level in response to HT. The mean HDL cholesterol increase in the IVS1-397 C/C group was over twice the increase for the remainder of the cohort (13.1 mg/dl vs. 6.0 mg/dl, $p = 0.004$)[45]. This difference persisted regardless of whether estrogen alone, or estrogen plus progestin were employed. Further analysis revealed that the HDL3 cholesterol fraction accounted for the majority of the total HDL cholesterol increase. The HDL3 fraction increased by 13.6 mg/dl for the IVS1-397 C/C group vs. 8.2 mg/dl for the combined C/T and T/T groups ($p = 0.04$)[45].

### The IVS1-397 C/C polymorphism, E-selectin and C-reactive protein

All subjects receiving HT experienced a significant drop in E-selectin levels vs. the placebo group. However, subjects with the IVS1-397 C/C polymorphism experienced a greater reduction in E-selectin vs. subjects with the other genotypes (24% vs. 14%, respectively; $p = 0.021$)[44].

C-reactive protein levels increased for all subjects receiving HT, with a 31% increase in comparison to placebo ($p = 0.03$). However, there was no difference in C-reactive protein response between women with the C/C genotype compared to other women[44].

## PROPOSED MECHANISM FOR VARIABLE GENETIC RESPONSE TO ESTROGEN: THE MYB TRANSCRIPTION FACTOR

The ER-α IVS1-397 C allele produces a sequence that resembles a binding site for the transcription factor B-myb. Luciferase reporter constructs containing the sequence spanning the ER-α IVS1-397 site were produced to investigate whether this was a functional myb binding site. Two different cell lines were then co-transfected with their reporter constructs and a myb expression vector. In cells transfected with the reporter construct containing the C allele, there was a ten-fold increase in luciferase activity compared with only a two-fold increase in cells with the T reporter construct[44]. This suggests that subjects with the ER-α IVS1-397 C/C genotype may have enhanced activation of the ER-α gene through interaction with the myb transcription factor. B-myb is known to be an estrogen-sensitive target gene. Thus, this could produce a signal-amplifying cascade, resulting in an enhanced response to estrogen in subjects with the C/C polymorphism.

## CONCLUSIONS

Mechanisms that define the influence of exogenous estrogen therapy on cardiovascular risk are complex and incompletely understood. Genetic factors appear to play a role. Women who carry the ER-α IVS1-397 C/C genotype experience an augmented increase in HDL cholesterol and a more profound drop in E-selectin than women with the T/C or T/T genotypes. No difference in C-reactive protein elevation was detected among the genotypes. The effect of this gene polymorphism on estrogen-sensitive clinical events is not yet known. However, if there is indeed an estrogen-sensitive phenotype defined by the presence or absence of certain ER-α polymorphisms, this suggests that genetic screening may ultimately assist clinicians and women to make better decisions about use of hormone therapy.

# References


1. Gerhard M, Walsh BW, Tawakol A, *et al.* Estradiol therapy combined with progesterone and endothelium-dependent vasodilation in postmenopausal women. *Circulation* 1998;98:1158–63
2. Herrington DM. Prevention of cardiovascular disease by estrogen. In Rubanyi GM, Kauffman R, eds. *Estrogen and the Vessel Wall.* Amsterdam, The Netherlands: Harwood Academic Publishers, 1998: 261–70
3. Hulley S, Grady D, Bush T, *et al.* Randomized trial of estrogen plus progestin for secondary prevention of coronary heart disease in postmenopausal women. *J Am Med Assoc* 1998;280:605–13
4. Rossouw JE, Anderson GL, Prentice RL, *et al.* for the Writing Group for the Women's Health Initiative Investigators. Risks and benefits of estrogen plus progestin in healthy postmenopausal women: principal results from the Women's Health Initiative randomized controlled trial. *J Am Med Assoc* 2002;288:321–33
5. Miller NE, Forde OH, Thelle DE, Mjos OD. The Tromso Heart Study. High-density lipoprotein and coronary heart disease: a prospective case-control study. *Lancet* 1977;1:965–8
6. Karathanasis SK, Ferris E, Haddad IA. DNA inversion within the apolipoproteins AI/CIII/AIV-encoding gene cluster of certain patients with premature atherosclerosis. *Proc Natl Acad Sci USA* 1987;84:7198–202
7. Badimon JJ, Badimon L, Fuster V. Regression of atherosclerotic lesions by high density lipoprotein plasma fraction in the cholesterol-fed rabbit. *J Clin Invest* 1990;85:1234–41
8. Castro GR, Fielding CJ. Early incorporation of cell-derived cholesterol into pre-beta-migrating high-density lipoprotein. *Biochemistry* 1988;27:25–9
9. Mackness MI, Abbott C, Arrol S, Durrington PN. The role of high-density lipoprotein and lipid-soluble antioxidant vitamins in inhibiting low-density lipoprotein oxidation. *Biochem J* 1993;294: 829–34
10. Manninen V, Elo O, Frick H, *et al.* Lipid alterations and decline in the incidence of coronary heart disease in the Helsinki Heart Study. *J Am Med Assoc* 1988;260:641–51
11. Robins SJ, Collins D, Wittes JT, *et al.* Relation of gemfibrozil treatment and lipid levels with major coronary events. VA-HIT: a randomized controlled trial. *J Am Med Assoc* 2001; 285:1585–91
12. Brown BG, Zhao X-Q, Chait A, *et al.* Simvastatin and niacin, antioxidant vitamins, or the combination for the prevention of coronary disease. *N Engl J Med* 2001;345:1583–92
13. Nabulsi AA, Folsom AR, White A, *et al.* Association of hormone-replacement therapy with various cardiovascular risk factors in postmenopausal women. The Atherosclerosis Risk in Communities Study Investigators. *N Engl J Med* 1993;328:1069–75
14. Manolio TA, Furberg CD, Shemanski L, *et al.* Associations of postmenopausal estrogen use with cardiovascular disease and its risk factors in older women. *Circulation* 1993;88:2163–71
15. Walsh BW, Li H, Sacks FM. Effects of postmenopausal hormone replacement with oral and transdermal estrogen on high density lipoprotein metabolism. *J Lipid Res* 1994;35:2083–93

16. The Writing Group for the PEPI Trial. Effects of estrogen or estrogen/progestin regimens on heart disease risk factors in postmenopausal women. The Postmenopausal Estrogen/Progestin Interventions (PEPI) Trial. *J Am Med Assoc* 1995;273:199–208
17. Schaefer EJ, Foster DM, Zech LA, *et al.* The effects of estrogen administration on plasma lipoprotein metabolism in premenopausal females. *J Clin Endocrinol Metab* 1983;57:262–7
18. Brinton EA. Oral estrogen replacement therapy in postmenopausal women selectively raises levels and production rates of lipoprotein A-I and lowers hepatic lipase activity without lowering the fractional catabolic rate. *Arterioscler Thromb Vasc Biol* 1996;16:431–40
19. Sudhir K, Chou TM, Chatterjee K, *et al.* Premature coronary artery disease associated with a disruptive mutation in the estrogen receptor gene in a man. *Circulation* 1997;96:3774–7
20. Applebaum-Bowden D, McLean P, *et al.* Lipoprotein, apolipoprotein, and lipolytic enzyme changes following estrogen administration in postmenopausal women. *J Lipid Res* 1989;30: 1895–906
21. Quintao EC, Nakandakare E, Oliveira HC, *et al.* Oral estradiol-17 beta raises the level of plasma high-density lipoprotein in menopausal women by slowing down its clearance rate. *Acta Endocrinol (Copenh)* 1991;125:657–61
22. Barbaras R, Puchois P, Grimaldi P, *et al.* Relationship in adipose cells between the presence of receptor sites for high density lipoproteins and the promotion of reverse cholesterol transport. *Biochem Biophys Res Commun* 1987;149:545–54
23. Cheung MC, Brown BG, Wolf AC, Albers JJ. Altered particle size distribution of apolipoprotein A-I-containing lipoproteins in subjects with coronary artery disease. *J Lipid Res* 1991; 32:383–94
24. Rader DJ, Ikewaki K, Duverger N, *et al.* Very low high-density lipoproteins without coronary atherosclerosis. *Lancet* 1993;342:1455–8
25. Gruchow HW, Anderson AJ, Barboriak JJ, Sobocinski KA. Postmenopausal use of estrogen and occlusion of coronary arteries. *Am Heart J* 1988;115:954–63
26. Bush TL, Barrett-Connor E, Cowan LD, *et al.* Cardiovascular mortality and noncontraceptive use of estrogen in women: results from the Lipid Research Clinics Program Follow-up Study. *Circulation* 1987;75:1102–9
27. Herrington DM, Reboussin DR, Brosnihan KB, *et al.* Effects of estrogen replacement on the progression of coronary-artery atherosclerosis. *N Engl J Med* 2000;343:522–9
28. Herrington DM, Vittinghoff E, Howard TD, *et al.* Factor V Leiden, hormone replacement therapy, and risk of venous thromboembolic events in women with coronary disease. *Arterioscler Thromb Vasc Biol* 2002;22:1012–17
29. Cushman M, Meilahn EN, Psaty BM, *et al.* Hormone replacement therapy, inflammation, and hemostasis in elderly women. *Arterioscler Thromb Vasc Biol* 1999;19:893–9
30. Ridker PM, Cushman M, Stampfer MJ, Tracy RP, Hennekens CH. Inflammation, aspirin, and the risk of cardiovascular disease in apparently healthy men. *N Engl J Med* 1997;336:973–9
31. Cushman M, Legault C, Barrett-Connor E, *et al.* Effect of postmenopausal hormones on inflammation-sensitive proteins. The Postmenopausal Estrogen/Progestin Interventions (PEPI) Study. *Circulation* 1999;100:717–22
32. van Baal WM, Kenemans P, Van der Mooren MJ, *et al.* Increased C-reactive protein levels during short-term hormone replacement therapy in healthy postmenopausal women. *Thromb Haemost* 1999;81:925–8
33. DeMeeus JB, Pourrat O, Gombert J, Magnin G. C-reactive protein levels at the onset of labour and at day 3 post-partum in normal pregnancy. *Clin Exp Obstet Gynecol* 1998;25:9–11
34. Kinlay S, Selwyn AP, Libby P, Ganz P. Inflammation, the endothelium, and the acute coronary syndromes. *J Cardiovasc Pharmacol* 1998;32 (Suppl 3):S62–6
35. Caulin-Glaser T, Watson CA, Pardi R, Bender JR. Effects of 17beta-estradiol on cytokine-induced endothelial cell adhesion molecule expression. *J Clin Invest* 1996;98:36–42
36. Simoncini T, De Caterina R, Genazzani AR. Selective estrogen receptor modulators: different actions on vascular cell adhesion molecule-1 (VCAM-1) expression in human endothelial cells. *J Clin Endocrinol Metab* 1999;84:815–18
37. Cid MC, Kleinman HK, Grant DS, *et al.* Estradiol enhances leukocyte binding to tumor necrosis factor (TNF)-stimulated endothelial cells via an increase in TNF-induced adhesion molecules E-selectin, intercellular adhesion molecule type 1, and vascular cell adhesion molecule type 1. *J Clin Invest* 1994;93:17–25
38. Winkler M, Kemp B, Hauptmann S, Rath W. Parturition: steroids, prostaglandin E2, and expression of adhesion molecules by endothelial cells. *Obstet Gynecol* 1997;89:398–402
39. van Baal WM, Kenemans P, Emeis JJ, *et al.* Long-term effects of combined hormone replacement therapy on markers of endothelial function and inflammatory activity in healthy postmenopausal women. *Fertil Steril* 1999;71:663–70
40. Hwang S-J, Ballantyne CM, Sharrett R, *et al.* Circulating adhesion molecules VCAM-1, ICAM-1, and E-selectin in carotid atherosclerosis and incident coronary heart disease cases: the Atherosclerosis Risk in Communities (ARIC) study. *Circulation* 1997;96:4219–25
41. Ridker PM, Rifai N, Pfeffer MA, *et al.* Inflammation, pravastatin, and the risk of coronary events

after myocardial infarction in patients with average cholesterol levels. Cholesterol and Recurrent Events (CARE) Investigators. *Circulation* 1998;98: 839–44

42. Belch JJ, Shaw JW, Kirk G, *et al.* The white blood cell adhesion molecule E-selectin predicts restenosis in patients with intermittent claudication undergoing percutaneous transluminal angioplasty. *Circulation* 1997;95:2027–31
43. Caulin-Glaser T, Farrell WJ, *et al.* Modulation of circulating cell adhesion molecules in postmenopausal women with coronary artery disease. *J Am Coll Cardiol* 1998;31:1555–60
44. Herrington DM, Howard TD, Brosnihan KB, *et al.* Common estrogen receptor polymorphism augments effects of hormone replacement therapy on E-selectin but not C-reactive protein. *Circulation* 2002;105:1879–82
45. Herrington DM, Howard TD, Hawkins GA, *et al.* Estrogen-receptor polymorphisms and effects of estrogen replacement on high-density lipoprotein cholesterol in women with coronary disease. *N Engl J Med* 2002;34:967–74

# Hormone replacement therapy: new pharmacological and endocrinological approaches

25

*M. Oettel*

## INTRODUCTION

More than 70 years ago, Adolf Butenandt[1] reported on the improvement in the health status of 20-month-old female rats treated with estrogen for 3 months. After this pioneering work, estrogen-containing medicines were first introduced in the late 1940s as treatments for the climacteric symptoms associated with menopause[2]. At that time, knowledge of the pharmacology and toxicology was relatively limited, but it was very quickly extended during the following decades. The first publications about the estrogen receptor appeared in 1966[3] and about the progesterone receptor in 1970[4]. The public acceptance of hormone replacement therapy (HRT) in postmenopausal women from the 1960s to this day is like a roller-coaster ride between ebullient enthusiasm and strong scepticism. At present, we are again going through a depressive phase, which has been caused by the recent findings – or better, their public interpretations – of the Premarin/medroxyprogesterone acetate (MPA) arm of the American large-scale Women's Health Initiative (WHI) randomized trial[5] (published in July 2002) and the British Million Women Study[6] (published in August 2003).

Despite the enormous mis- and over-interpretations of these two studies, the pharmaceutical industry will continue research and development work in this field. At present, research into especially the molecular biological background of the steroid hormone action on different cells and tissues, including the estrogen and progestin signaling pathways, is being carried out intensively, giving rise to original approaches to the development of new hormonal regimens for postmenopausal women.

From a pharmacological and endocrinological point of view, we have strictly to distinguish between the effects of estrogens and those of progestins. Progestins must be administered in addition to the estrogens in women with a uterus to avoid a clearly increased risk of endometrial cancer[7]. To make it more difficult, with respect to neither the estrogens nor the progestins can we speak of uniform, comparable effects of the two pharmacological classes. Different estrogens and/or progestins may produce different results in clinical trials. Therefore, it also appears inappropriate to claim that the unwanted side-effects of the 'estrogens' or of the 'progestins' are a homogeneous class effect. In other words, an estrogen is not an estrogen as well as a progestin is not a progestin. Because the study arm with conjugated estrogens only (hysterectomized women) was not terminated, the presently known results of the WHI study have to be related mainly to the administration of the chosen progestin MPA, underlining the importance of the progestin component. But let us start with the estrogens.

## THE ESTROGENIC COMPONENT OF HRT

Originally identified as reproductive hormones, estrogens and progestins are now generally thought also to play important roles in non-reproductive tissues. Can we explain this by the evolution of steroid receptors within phylogenesis? To begin with, we can state that estrogen receptors (ER) $\alpha$ and $\beta$, androgen receptors, progesterone receptors, glucocorticoid receptors and mineralocorticoid receptors are not found outside the vertebrates[8], i.e. steroid receptors are principally vertebrate receptors. Within the vertebrates, the two estrogen receptors are definitely the oldest (Table 1[9]). From this, we can derive the fact that the target tissues for estrogens must be very multifarious, starting with the bone (vertebra or skeleton of symmetric animals) and then influencing all subsequently occurring organ systems like the cardiovascular system, central nervous system, and reproductive system. This could also explain why comparatively very low estrogen dosages are sufficient for bone protection. On the other hand, the specific regulation of physiological processes by progesterone is a relatively recent phylogenetic innovation[10] and is focused more on oviduct and oviposition in birds and uterus, pregnancy maintenance, and breast tissue in mammals. For the pharmacologists, this could imply that it is easier to find dissociated, tissue-specific estrogens than favorably dissociated progestins (e.g. without unwanted effects on the mammary gland).

## The human estrogens

The human estrogens are the estrogenic key steroid, 17β-estradiol, its oxidized form, the '17β-estradiol reservoir' estrone, and the impeded estrogen, estriol. In comparison to that of young, cyclic women in their follicular phase (corresponding to 100%), the daily production rate in postmenopausal women decreases to approximately 6–10% for 17β-estradiol and to approximately 60–80% for estrone, whereas there are no differences for estriol[11]. It is therefore obvious that 17β-estradiol (E2) or a suitable E2 ester should be administered for replacement in the presence of clear clinical symptoms of estrogen deficiency. E2 is the most suitable and tailorable human estrogen for this indication. For the reduction of bone turnover (see above-mentioned estrogen receptors as the phylogenetic first steroid receptors in vertebrates, i.e. the first animals with bones), the extremely low oral daily dose of 0.25 mg micronized E2 is sufficient[12]. This ultra-low dose of E2 decreases markers of bone turnover to the same degree as 0.5 mg/day or 1.0 mg/day of E2, with an adverse effect profile that was equivalent to placebo[13]. Another step forward in reducing the E2 dose has been made by Schering/Berlex Laboratories. A once-a-week transdermal patch delivers only 0.014 mg of E2 each day (Menostar®) and is still effective in the prevention of osteoporosis. This dosage provides nearly 50% less estrogen per day than the lowest-dose transdermal estrogen product currently available for the prevention of the important bone disease. The patch will not require a concomitant progestin, even for women with an intact uterus.

On the other hand, it must be considered that other tissues need much higher E2 doses for relieving symptoms of estrogen deficiency (e.g. hot flushes, mood swings). In the near future, the individualization of HRT will be enhanced by tailoring the dosages of E2, including new routes of administration and new pharmaceutical formulations, such as nasal[14] and intravaginal administration[15].

It remains an open question whether specific pharmacological interventions for influencing esterification, ester breakage, and reprocessing of the natural, endogenous E2 fatty acid esters can provide alternatives or additional pharmacological benefits for exogenous estrogen administration[16–18].

Our knowledge of the associations between estrogen receptor α gene polymorphisms and clinical and toxicological effects of estrogens will

**Table 1** Evolution of steroid receptors[8–10]

| *Steroid receptor* | *First phylogenetic appearance* | *First evolutionary target* |
|---|---|---|
| Progesterone receptor | birds, mammals | oviduct, oviposition, uterus, mamma |
| Mineralocorticoid receptor | tetrapods | osmolarity, marine → fresh water, 'inner ocean' |
| Estrogen receptor | Atlantic croaker | ? |
| Androgen receptor | teleosts | sexual dimorphisms |
| Estrogen receptor α and β, CR | vertebrates | bone, stress |

CR, cortisol receptor

no doubt also be essentially extended in the future, thus contributing to a refining and tuning of the right dose[19–21].

## The animal estrogens

*Conjugated estrogens*

Conjugated equine estrogens (CEE) are a complex urinary extract of pregnant mare's urine and contain at least ten estrogens in their sulfate ester form; these are the ring B saturated estrogens, estrone (E1), 17β-estradiol (17β-E2), and 17α-estradiol (17α-E2), and the ring B unsaturated estrogens, equilin (Eq), 17β-dihydroequilin (17β-Eq), 17α-dihydroequilin (17α-Eq), equilenin (Eqn), 17β-dihydroequilenin (17β-Eqn), 17α-dihydroequilenin (17α-Eqn), and $\Delta^{8,9}$-dehydroestrone ($\Delta^{8,9}$-dehydro-E1). CEE is the most widely prescribed estrogenic formulation for HRT. Precise pharmacokinetic studies of the oral formulation have been difficult. Some equine derivatives have a half-life of several days[22].

Several ring B unsaturated conjugated estrogens have been shown to have a nearly two-fold higher affinity for the ERβ, and experimental data have indicated that $\Delta^{8,9}$-dehydroestrone exhibits tissue-selective effects[23]. However, it is not known now whether certain components of CEE will be marketed as single-agent drugs. Nevertheless, certain equine estrogens are lead compounds in the search for new, tissue-specific estrogens.

*17α-Estradiol*

This weak estrogenic epimer of 17β-estradiol is the main endogenous estrogen in cows. 17α-E2 shows low relative binding to ERα (~ 23%), preferring binding to ERβ[23] and 10–100 times lower 'classical' genomic action (e.g. on the rodent uterus *in vivo* and on human breast cancer cells *in vitro*). In principle, endogenous 17α-E2 can be formed by aromatization of epi-testosterone. However, we only succeeded in sporadically detecting 17α-E2 in the serum of untreated men and men treated orally with 17α-E2 using gas chromatography/liquid mass chromatography. The reason was an enormous first-pass effect in the liver[24]. This caused us to develop better designed, more stable derivatives of 17α-E2. These compounds showed an excellent pharmacodynamic profile *in vitro* as well as *in vivo*. Unfortunately, in our own clinical studies with one of these steroids (J 861), the desired dissociation was not seen between strong estrogenic action on the central nervous and cardiovascular systems and failing or very low estrogenic activities on the uterus[25].

## The plant estrogens

Given the positive effects of lower-dose estrogen, it could be plausible and logical to look for substances that have less affinity for the estrogen receptor than 17β-E2 and use other signaling pathways in the hope of identifying herbs or nutritional supplements that reduce menopausal symptoms and, perhaps, benefit bone without the adverse effects associated with HRT. By integrating ancient medical and botanical knowledge with modern technologies of molecular biology, it is anxiously hoped to find several options to reduce the effects of estrogen deficiency on postmenopausal women[26].

The so-called phytoestrogens are non-steroidal plant compounds. The most common types of phytoestrogens are coumestans, lignans and isoflavones. The major dietary isoflavones, genistein and daidzein, are found almost exclusively in legumes, including soy. These compounds have definitely weak 'classical', genomic estrogenic activity[27]. Other signaling pathways within the target cell are being discussed, e.g. the inhibition of tyrosine kinase[28].

Phytoestrogens are thought to have estrogenic and non-estrogenic or antiestrogenic effects, like selective estrogen receptor modulators (SERMs), depending on the respective tissue and receptor availability. Some of these plant estrogens, including genistein and also silymarin, appear to have greater affinity for ERβ, as opposed to ERα[29]. This may explain the anticipated positive effects on the central nervous system, blood vessels, and bone, whilst conversely little or no effect on breast and endometrial tissue[30].

Epidemiological data suggest that phytoestrogens could have a preventive effect against various estrogen-related diseases/symptoms, such as breast cancer, menopausal symptoms, cardiovascular diseases and osteoporosis. To prove these assumptions, available controlled clinical trials have been critically reviewed. In particular, soy isoflavones have been studied extensively[31]. However, there is no scientific evidence so far for an effect of phytoestrogens on menopausal symptoms and risk factors for breast cancer. On the other hand, isoflavones containing soy protein can lower the serum levels of total cholesterol, low density lipoprotein (LDL) cholesterol and triglycerides[32]. There is relatively strong evidence for a preventive effect of soy isoflavones on postmenopausal bone loss of the lumbar spine. However, the heterogeneity of the published clinical studies performed to date means it is difficult to make a definitive statement[30]. In addition, the pharmacological background for bone-protective effects of soy phytoestrogens has remained unclear to date[33].

## The selective estrogen receptor modulators

The clinical development of non-steroidal antiestrogens over the past 40 years has resulted in the first agents (clomiphene and tamoxifen) for the induction of ovulation in subfertile women, the first antiestrogen (tamoxifen) specifically for the treatment of ER-positive breast cancer, the first chemopreventive (tamoxifen) to reduce the incidence of breast cancer in high-risk pre- and postmenopausal women, and the first SERM (raloxifene) for the treatment and prevention of osteoporosis, but with breast and uterine safety[34]. SERMs are mostly non-steroid molecules that maintain some of the desirable agonist properties of estrogens, e.g. on bone tissue and the cardiovascular system, but not their stimulating effects on the gynecological sphere[35]. The discovery by Jordan and co-workers in 1987[36], that the 'antiestrogens' tamoxifen and raloxifene showed estrogenic effects in preventing bone loss in ovariectomized rats, revolutionized the way in which we have come to think of nuclear receptor functioning. Since that time, broad insights have been garnered into both the mechanisms involved in the primary, ligand-activated nuclear transcription pathway as well as other, non-traditional pathways via which estrogens may exert their effects[37]. However, the different molecular biological details of the mode of action of SERMs are not being treated in greater detail here (for review see reference 38). For example, Martini and Katzenellenbogen[39] recently identified a selective repressor protein of estrogen receptor activity.

From the clinical point of view, treatments with SERMs, such as tamoxifen and raloxifene, may provide partial benefits with respect to the risk of breast cancer, some cardiovascular risk factors (LDL-cholesterol, fibrinogen), and bone loss, but may be associated with increases in subclinically worsening prolapse[40], in endometrial cancer (tamoxifen), and hot flushes (raloxifene), and their effect on heart disease is uncertain[38]. Therefore, a variety of SERMs are now being examined for potential use in the prevention and treatment of postmenopausal conditions. In the near future, the armamentarium of clinically useful SERMs will be broadened.

## The ligands for estrogen receptor isotypes α and β

The discovery of a second estrogen receptor isotype ERβ has provided additional possibilities for the treatment of estrogen deficiency. The initially great expectations are based on the observation that ERα and ERβ are unequally distributed in various tissues. These results give hope that tissue-specific effects can be achieved with ER isotype-selective ligands. Subsequently, the question arose which physiological responses are attributable to either ERα or ERβ or both receptors[41]. To answer these questions, mRNA and protein expression of the receptors in numerous tissues have been studied[42–44]. Dominant expression of the respective ER isotypes in certain tissues suggests a distinct physiological role. ERα has a broad expression pattern and is most abundant in uterus, vagina, liver, and pituitary. ERβ is expressed in rat ovary, prostate, epididymis, lung, hypothalamus and bladder[45]. Low expression of ERβ was observed in all uterine tissues[46].

The hoped-for physiological importance of ERα and ERβ has also been documented using ERα knockout mice. The most commonly recognized estrogenic responses (uterine weight, vaginal cornification, etc.) are obliterated in ERα knockout mice which can be considered to be ERβ-dominant[47,48]. However, the ovary secretes high levels of estrogen. The ERβ knockout, by contrast, has ovarian anomalies[49]. Therefore, specific agonists or antagonists for ERα and ERβ might potentially be important therapeutic agents. However, the complex situation with selective targeting of ERα and ERβ is that the distribution of the receptors may be exclusively ERα or ERβ at some target sites, but other sites may contain a combination of the receptor types, leading to compensatory mechanisms. As a start, the drug discovery process is exploiting relative receptor affinities as a means of establishing drug selectivity. In this context, Craig V. Jordan postulates that, if the ligand has an approximately 1000-fold (!) excess affinity for one receptor over another, this may provide therapeutic selectivity if pharmacokinetics can be controlled[34].

The other complicating situation is that agonist ligands at ERα and ERβ may have selectivity of action based on the perturbation of their respective complexes. In other words, all estrogens may not be the same, and different classes of estrogens that exist by complexing ERα may produce agonist as well as antagonist actions at ERβ sites, based on the structure of the complex. Incidentally, this is one of the key messages of this review: an estrogen is not an estrogen. Clinical findings obtained with one estrogen cannot be translated to the situation with another estrogen. One of the reasons for this is the recognition that the ERβ gene has an impaired AF-1 domain compared with ERα, so that the necessary synergy with the AF-2 coactivator binding site is dramatically reduced[50]. Progress in receptor selectivity will be evaluated on the basis of modern techniques for studying both structure–function relationships and comparing with the well-known methodology for estimating relative receptor affinity.

An example of the pharmaceutical industry's efforts to find potent selective ligands for the two estrogen receptors from structure-based design comes from Hillisch and colleagues[41]. Based on the crystal structure of the ERα ligand-binding domain (LBD) and a homology model of the ERβ LBD, the group has found steroidal ligands that exploit the differences in size and flexibility of the two ligand-binding cavities. To unravel the physiological roles of the two receptors, *in vivo* experiments with rats were conducted using the found ERα and ERβ selective agonists in comparison to 17β-estradiol. The ERα agonist induced uterine growth and caused bone-protective effects, reduced plasma levels of luteinizing hormone and follicle stimulating hormone (FSH) and increased angiotensin I, while the ERβ agonist did not lead at all, or only at high doses, to such effects despite high plasma levels. It can thus be concluded that estrogen effects on the uterus, pituitary, bone and liver are primarily mediated via ERα. The simultaneous administration of the ERα and ERβ ligands did not lead to an attenuation of ERα-mediated effects on the uterus, pituitary and liver parameters.

In the near future, we will know more about the specific pharmacodynamic profile, for example of selective ERβ ligands. Only then will it be possible to make more exact assessments of their value in medical use and the approximate launch date of specific estrogen receptor ligands for HRT.

## Pharmacological interactions with estrogen-transforming enzymes

Two principal pathways are involved in the last steps of E2 formation: the 'aromatase pathway', which transforms androgens, mainly androstenedione, into estrogens, and the 'sulfatase pathway', which converts estrone sulfate into estrone by estrone sulfatase (EC:3.1.6.2). The final step of estrogen genesis is the conversion of the weak estrone to the potent biologically active E2 by the action of a reductive 17β-hydroxysteroid dehydrogenase type 1 activity (17β-HSD-1; EC:1.1.1.62)[51].

### *Induction of aromatase*

The number of primordial follicles, and hence granulosa cells, tends towards zero at the menopause[52]. Thus, one of the most important synthetic sites for the biosynthesis of estrogens is no longer available and the postmenopausal woman now gains insufficient amounts of estrogen only from the aromatization of androgens in the periphery, mainly from the fatty tissue. It might, therefore, be a logical approach to increase the endogenous estrogen biosynthesis by an induction or amplification of the aromatase activity. Circulating steroidal androgenic precursors are essential substrates for extragonadal estrogen biosynthesis via aromatase. However, the levels of $C_{19}$-precursors decline markedly with advancing age in women, possibly from the mid- to the late reproductive years. This may explain why women are at increased risk for bone mineral loss and fracture and possibly decline in cognitive function compared with men. Aromatase expression in these various sites is regulated - under the control of only one gene, but of different tissue-specific promoters - by different cohorts of transcription factors. Thus, in principle, it should be possible to develop selective aromatase modulators that block aromatase expression in unwanted target tissues (for example, in breast and uterus), but allow unimpaired estrogen biosynthesis in other tissues such as bone or the central nervous system[53].

As well as the androgens as natural substrates for aromatase, a number of other inductors or modulators of aromatase activity are well known: glucocorticoids[54], 17α-E2[55], FSH[56,57], growth factors like insulin growth factor-1 (IGF-I)[58,59] and transforming growth factor-α (TGFα)[60], some nucleotides[61,62], prostaglandin $E_2$ ($PGE_2$)[63], and even pesticides[64]. In spite of that, it can be assessed that an aromatase inductor for the treatment of climacteric symptoms will not be launched in the short or medium term.

*Inhibition of estrone sulfatase*

There is convincing evidence that, like the aromatase pathway, the estrone sulfatase pathway, i.e. hydrolysis of estrone sulfate to estrone, plays an important role in the *in situ* production of bioactive estrogens in breast tumors, accounting for the higher estrogen levels in breast tumors of postmenopausal women than those in plasma from the same individuals[65]. Thus, estrogen derivatives as well as non-estrogens as inhibitors of estrone sulfatase are welcomed as a new approach to estrogen replacement in the hope of a significant reduction of the breast cancer risk. Although several groups have found effective inhibitors of estrone sulfatase, no compound has advanced far enough in clinical trials as to give us reason to expect a medicinal product with this very original mode of action for HRT in the near future[66-74].

*Cell technological and stem cell approaches for enhancing endogenous estrogens*

Although the conditions for cultivation and storage of granulosa cells have long been known[75,76], no practical procedures for the removal of granulosa cells or parts of ovaries (autografts) in premenopausal women and subsequent long-term storage and retransfer after menopause are known. The same observation applies to stem cell technology.

However, granulosa and germinal epithelium appear to be derived from different progenitor cells[77]. This could mean that stem cell technology for obtaining granulosa cells is not related to interference with the germline.

## THE PROGESTATIONAL COMPONENT OF HRT

At present, at least 22 different progestins are on the market (Figure 1). Almost all of them are also

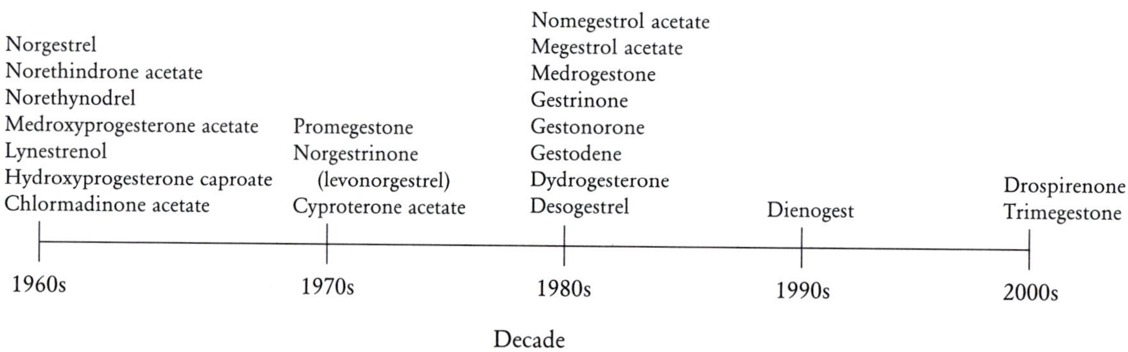


**Figure 1** Launch of progestins

**Table 2** The history of medical indications for progestins

| | |
|---|---|
| 1934 | Replacement therapy in oophorectomized women (Kaufmann) |
| 1937 | Treatment of oligo- and hypomenorrhea (von Kehrer) |
| 1938 | Treatment of anovulation (Clauberg) |
| 1953 | Treatment of menorrhagia (Kaufmann) |
| 1956 | Female contraception with norethynodrel (Pincus) |
| 1969 | Endometriosis (Kistner) |
| 1970s | Postmenopausal hormone replacement therapy |
| 1980s | Male contraception |
| 1990s | Premenstrual syndrome |
| 2000s | Endometriosis and leiomyoma (SPRMs and/or tissue-selective progestins) |

SPRM, selective progesterone receptor modulator

used as progestational components for HRT. Table 2 shows the history of medical indications for progestins. Interestingly, replacement therapy in oophorectomized women was considered as the first indication for progestins as early as in 1934. Progestins have been administered together with estrogens for the prevention of endometrial hyperplasia from the 1970s.

## A progestin is not a progestin

The group of progestins is so heterogeneous regarding its pharmacodynamic as well as pharmacokinetic profile that one cannot speak of a uniform pharmacological class at all. The reason is that the only pharmacological feature common to all progestins is the secretory transformation of the estrogen-primed rabbit endometrium. All other actions differ so much that it is not justified to compare the clinical results of one progestin with those of another progestin.

Examples of the huge variety of actions of progestins include those below[78-84]:

(1) Binding at steroid receptors other than the progesterone receptor and therefore activation of several gene transcriptions and hence, very different estrogenic or antiestrogenic, glucocorticoid or antiglucocorticoid, mineralocorticoid or antimineralocorticoid activities;

(2) Signaling pathways other than the 'classical' nuclear progesterone receptor[85-87];

(3) Androgenic or antiandrogenic effects including effects on the ovarian, adrenal, and dermal steroid biosynthesis and steroid metabolism[88];

(4) Strong or weak inhibition of gonadotropin secretion[25,83];

(5) Very different endothelial actions[89-93];

(6) Extremely varying effects on different functions of the central nervous system; depending on dosage, regimen, and respective pharmacodynamic profile, progestins attenuate the genomic as well as the non-genomic estrogen effects on the central nervous system[94,95];

(7) Different actions on hepatic functions despite absence of the progesterone receptor in the liver[96,97];

(8) Angiogenic as well antiangiogenic effects[98,99];

(9) Proliferative vs. antiproliferative actions on mammary tissues[100].

There are also enormous differences in the pharmacokinetics of the various progestins. For example, the terminal half-lives may range from 7 h (norethindrone acetate) to more than 70 h (chlormadinone acetate). This correlates very well with the strongly differing metabolic stability in human liver microsomal preparations *in vitro*[101]. The plasma distribution volumes vary from 3.7 (drospirenone) to 46.2 (dienogest) l/kg and the relative binding to sex hormone binding globulin (SHBG) from zero (dienogest, drospirenone) to 75.3% (gestodene). Finally, the progestins may be on the market as active drugs or as prodrugs (e.g. ethynodiol diacetate vs. norethindrone; desogestrel vs. 3-ketodesogestrel).

The 19-norprogestins without the 17α-ethinyl group (dienogest, drospirenone, trimegestone) introduce a new stage. These progestins combine features of modern norprogestins and natural 17α-hydroxyprogesterone derivatives[25,102-104]. The expected pharmacodynamic profile of a progestin of the future includes:

(1) Antiproliferative action on mammary gland and endometrium;

(2) No unwanted effects on the cardiovascular system and on liver functions;

(3) Antiandrogenic action on the skin;

(4) No influence on libido;

(5) Bone protection;

(6) No antiestrogenic action on the central nervous system.

However, among the many progestins for HRT already on the market, there exists no compound of first choice. Therefore, the development of new generations of progestins to improve the selectivity profile of these compounds will be a great challenge. Perhaps also, non-steroidals will play a greater part in the future. For example, the naturally occurring progestational plant substances, like the flavonoid apigenin from chamomile or some procyanidines from grape-seed extracts, could be lead structures for the chemists[105]. Beyond this, there exists no correlation between progestational and antiproliferative activities of progestins. Therefore, directed progestin development with concomitant anti-proliferative benefit could be envisaged (W. Römer, personal communication).

## Selective progesterone receptor modulators

Modern techniques of quantitative structure-activity relationships (QSAR) have made it possible to develop specific receptor modulators also with the progestins[106-108]. A wanted tissue-specific progestin would counteract the stimulatory effect of estrogens on the uterus, while not interfering with the estrogen's other actions, e.g. bone activity. Will selective progesterone receptor modulators (SPRMs) be the future HRT component to counteract the proliferative effects of estrogens on endometrium and simultaneously on the different mammary gland tissues? Both steroidal and non-steroidal SPRMs are in the phase of preclinical development. Therefore, the evaluation of their therapeutic potential is difficult at present[80]. Most advanced in clinical trials in premenopausal as well as postmenopausal women are the so-called mesoprogestins asoprisnil (J 867) and asoprisnil ecamate (J 956). These compounds belong to a group of 11β-phenyl ring-substituted steroids that have both antiprogestational and progestational activities[109,110]. Here, too, a clear statement on the therapeutic significance of the mesoprogestins cannot be made at present.

## Selective ligands for progesterone receptor isoforms A and B

Receptors for progesterone are expressed as two distinct isoforms, PR-A and PR-B, that arise from a single gene but with alternate promoters[111]. The expression of both isoforms is conserved in rodents and humans and overlaps spatiotemporally in female reproductive tissues. However, the ratios of the individual isoforms vary in reproductive tissues as a consequence of developmental and hormonal status and during carcinogenesis. Briefly, the PR-A isoform is necessary for uterine blastocyst implantation, and ablation of PR-A results in abnormal progesterone-dependent uterine epithelial proliferation. On the other hand, the PR-A isoform is not required for eliciting mammary gland morphogenic response to progesterone in rodents[112,113].

*In vitro* evidence reveals that PR-A inhibits PR-B function and the cellular ratio of PR-A : PR-B is likely to be an important determinant of the progesterone action on a given tissue[114]. One may easily imagine that these pharmacological findings greatly stimulate researchers in the pharmaceutical industry. For example, Larrea and colleagues[115] have found that gestodene is a relatively more potent transcriptional activator of PR-A than either norethindrone or progesterone. However, our knowledge obtained with this original pharmacological approach does not yet allow a reliable statement to be made on the therapeutic-clinical potential of specific ligands of the two PR isoforms.

## CONCLUDING REMARKS

This review only refers to the many new pharmacological possibilities to be expected for estrogen replacement with or without progestins for the treatment of postmenopausal symptoms, from the personal point of view of an employee of the pharmaceutical industry. As shown in this paper, a great number of basic endocrine pharmacological approaches exist that are being followed by different companies in a very persistent and costly way. From the point of view of clinical research, the old question still remains to be answered: how can suitable markers be used to recognize postmenopausal women who are still healthy but have a specific risk factor, in good time to include them in placebo-controlled studies?

However, the clinical and practical relevance of the different relatively mature or relatively immature approaches, in most cases, is still not clear. Therefore, it will be essential during the next few years to use the existing therapeutic armamentarium better than before. Key words for this statement include qualified clinical experience on a rational basis, individualization including tailoring of estradiol dose, greater emphasis on pharmacokinetics, new pharmaceutical formulations (e.g. intrauterine progestin insertion) and, last but not least, permanent information and education of the patients, the physicians, and the public.

# References


1. Butenandt A. Untersuchungen über das weibliche Sexualhormon. Abhandlung der Ges. der Wiss. zu Göttingen, III. Folge, Heft 2, Tafel IV, 1931
2. McDonnell DP. Mining the complexities of the estrogen signalling pathways for novel therapeutics. *Endocrinology* 2003;144:4237–40
3. Toft DO, Gorski J. A receptor molecule for estrogens: isolation from the rat uterus and preliminary characterization. *Proc Natl Acad Sci USA* 1966;55:1574–81
4. O'Malley BW, Sherman MR, Toft DO. Progesterone 'receptors' in the cytoplasm and nucleus of chick oviduct target tissue. *Proc Natl Acad Sci USA* 1970;67:501–8
5. National Institutes of Health. NIH news release. NHLBI stops trial of estrogen plus progestin due to increased breast cancer risk, lack of overall benefit. www.nhlbi.nih.gov/new/press/02-07-09.htm (accessed 2002 Aug 27)
6. Million Women Study Collaborators. Breast cancer and hormone-replacement therapy in the Million Women Study. *Lancet* 2003;362:419–27
7. Newcomb PA, Trentham-Dietz A, Egan KM, *et al.* Fracture history and risk of breast and endometrial cancer. *Am J Epidemiol* 2001;153:1071–8
8. Thornton JW, Need E, Crews D. Resurrecting the ancestral steroid receptor: ancient origin of estrogen signaling. *Science* 2003;301:1714–17
9. McLachlan JA. Environmental signaling: What embryos and evolution teach us about endocrine disrupting chemicals. *Endocr Rev* 2001;22:319–41
10. Thornton JW. Evolution of vertebrate steroid receptors from an ancestral estrogen receptor by ligand exploitation and serial genome expansions. *Proc Natl Acad Sci USA* 2001;98:5671–6
11. Gruber CJ ,Tschugguel W, Schneeberger C, *et al.* Production and actions of estrogens. *N Engl J Med* 2002;346:340–52
12. Prestwood KM, Kenny AM, Kleppinger A, *et al.* Ultralow-dose micronized 17β-estradiol and bone density and bone metabolism in older women. *J Am Med Assoc* 2003;290:1042–8
13. Prestwood KM, Kenny AM, Unson C, *et al.* The effect of low dose micronized 17β-estradiol on bone turnover, sex hormone levels, and side effects in older women. *J Clin Endocrinol Metab* 2000;85:4462–9
14. Wattanakumtornkul S, Pinto AB, Williams DB. Intranasal hormone replacement therapy. *Menopause* 2003;10:88–98

15. Speroff L. Efficacy and tolerability of a novel estradiol vaginal ring for relief of menopausal symptoms. *Obstet Gynecol* 2003;102:823-34
16. Fernández-Real JM, Sanchis D, Ricart W, *et al.* Plasma oestrone-fatty acid ester levels are correlated with body fat mass in humans. *Clin Endocrinol* 1999;50:253-60
17. Paris A, Goutal I, Richard J, *et al.* Uterotrophic effect of a saturated fatty acid 17-ester of estradiol-17beta administered orally to juvenile rats. *APMIS* 2001;109:365-75
18. Cullel-Young M, Del Fresno M. Oleoyl-estrone. *Drugs Future* 2002;27:648-54
19. Herrington DM, Howard TD, Hawkins GA, *et al.* Estrogen-receptor polymorphisms and effects of estrogen replacement on high-density lipoprotein cholesterol in women with coronary disease. *N Engl J Med* 2002;346:967-74
20. Herrington DM, Howard TD, Brosnihan KB, *et al.* Common estrogen receptor polymorphism augments effects of hormone replacement therapy on E-selectin but not C-reactive protein. *Circulation* 2002;105:1879-82
21. Shearman AM, Cupples LA, Demissie S, *et al.* Association between estrogen receptor α gene variation and cardiovascular disease. *J Am Med Assoc* 2003;290:2263-70
22. DeLignière B, Silberstein S. Pharmacodynamics of oestrogens and progestogens. *Cephalalgia* 2000; 20:200-7
23. Bhavnani BR. Estrogens and menopause: pharmacology of conjugated equine estrogens and their potential role in the prevention of neurodegenerative diseases such as Alzheimer's. *J Steroid Biochem Molec Biol* 2003;85:473-82
24. Hobe G, Schön R, Goncharov N, *et al.* Some new aspects of 17α-estradiol metabolism in man. *Steroids* 2002;67:883-93
25. Oettel M, Holz C. Hybrid progestins: the example of dienogest. In Sitruk-Ware R, Mishell DR, eds. *Progestins and Antiprogestins in Clinical Practice.* New York: Marcel Dekker, 2000:163-77
26. Prestwood KM. The search for alternative therapies for menopausal women: estrogenic effects of herbs. *J Clin Endocrinol Metab* 2003;88:4075-6
27. Jefferson WN, Newbold RR. Potential endocrine-modulating effects of various phytoestrogens in the diet. *Nutrition* 2000;16:659-62
28. Makarevich A, Sirotkin A, Taradajnik T, *et al.* Effects of genistein and lavendustin on reproductive processes in domestic animals *in vitro.* *J Steroid Biochem Molec Biol* 1997;63:329-37
29. Seidlova-Wuttke S, Becker T, Christoffel V, *et al.* Silymarin is a selective estrogen receptor β (ERβ) agonist and has estrogenic effects in the metaphysis of the femur but no antiestrogenic effects in the uterus of ovariectomized (ovx) rats. *J Steroid Biochem Molec Biol* 2003;86:179-88
30. Huntley AL, Ernst E. Soy for the treatment of perimenopausal symptoms - a systematic review. *Maturitas* 2003;in press
31. Zitterman A. Phytoöstrogene. *Zentralbl Gynäkol* 2003;125:195-201
32. Anderson JW, Johnstone BM, Cook-Newell ME. Meta-analysis of the effects of soy protein intake on serum lipids. *N Engl J Med* 1995;333:276-82
33. Register TC, Jayo M J, Anthony MS. Soy phytoestrogens do not prevent bone loss in postmenopausal monkeys. *J Clin Endocrinol Metab* 2003;88:4362-70
34. Jordan VC. Antiestrogens and selective estrogen receptor modulators as multifunctional medicines. 2. Clinical considerations and new agents. *J Med Chem* 2003;46:1081-111
35. Trémollières F, Lopes P. Les modulateurs spécifiques des récepteurs oestrogéniques (SERMs). *Presse Med* 2002;31:1323-8
36. Jordan VC, Phelps E, Lindgren JU. Effects of anti-estrogens on bone in castrated and intact female rats. *Breast Cancer Res Treat* 1987;10:31-5
37. Miller CP. SERMs: evolutionary chemistry, revolutionary biology. *Curr Pharm Dev* 2002;8: 2089-111
38. Riggs BL, Hartmann LC. Selective estrogen-receptor modulators - mechanisms of action and application to clinical practice. *N Engl J Med* 2003;348:618-29
39. Martini PGV, Katzenellenbogen BS. Modulation of estrogen receptor activity by selective coregulators. *J Steroid Biochem Molec Biol* 2003;85: 117-22
40. Vardy MD, Lindsay R, Scotti RJ, *et al.* Short-term urogenital effects of raloxifene, tamoxifen, and estrogen. *Am J Obstet Gynecol* 2003;189:81-8
41. Hillisch A, Peters O, Kosemund D, *et al.* Dissecting physiological roles of receptor α and β with potent selective ligands from structure-based design. *Proc Natl Acad Sci USA*, submitted
42. Dechering K, Boersma C, Mosselman S. Estrogen receptors α and β: two receptors of a kind? *Curr Med Chem* 2000;7:561-76
43. Nilsen J, Brinton RD. Impact of progestins on estrogen-induced neuroprotection: synergy by progesterone and 19-norprogesterone and antagonism by medroxyprogesterone acetate. *Endocrinology* 2002;143:205-12
44. Pettersson K, Gustafsson JA. Role of estrogen receptor beta in estrogen action. *Annu Rev Physiol* 2001;63:165-92
45. Kuiper GG, Gustafsson JA. The novel estrogen receptor-beta subtype: potential role in the cell- and promoter-specific actions of estrogens and anti-estrogens. *FEBS Lett* 1997;410:87-90
46. Frasor J, Barnett DH, Danes JM, *et al.* Response-specific and ligand dose-dependent modulation of estrogen receptor (ER) alpha activity by

ERbeta in the uterus. *Endocrinology* 2003;144: 3159-66

47. Lubahn DB, Moyer JS, Golding TS, *et al.* Alteration of reproductive function but not prenatal sexual development after insertional disruption of the mouse estrogen receptor gene. *Proc Natl Acad Sci USA* 1993;90:11162-66
48. Couse JF, Lindzey J, Grandien K, *et al.* Tissue distribution and quantitative analysis of estrogen receptor-alpha (ERalpha) and estrogen receptor-beta (ERbeta) messenger ribonucleic acid in the wild-type and ERalpha-knockout mouse. *Endocrinology* 1997;138:4613-21
49. Krege JH, Hodgin JB, Couse JF, *et al.* Generation and reproductive phenotypes of mice lacking estrogen receptor beta. *Proc Natl Acad Sci USA* 1998;95:15677-82
50. McInerney EM, Weis KE, Sun J, *et al.* Transcription activation by the human estrogen receptor subtype beta (ER beta) studied with ER beta and ER alpha receptor chimeras. *Endocrinology* 1998;139:4513-22
51. Pasqualini JR, Caubel P, Friedman AJ, *et al.* Norelgestromin as a selective estrogen enzyme modulator in human breast cancer cell lines. Effect on sulfatase activity in comparison to medroxyprogesterone acetate. *J Steroid Biochem Molec Biol* 2003;84:193-8
52. Block E. Quantitative morphological investigations of the follicular system in women. Variation at different ages. *Acta Anat* 1952;14:108-23
53. Simpson ER, Davis SR. Minireview: aromatase and the regulation of estrogen biosynthesis - some new perspectives. *Endocrinology* 2001;142:4589-94
54. Simpson ER, Ackerman GE, Smith ME, *et al.* Estrogen formation in stromal cells of adipose tissue of women: induction by glucocorticoids. *Proc Natl Acad Sci USA* 1981;78:5690-4
55. Hoffmann R, Niiyama S, Huth A, *et al.* 17α-estradiol induces aromatase activity in intact human anagen hair follicles *ex vivo*. *Exp Dermatol* 2002;11:376-80
56. Hillier SG, DeZwart FA. Evidence that granulosa cell aromatase induction/activation by follicle-stimulating hormone is an androgen receptor-regulated process *in-vitro*. *Endocrinology* 1981;109: 1303-5
57. Chan WK, Tan CH. Induction of aromatase activity in porcine granulosa cells by FSH and cyclic AMP. *Endocr Res* 1987;13:285-99
58. Adashi EY, Resnick CE, Brodie AMH, *et al.* Somatomedin-C-mediated potentiation of follicle-stimulating hormone-induced aromatase activity of cultured rat granulosa cells. *Endocrinology* 1985;117:2313-20
59. Costrici N, Lunenfeld B, Pariente C, *et al.* Induction of aromatase in human granulosa cells by both follicle stimulating hormone and insulin-like growth factor-I involves tyrosine phosphorylation. *Gynecol Endocrinol* 1994;8:183-9
60. Gangrade BK, Davis JS, May JV. A novel mechanism for the induction of aromatase in ovarian cells *in vitro*: role of transforming growth factor alpha-induced protein tyrosine kinase. *Endocrinology* 1991;129:2790-2
61. Bellino FL, Hussa RO. Estrogen synthetase stimulation by dibutyryl cyclic adenosine 3′,5′-monophosphate on human choriocarcinoma cell culture: the relative biosynthetic rate of the nicotinamide adenine dinucleotide phosphate (reduced form)-cytochrome c reductase component. *Endocrinology* 1982;111:1038-44
62. Schmidt M, Löffler G. Induction of aromatase activity in human adipose tissue stromal cells by extracellular nucleotides. *Eur J Biochem* 1998; 252:147-54
63. Brueggemeier RW, Richards JA, Joomprabutra S, *et al.* Molecular pharmacology of aromatase and its regulation by endogenous and exogenous agents. *J Steroid Biochem Molec Biol* 2001;79:75-84
64. Sanderson JT, Boerma J, Lansbergen GWA, *et al.* Induction and inhibition of aromatase (CYP19) activity by various classes of pesticides in H295R human adrenocortical carcinoma cells. *Toxicol Appl Pharmacol* 2002;182:44-5
65. Chatterton RT, Geiger AS, Gann PH, *et al.* Formation of estrone and estradiol from estrone sulfate by normal breast parenchymal tissue. *J Steroid Biochem Molec Biol* 2003;86:159-66
66. Schwarz S, Weber G, Kühner F. Sulfamate des 17α-Äthinylestradiols. *Z Chem* 1970;10:299-300
67. Stölzner W. Tierexperimenteller Beitrag zur Entwicklung estrogener Wirkstoffe. Dissertation (Promotion B), Friedrich-Schiller-Universität Jena, 1989
68. Elger W, Schwarz S, Hedden A, *et al.* Sulfamates of various estrogens are prodrugs with increased systemic and reduced hepatic estrogenicity at oral application. *J Steroid Biochem Molec Biol* 1995; 55:395-403
69. Elger W, Palme HJ, Schwarz S. Novel oestrogen sulfamates: a new approach to oral hormone therapy. *Exp Opin Invest Drugs* 1998;7:575-89
70. Woo LWL, Howarth NM, Purohit A, *et al.* Steroidal and nonsteroidal sulfamates as potent inhibitors of steroid sulfatase. *J Med Chem* 1998; 41:1068-83
71. Römer W, Oettel M, Schwarz S. Scavestrogen sulfamates: correlation between estrone sulfatase inhibiting and antioxidant effects. *Can J Physiol Pharmacol* 1998;76:99-109
72. Barth A, Römer W, Oettel M. Influence of subchronic administration of oestrone-3-O-sulphamate on oestrone sulphatase activity in liver, spleen, and white blood cells of ovariectomized rats. *Arch Toxicol* 2000;74:366-71

73. Winum JY, Vullo D, Casini A, *et al.* Carbonic anhydrase inhibitors. Inhibition of cytosolic isozymes I and II and transmembrane, tumor-associated isozyme IX with sulfamates including EMATE also acting as steroid sulfatase inhibitors. *J Med Chem* 2003;46:2197-204
74. Raobaikady B, Purohit A, Chander SK, *et al.* Inhibition of MCF-7 breast cancer cell proliferation and *in vivo* steroid sulphatase activity by 2-methoxyoestradiol-bis-sulphamate. *J Steroid Biochem Molec Biol* 2003;84:351-8
75. McAllister JM, Mason JI, Byrd W, *et al.* Proliferating human granulosa-lutein cells in long term monolayer culture: expression of aromatase, cholesterol side-chain cleavage, and 3β-hydroxysteroid dehydrogenase. *J Clin Endocrinol Metab* 1990;71:26-33
76. Baird DT, Webb R, Campbell BK, *et al.* Long-term ovarian function in sheep after ovariectomy and transplantation of autografts stored at −196°C. *Endocrinology* 1999;140:462-71
77. Boland NI, Gosden RG. Clonal analysis of chimaeric mouse ovaries using DNA *in situ* hybridization. *J Reprod Fertil* 1994;100:203-10
78. Skouby SO. The rationale for a wider range of progestogens. *Climacteric* 2003;3(Suppl 2):14-20
79. Kuhl H. Neue Gestagene - ihre Vor- und Nachteile. *Therapeutische Umschau* 2001;58:527-33
80. Oettel M, Elger W, Gräser T, *et al.* What is past is prologue: estrogen/progestin replacement tomorrow. *Gynecol Endocrinol* 2001;15(Suppl 4): 68-90
81. Oettel M, Gräser T, Hoffmann H. Why dienogest as a progestogenic component of postmenopausal nonandrogenic hormone replacement therapy? *Drugs Today* 2001;37(Suppl G):3-15
82. Fylstra DL. Postmenopausal hormone replacement therapy: does the progestin make a difference? *J South Carolina Med Assoc* 2002;98:12-19
83. Sitruk-Ware R. Progestogens in hormonal replacement therapy: new molecules, risks, and benefits. *Menopause* 2002;9:6-15
84. Sitruk-Ware R. Progestins in hormonal replacement therapy (HRT): new molecules, risks and benefits. *Ann Endocrinol* 2003;64:178
85. Falkenstein E, Norman AW, Wehling M. Mannheim classification of nongenomically initiated (rapid) steroid action(s). *J Clin Endocrinol Metab* 2000;85:2072-5
86. Zhu Y, Bond J, Thomas P. Identification, classification, and partial characterization of genes in humans and other vertebrates homologous to a fish membrane progestin receptor. *PNAS* 2002; 100:2237-42
87. Sager G, Orbo A, Jaeger R, *et al.* Non-genomic effects of progestins - inhibition of cell growth and increased intracellular levels of cyclic nucleotides. *J Steroid Biochem Molec Biol* 2003;84:1-8
88. Raudant D, Rabe T. Progestogens with anti-androgenic properties. *Drugs* 2003;63:463-92
89. Seeger H, Mück AO, Lippert TH. Einfluss von Östradiol und der Gestagene Chlormadinonazetat, Dienogest und Norethisteron auf den Kalzium-Influx in menschlichen Aortenmuskelzellen: Vergleich bei ruhenden und aktivierten Zellen. *J Menopause* 1996;3:32-4
90. Sitruk-Ware R. Progestins and cardiovascular risk markers. *Steroids* 2000;65:651-8
91. Rosano GMC, Fini M. Comparative cardiovascular effects of different progestins in menopause. *Int J Fertil* 2001;46:248-56
92. Tatsumi H, Kitawaki J, Tanaka K, *et al.* Lack of stimulatory effect of dienogest on the expression of intercellular adhesion molecule-1 and vascular cell adhesion molecule-1 by endothelial cell as compared with other synthetic progestins. *Maturitas* 2002;42:287-94
93. Perusquia M, Villalón CM, Navarette E, *et al.* Vasodilating effect of norethisterone and its 5α metabolites: a novel nongenomic action. *Eur J Pharmacol* 2003;475:161-9
94. Nilsson S, Makela S, Treuter E, *et al.* Mechanisms of estrogen action. *Physiol Rev* 2001;81: 1535-65
95. Saletu G, Anderer P, Gruber G, *et al.* Insomnia related to postmenopausal syndrome and hormone replacement therapy: sleep laboratory studies on baseline differences between patients and controls and double-blind, placebo-controlled investigations on the effects of a novel estrogen-progestogen combination (Climodien®, Lafamme®) versus estrogen alone. *J Sleep Res* 2003;12:1-16
96. Brambilla G, Martelli A. Are some progestins genotoxic liver carcinogens? *Mutation Res* 2002; 412:155-63
97. Boada LD, Zumbado M, del Rio I, *et al.* Steroid hormone progesterone induces cell proliferation and abnormal mitotic processes in rat liver. *Arch Toxicol* 2002;75:707-16
98. Nakamura M, Katsuki Y, Shibutani Y, *et al.* Dienogest, a synthetic steroid, suppresses both embryonic and tumor-cell-induced angiogenesis. *Eur J Pharmacol* 1999;386:33-40
99. Hague S, MacKenzie IZ, Bicknell R, *et al.* *In-vivo* angiogenesis and progestogens. *Hum Reprod* 2002;17:786-93
100. Katsuki Y, Shibutani Y, Aoki D, *et al.* Dienogest, a novel synthetic steroid, overcomes hormone-dependent cancer in a different manner than progestins. *Cancer* 1997;79:169-76
101. Kuhnz W, Gieschen H. Predicting the oral bioavailability of 19-nortestosterone progestins *in vivo* from their metabolic stability in human liver microsomal preparations *in vitro*. *Drug Metab Dispos* 1998;26:1120-7

102. Krattenmacher R. Drospirenone: pharmacology and pharmacokinetics of a unique progestogen. *Contraception* 2000;62:29–38
103. Wahab M, Al-Azzawi F. Trimegestone: expanding therapeutic choices for the treatment of the menopause. *Expert Opin Investig Drugs* 2001;10:1737–44
104. Thorneycroft ICH. Evolution of progestins. Focus of the novel progestin drospirenone. *J Reprod Med* 2003;47(Suppl):975–80
105. Zand RSR, Jenkins DJA, Diamandis EP. Effects of natural products and nutraceuticals on steroid hormone-regulated gene expression. *Clin Chim Acta* 2001;312:213–19
106. Hillisch A. Tissue specific-drug targeting. Oral presentation to the Bregenz Summer School Endocrinology, July 27-31, 2003
107. Chen HF, Li Q, Yao X, *et al.* 3D-QSAR and docking study of the binding mode of steroids to progesterone receptor active site. *QSAR Comb Sci* 2003;22:604–13
108. Mordasini T, Curioni A, Bursi R, *et al.* The binding mode of progesterone to its receptor deduced from molecular dynamics simulations. *ChemBioChem* 2003;4:155–61
109. Elger W, Bartley J, Schneider B, *et al.* Endocrine pharmacological characterization of progesterone antagonists and progesterone receptor modulators with respect to PR-agonistic and antagonistic activity. *Steroids* 2000;65:713–23
110. Chwalisz K, Garg R, Brenner RM, *et al.* Selective progesterone receptors modulators (SPRMs): a novel therapeutic concept in endometriosis. *Ann NY Acad Sci* 2002;955:373–88
111. Saner KJ, Welter BH, Zhang F, *et al.* Cloning and expression of a novel, truncated, progesterone receptor. *Mol Cell Endocrinol* 2003;200:155–63
112. Conneely OM, Jericevic BM. Progesterone regulation of reproductive function through functionally distinct progesterone receptor isoforms. *Rev Endocr Metab Disord* 2002;3:201–9
113. Fang X, Wong S, Mitchell BF. Messenger RNA for progesterone isoforms in the late-gestation rat uterus. *Am J Physiol Endocrinol Metab* 2002; 283:E1167–72
114. Arnett-Mansfield RL, deFazio A, Wain GV, *et al.* Relative expression of progesterone receptors A and B in endometrioid cancers of the endometrium. *Cancer Res* 2001;61:4576–82
115. Larrea F, Garcia-Becerra R, Lemus AE, *et al.* A-ring reduced metabolites of 19-nor synthetic progestins as subtype selective agonists for ER alpha. *Endocrinology* 2001;142:3791–9

# 26 Future perspectives in hormone replacement therapy and menopause research

*A. R. Genazzani and M. Gambacciani*

## INTRODUCTION

The rates of osteoporosis, cardiovascular disease, dementia, and the decline of quality of life among elderly people in the next century will be greatly determined by the success of possible preventive measures. Postmenopausal estrogen deficiency is a causal or a contributing factor of different conditions and diseases that can induce a worsening of women's health and quality of life. Menopause is not a disease, and the vast majority of women do not need therapies, but some of them need hormone replacement. However, randomized clinical trials have clearly indicated that postmenopausal hormone replacement therapy (HRT) is not a remedy that can be dispensed to everyone[1,2]. The research should be aimed at different goals.

## THE MEANING OF HORMONE REPLACEMENT THERAPY

Hormones are not drugs and are not meant to cure. The administration of hormones after menopause is not a therapy for a disease. That is why the North American decision to change the wording of hormone replacement therapy to hormone therapy is misleading[3]. HRT, by definition, can only prevent and/or to some extent reverse the clinical and metabolic effects of estrogen deprivation. When a disease is already present, the role of hormones is secondary to that of other specific agents for the cardiovascular apparatus (statins, beta-blockers, etc.) or for the bone (raloxifene, bisphosphonates)[3]. Thus, focusing our attention on HRT, we need to improve our knowledge and skills in replacing the appropriate amount of hormones in suitable women at the proper time.

## PERSONALIZATION: TAILORING HRT DOSES AND COMBINATIONS

After the menopause, women are not completely estrogen-depleted. Postmenopausal women are estrogen-deficient: the extent and the clinical relevance of this deprivation and its effects on different tissues, organs and apparatuses depend on the time since menopause, type of menopause, and body weight. Different age groups, at different times since menopause, need progressively lower doses of hormones. In clinical practice, no-one prescribes a product specifically designed and studied for perimenopausal women to a population that is 30 years older[4-6]. In this way, investigations should focus on the use of different estrogen–progestin doses and combinations in the age groups and conditions specific for women usually seeking medical assistance for menopause-related problems[4-6].

## DECREASING THE CARDIOVASCULAR RISK

The choice of the correct HRT dose and the timing of treatment is relevant particularly for the effects on cardiovascular events. The early arm in the increased cardiovascular events described in the Women's Health Initiative (WHI) and Heart and Estrogen/progestin Replacement Study (HERS) seems to be related to the deferred hormone treatment and to the specific characteristics of the populations in terms of age and cardiovascular disease risk factors[1,2,5,6]. A recent analysis of four large, placebo-controlled, randomized clinical trials conducted in over 7000 postmenopausal women, aged 50–59 years, indicates that HRT is not associated with increased risk of coronary heart disease within the 1st year of treatment[7]. The aim of these trials was to evaluate the vasomotor relief and endometrial safety, in postmenopausal women aged 50–59 years treated with HRT, including conjugated equine estrogens, conjugated equine estrogens plus medroxyprogesterone acetate, conjugated equine estrogens with trimegestone, 17β-estradiol with trimegestone, or 17β-estradiol with norethisterone acetate. During the 1st year of therapy in all cohorts, no cardiovascular-related deaths occurred. One subject in the active treatment groups had a myocardial infarction (equivalent to an annual rate of 0.17 per 1000 patient-years). Two women in the placebo groups had myocardial infarctions (equivalent to 3.7 events per 1000 patient-years). The expected annualized rate of myocardial infarctions among the general population of women ages 50–59 years is 1.4 per 1000 women. The annualized rate in the study for stroke was 0.87 per 1000 patient-years among women on active agents and 0 for placebo (expected rate for the general population in this age-group is 0.8). Deep vein thrombosis occurred among the actively treated women at a rate of 1.04 per 1000 patient-years, with an expected rate of 0.76 or greater. No deep vein thrombosis was reported among placebo subjects. The increase in deep vein thrombosis with hormone therapy is consistent with previous data[8]. These findings suggest that the results of early coronary heart disease risk observed in the HERS and WHI might not be applicable to healthy, younger postmenopausal women who seek treatment for menopausal symptoms. Thus, clinicians who use HRT to treat the symptoms of menopause in healthy, early postmenopausal women should not be concerned about the risks of cardiovascular events.

It is relevant that the early arm for cardiovascular events evidenced in the HERS and WHI was not evident in statin-treated women. Thus, if women at high risk for cardiovascular events are properly treated, they can receive adequate HRT, when indicated. Future research on different schedules, route of administrations and combinations should take into account the possible concomitant use of specific cardiovascular drugs, particularly statins. The statin ability to stabilize the atherosclerotic plaques may be essential in reducing the potential harmful effect of the prothrombotic action of estrogen in women who already have atherosclerotic lesions. Further research in women treated with statins is needed to give further information on the optimal dose and combination for hormone replacement in symptomatic postmenopausal women.

In this regard, any alternative intervention to HRT must be proven to be safe and effective for specific symptoms and/or risk profiles, avoiding inappropriate enthusiasms with products of unproven efficacy and safety[9].

## THE EARLY INITIATION MODEL

Maintaining constant estrogen levels during menopausal transition, tapering the estrogen dose in the postmenopausal years and always using the minimum effective dose are the markers of a management that is opposite to that used in the HERS and WHI trials where elderly postmenopausal women were treated with the standard HRT dose even after a 10–15-year period of untreated hypoestrogenism. It is imperative to underline that we cannot treat with the same dosage and schedule women with an age varying from 50 to 79 years, with a drug that was studied and approved for the treatment of early postmenopausal women[10]. If a given dose is suitable at 50 years, it is definitely an overdose at 70–79 years.

Primarily, women seek HRT for symptomatic relief of hot flushes. The hot flushes themselves reveal the brain's susceptibility to estrogen reduction and a myriad of additional negative effects[11]. Estrogen has a positive effect on neurofunction, improving neurotransmission, neuroprotection, neurite branching synaptogenesis, cerebral blood flow and trophic factor expression[11]. Its depletion may impair memory and cognitive function and accelerate the onset of Alzheimer's disease[11]. According to the Cache County Study[12], early initiation and continuation of HRT after menopause may halt degeneration and provide some cognitive protection. Conversely, no neurocognitive protection was evident when HRT was started 10–15 years after menopause[12]. This defensive brain effect depends on the duration of treatment and how early treatment is initiated. Accordingly, the need for long-term treatment with a safe HRT combination is not contradicted by the negative WHI results, where elderly women started the treatment many years after menopause[13]. The same concept can be applied to the prevention of cardiovascular disease: starting standard HRT 10–15 years after the menopause is a nonsense in order to prevent the atherosclerotic process that is already present[6-8]. An earlier initiation can reduce the progression of the atherogenesis, a later hormone intervention can only be dangerous in term of procoagulant effects in patients with atherosclerotic plaques[6-8].

## THE ROLE OF LOWER HRT DOSES

Lower estrogen doses than the gold standard of 0.625 mg/day oral conjugated estrogens or equivalent doses of other estrogens can relieve vasomotor symptoms and prevent bone loss[14-25]. The attention of clinical researchers should focus on the efficacy of early initiation and continuation of low-dose HRT on osteoporotic fractures and other health outcomes. However, the safety of the standard higher doses used in the past as well as in the HERS and WHI should no longer vaguely refer to newer HRT schedules with lower dosages. The choice of different estrogen doses may at least in part reduce the stimulation of breast tissue, since we know that breast cancer risk can be related to the endogenous estradiol levels. Thus, it is reasonable to speculate that, by using lower estrogen doses, we can also decrease the breast stimulation while maintaining the clinical effect and the bone-sparing action of HRT. However, data on this point are missing. Long-term prospective trials will clarify the safety of lower-dose HRT, particularly in terms of breast cancer risk.

An ultra-low-dose estrogen preparation, releasing 0.014 mg/day of 17β-estradiol (Menostar™), has been presented. In a 2-year, randomized, multicenter, placebo-controlled clinical trial of 417 postmenopausal women 60–80 years old, its efficacy was reported in the prevention of postmenopausal osteoporosis (http://www.fda.gov/cder/foi/label/2004/21674_menostar_lbl.pdf). The US Food and Drug Administration (FDA) approved this once-a-week patch for marketing in the United States for osteoporosis prevention. In this study, there was no difference in the incidence of breast cancer, blood clots or cardiovascular events in the active group vs. the placebo group. A progestin is generally required for women with a uterus when they use standard, higher doses of estrogen. However, in this 2-year clinical study, the very low dose of estrogen in Menostar did not increase the risk of endometrial hyperplasia among women with a uterus. Therefore, this patch does not require a daily concomitant progestin to protect against endometrial cancer among women with an intact uterus. With this patch, women's estrogen can return to the lowest physiological level proven to prevent bone loss to date.

Menostar therapy also resulted in consistent, statistically significant suppression of bone turnover, as reflected by changes in serum and urine markers of bone formation (osteocalcin and bone-specific alkaline phosphatase) and bone resorption (carboxyterminal telopeptide of type 1 collagen (ICTP) and the urinary deoxypryridoline/creatinine ratio).

The extent of estrogen deficiency in postmenopausal women may pre-determine osteoporosis risk. Women with low-estrogen syndrome, or those with trace or undetectable estrogen levels (estradiol levels $< 5$ pg/ml), are at a 2.5 times greater relative risk for osteoporosis and debilitating bone and hip fractures compared to other postmenopausal women. In severely estrogen-depleted women, presenting endogenous estradiol levels $< 5$ pg/ml), Menostar was more effective in inducing an increase in BMD at lumbar spine and total hip sites.

## CLARIFYING THE PROTECTIVE EFFECTS OF HRT ON COLORECTAL CANCER

Gender differences in the incidence and biological history of colon cancer have been observed. In particular, more favorable colon cancer incidence and mortality trends have been reported in females compared to males. Observational studies demonstrate that current use of HRT reduces the risk for colorectal adenoma and colon cancer by 30–40 %[26]; this protection is substantially reduced when HRT is stopped, while surgical menopause doubles the risk of colorectal adenoma[26]. The protective effect of HRT on colon cancer has been confirmed by the WHI[1]. Colon cancer protection by HRT is linked to the duration of use, with higher protection in women receiving HRT for more than 5 years[26]. Thus, available data suggest a reduced risk of colorectal adenoma and colon cancer in HRT current users. The protective role of estrogens in colon carcinogenesis is still under study. Estrogen receptors have been identified in normal colon in both sexes, and decreased levels are associated with colonic tumorigenesis in the female. It has been demonstrated that the estrogen receptor (ER) gene is methylated in 90% of colon cancer tissues. Methylation of DNA is equivalent to gene silencing, with inactivation of a number of genes downstream. Methylation-associated inactivation of the ER gene in aging colon rectal mucosa could be one of the earliest events in colorectal carcinogenesis. *In vitro* estrogens reduce the ER-gene methylation and inhibit cell proliferation. Estrogens may influence microsatellite instability which occurs in approximately 10–15% of colon tumors. Moreover, estrogens have been shown to increase the expression of vitamin D receptors (VD-R) in a variety of tissues; 1,25-dihydroxyvitamin D and several of its analogs are known to be potent antineoplastic and prodifferentiative agents in several cell types, including colon-derived cells. The protective effect of estrogens against dimethylhydrazine-induced colon carcinogenesis in mice is associated with reduced methylation of the VD-R gene and with up-regulation of both VD-R gene transcription and protein expression. Therefore, increased VD-R activity may be one of the mechanisms by which estrogens protect against colon carcinogenesis. Moreover, exogenous estrogens and progestins decrease bile acid production, thus reducing its chronic irritative effect on the mucosa.

## AVOID THE EXCESS IN BREAST CANCER RISK

The real dilemma in the long-term use of HRT is the possible promotion of breast cancer. The most important data of the WHI and what prematurely terminated the study was the effect of HRT on increased risk of invasive breast cancer. Although the risk exceeded the set limit, in reality it is not statistically significant, with a lower boundary of 1.00[27]. This suggests a small increase in risk with HRT use for 5 years. Additionally, the hazard ratio for previous non-users of HRT was only 1.06; thus the increase in risk was almost entirely in the previous-user population. Notwithstanding, this is the major concern and we as clinicians must seek newer strategies to eliminate this trend. As well as the reduction of cumulative estrogen dose, the options can be different.

The overall results reveal that the estrogen–progestin combinations increased the rate of breast cancer after 5 years of use, while estrogen replacement alone had no remarkable effects. The combination of different progestins as well as the use of different routes of hormone administration may play a role in the ultimate breast effect[28]. The flaws of the Million Women Study (MWS) make this observational study unreliable to ascertain the real effect of different doses and combinations of HRT on breast cancer risk[29,30]. We need more accurate data on the critical issue of the dose effect. All the literature preceding the WHI study was even more pessimistic in terms of breast cancer risk in HRT-treated women[31-33].

## CLARIFY THE PROGESTIN ROLE

The critical issue seems to be the progestin that is added to the estrogen therapy with the sole aim of protecting the endometrium. Various progestins have different risk/benefit profiles. The impact of combined estrogen and progestin on risk of breast cancer has been controversial. Although protective effects analogous to those for endometrial cancer have been hypothesized for breast cancer, cyclical use of progestin to simulate normal menstrual cycles increases mitotic activity in the breast[34,35]. However, data on the effects of the addition of progestins to estrogens on the risk of breast cancer are conflicting. In early reports, an estrogen–progestin regimen was reported to reduce breast cancer risk[36]. Conversely, the WHI confirms the small increased breast cancer risk with combined CEE/MPA therapy, as identified in previous observational studies[7]. Conversely, in the estrogen-only arm of the WHI trial, the use of conjugated estrogens in postmenopausal women with prior hysterectomy over an average of 6.8 years was associated with an insignificant 23% reduction in breast cancer risk; this clearly requires further investigation[38]. Therefore, it is clear that our efforts should be directed to protect not only the endometrium but also the breast from the unwanted proliferation with a compound that is definitely different from medroxyprogesterone acetate. Other progestins may share the same dangerous effects on the breast, according to the MWS, but the flaws of this observational study make unreliable the ultimate results. The MWS does not give any information on the use of different progestins such as dydrogesterone, trimegestone, cyproterone acetate, natural micronized progesterone. Different progestins could have different outcomes, but the data are missing.

In relation to the use of ultra-low-dose estrogen preparations and endometrium protection, as for the Menostar experience, no significant endometrium proliferation was evident. However, it is recommended that women who have a uterus and who are treated with Menostar receive a progestin for 14 days every 6–12 months and undergo an endometrial biopsy at yearly intervals, or as clinically indicated.

## SMOKING-ASSOCIATED CANCERS AND HRT

Exogenous estrogens and progestins can protect the chronic irritative effect on the mucosae. This mechanism has been proposed for the protective effect that HRT seems to exert on smoking-associated cancers. In a population-based cohort of 29 508 Swedish women aged 25–65 years (oral cavity, pharynx, hypopharynx, esophagus, larynx, lung, bladder, and uterine cervix), the use of HRT was associated with a significantly reduced risk of smoking-associated cancers. The effect seems to be related to the time of HRT use, and is specific for smokers. In fact, in non-smokers, the rate of these tumors was not affected by the use of HRT[39]. The authors refer this promising protective effect of hormones to the possible action on degenerating mucosae for the chronic smoking-induced inflammatory processes[39]. Due to the number of women that are currently smoking, this possibility should be explored in larger prospective trials.

## NEW COMBINATIONS: THE ROLE OF SERMS

Different molecules should be studied in depth for their actions on the breast and cardiovascular system, and their specific mechanisms of actions should be elucidated. Selective estrogen receptor modulators (SERMs) are a promising family of molecules and some of these compounds have positive effects on breast cancer prevention as well as on cardiovascular risk parameters. Tamoxifene administration in the NSABP P1 trial was not associated with an increased incidence of adverse events, including endometrial cancer and venous thromboembolic events in women aged 50 or younger[40]. This observation suggests that, in the presence of adequate circulating estradiol levels, tamoxifen does not act as an estrogen agonist at these target tissues. In addition, the combination of HRT and tamoxifen does not adversely influence their biological effects on cardiovascular risk factors, bone density and clotting factors[42,43]. Altogether, these considerations provide a strong rationale for further investigations of the combination of tamoxifen and HRT in an attempt to reduce the risk, maintaining the benefits of both therapies. A large multicenter, placebo-controlled, phase III trial in postmenopausal healthy women on HRT, called the HOT Study, is currently ongoing to test whether the combination of HRT and low-dose tamoxifen (5 mg/day) retains the benefits while reducing the risks of either agent, so maintaining a high compliance rate. The addition of a SERM, such as tamoxifen, capable of reducing this growth-promoting effect on the breast could therefore be useful for women's health maintenance. However, one of the major concerns about tamoxifen is the increased risk of endometrial cancer, and thus the simultaneous progestin administration in the HRT combination is mandatory to neutralize the agonistic activity on the endometrium of both tamoxifen and estrogen. A step forward could be the use of a more 'selective' second- or third-generation SERM that is able to act as an anti-estrogen on both the endometrium and breast tissue, thus avoiding the use of progestins.

A randomized, double-blind, placebo-controlled, parallel treatment trial of raloxifene and placebo was carried out in a group of 91 postmenopausal women with at least two signs of vaginal atrophy. Patients were treated with a 17β-estradiol ring and randomized to receive concomitant raloxifene 60 mg/day or placebo for 6 months[43]. The results of this trial demonstrate that concomitant administration of raloxifene does not alter the effects of the 17β-estradiol ring on alleviating signs and symptoms of genitourinary atrophy in postmenopausal women. However, appropriate clinical trials should be performed before prescribing systemic estrogen administration in association with raloxifene.

A novel SERM (EM-652) has been reported to block the effects of estrogen administration on breast tissue and uterine weight, as well as the endometrium stimuli in castrated estrogen-replete animals[44]. Conversely, this novel SERM did not alter the cholesterol-lowering action and the bone-sparing effects of estradiol[44]. The possible use of estrogen alone in adjunction with SERMS to protect both the endometrium and the breast is currently being investigated in randomized clinical trials. These large ongoing trials should provide us in the near future with answers on the possible use of SERM as possible and safer alternatives to progestins for the long-term estrogen treatment of postmenopausal women.

## CONCLUSIONS

Menopause is a generic clinical sign, but it is not a non-specific clinical condition. Each single woman has her own menopause. It is important to treat each woman as a biologically unique patient. Thus, we have to emphasize the need for individualized treatment programs, according to personalized patient profiles. Different doses and combinations for different populations of women must be fully explored, taking into account not only efficacy but first the safety. Early intervention with personalized low-dose HRT should be explored as the first-line intervention. Combinations with specific cardiovascular drugs may offer a safe and effective strategy for the reduction of cardiovascular risk in women with specific cardiovascular risk factors. Estrogen administration in association with raloxifene warrants further studies. Long-term estrogen replacement must be explored and original combinations with new progestins and innovative SERMs will offer novel opportunities.

# References


1. Writing Group for the Women's Health Initiative Investigators. Risks and benefits of estrogen plus progestin in healthy postmenopausal women - principal results from the Women's Health Initiative randomised trial. *J Am Med Assoc* 2002; 288:321–33
2. Grady D, Herrington D, Bittner V, *et al.* Cardiovascular disease outcomes during 6.8 years of hormone therapy: Heart and Estrogen/progestin Replacement Study follow-up (HERS II). *J Am Med Assoc* 2002;288:49–57
3. Gambacciani M, Genazzani AR. The missing R. *Gynecol Endocrinol* 2003;17:91–4
4. Sociodemographic and clinical factors associated with HRT use in women attending menopause clinics in Italy. *Climacteric* 2000;3:241–7
5. Gambacciani M, Rosano GM, Monteleone P, Fini M, Genazzani AR. Clinical relevance of the HERS trial. *Lancet* 2002;360:64
6. Genazzani AR, Gambacciani M. A personal initiative for women's health: to challenge the Women's Health Initiative. *Gynecol Endocrinol* 2002;16:255–7
7. Lobo R, Pickar J. Evaluation of cardiovascular event rates with hormone therapy in healthy postmenopausal women. Presented at the *51st Annual Meeting of the American College of Obstetricians and Gynecologists*, 2003, Poster 7
8. Genazzani AR, Gambacciani M. Controversial issues in climacteric medicine. I. Cardiovascular disease and hormone replacement therapy. *Climacteric* 2000;3:233–40
9. MacLennan AH. The four harms of harmless therapies. *Climacteric* 1999;2:73–4

10. The Writing Group for the PEPI. Effects of hormone therapy on bone mineral density: results from the postmenopausal estrogen/progestin interventions (PEPI) trial. *J Am Med Assoc* 1996;276: 1389–96
11. Genazzani AR, Gambacciani M, Simoncini T, Schneider HPG. Controversial issues in climacteric medicine. III: Hormone replacement therapy in climacteric and aging brain. *Climacteric* 2003;6: 188–203
12. Zandi PP, Carlson MC, Plassman BL, *et al.* Hormone replacement therapy and incidence of Alzheimer disease in older women: The Cache County Study. *J Am Med Assoc* 2002;288:2123–9
13. Shumaker SA, Legault C, Rapp SR, *et al.* Estrogen plus progestin and the incidence of dementia and mild cognitive impairment in postmenopausal women: the Women's Health Initiative Memory Study: a randomized controlled trial. *J Am Med Assoc* 2003;289:2651–62
14. Utian WH, Shoupe D, Bachmann G, *et al.* Relief of vasomotor symptoms and vaginal atrophy with lower doses of conjugated equine oestrogens and medroxyprogesterone acetate. *Fertil Steril* 2001; 75:1065–79
15. Lindsay R, Gallagher JC, Kleerekoper M, Pickar JH. Effect of lower doses of conjugated equine estrogens with and without medroxyprogesterone acetate on bone in early postmenopausal women. *J Am Med Assoc* 2002;287:2668–76
16. Gambacciani M, Monteleone P, Genazzani AR. Low-dose hormone replacement therapy: effects on bone. *Climacteric* 2002;5:135–9
17. Ettinger B. Personal perspective on low-dosage estrogen therapy for postmenopausal women. *Menopause* 1999;6:273–6
18. Lobo RA, Whitehead MI. Is low-dose hormone replacement therapy for postmenopausal women efficacious and desirable? *Climacteric* 2001;4:110–19
19. Gambacciani M, Genazzani AR. Hormone replacement therapy: the benefits in tailoring the regimen and dose. *Maturitas* 2001;40:195–201
20. Stevenson JC, Teter P, Lees B. 17beta-estradiol (1 mg/day) continuously combined with dydrogesterone (5, 10 or 20 mg/day) increases bone mineral density in postmenopausal women. *Maturitas* 2001;38:197–203
21. Lees B, Stevenson JC. The prevention of osteoporosis using sequential low-dose hormone replacement therapy with estradiol-17 beta and dydrogesterone. *Osteoporos Int* 2001;12:251–8
22. Delmas PD, Pornel B, Felsenberg D, *et al.* A dose-ranging trial of a matrix transdermal 17β-estradiol for the prevention of bone loss in early postmenopausal women. *Bone* 1999;24:517-23
23. Genazzani AR, Gambacciani M. Hormone replacement therapy: the perspectives for the 21st century. *Maturitas* 1999;32:11–17
24. Archer DF, Dorin M, Lewis V, Schenider DL, Pickar JH. Effects of lower doses of conjugated equine estrogens and medroxyprogesterone acetate on endometrial bleeding. *Fertil Steril* 2001;75:1080–7
25. Gambacciani M, Ciaponi M, Cappagli B, *et al.* Effects of low-dose, continuous combined estradiol and norethisterone acetate on menopausal quality of life in early postmenopausal women. *Maturitas* 2003;44:157–63
26. Genazzani AR, Gadducci A, Gambacciani M. Controversial issues in climacteric medicine. II. Hormone replacement therapy and cancer. *Climacteric* 2001;4:181–93
27. Chlebowski RT, Hendrix SL, Langer RD, *et al.* Influence of estrogen plus progestin on breast cancer and mammography in healthy postmenopausal women: The Women's Health Initiative randomized trial. *J Am Med Assoc* 2003;289:3243–53
28. de Lignieres B, de Vathaire F, Fournier S, *et al.* Combined hormone replacement therapy and risk of breast cancer in a French cohort study of 3175 women. *Climacteric* 2002;5:332
29. Million Women Study Collaborators, Breast cancer and hormone-replacement therapy in the Million Women Study. *Lancet* 2003;362:419–27
30. Gambacciani M, Genazzani AR. The study with a million women (and hopefully fewer mistakes). *Gynecol Endocrinol* 2003;17:359–62
31. Collaborative Group on Hormonal Factors in Breast Cancer. Breast cancer and hormonal therapy: collaborative reanalysis of data from 51 epidemiological studies of 52 705 women with breast cancer and 108 411 women without breast cancer. *Lancet* 1997;350:1047–59
32. Schairer C, Lubin J, Troisi S, *et al.* Menopausal estrogen and estrogen-progestin replacement therapy and breast cancer risk. *J Am Med Assoc* 2000;283:485–91
33. Ross RK, Paganini-Hill A, Wan PC, Pike MC. Effect of hormonal replacement therapy on breast cancer risk: estrogen versus estrogen plus progestogen. *J Natl Cancer Inst* 2000;92:328–32
34. Pike MC, Peters RK, Cozen W, *et al.* Estrogen-progestin replacement therapy and endometrial cancer. *J Natl Cancer Inst* 1997;89:1110–16
35. Pike MC, Spicer DV, Dahnoush L, Press MF. Estrogens, progestogens, normal breast cell proliferation, and breast cancer risk. *Epidemiol Rev* 1993; 15:48–65
36. Gambrell RD Jr, Maier RC, Sanders BI. Decreased incidence of breast cancer in postmenopausal estrogen-progestogen users. *Obstet Gynecol* 1983;62: 435–43
37. Colditz GA, Rosner B, for the Nurses' Health Study Research Group. Use of estrogen plus progestin is associated with greater increase in breast cancer risk than estrogen alone. *Am J Epidemiol* 1998;147 (Suppl):64S

38. Anderson GL, Limacher M, Assaf AR, *et al.* for the Women's Health Initiative Steering Committee. Effects of conjugated equine estrogen in postmenopausal women with hysterectomy: the Women's Health Initiative randomized controlled trial. *J Am Med Assoc* 2004;291:1701–12
39. Olsson H, Bladström A, Ingvar C. Are smoking-associated cancers prevented or postponed in women using hormone replacement therapy? *Obstet Gynecol* 2003;102:565–70
40. Fisher B, Costantino JP, Wickerham DL, *et al.* Tamoxifen for prevention of breast cancer: report of the National Surgical Adjuvant Breast and Bowel Project P-1 Study. *J Natl Cancer Inst* 1998;90: 1371–88
41. Chang J, Powles TJ, Ashley SE, *et al.* The effect of tamoxifen and hormone replacement therapy on serum cholesterol, bone mineral density and coagulation factors in healthy postmenopausal women participating in a randomised, controlled tamoxifen prevention study. *Ann Oncol* 1996;7: 671–5
42. Decensi A, Robertson C, Rotmensz N, *et al.* Effect of tamoxifen and transdermal hormone replacement therapy on cardiovascular risk factors in a prevention trial. Italian Chemoprevention Group. *Br J Cancer* 1998;78:572–8
43. Pinkerton JV, Shifren JL, La Valleur J, *et al.* Influence of raloxifene on the efficacy of an estradiol-releasing ring for treating vaginal atrophy in postmenopausal women. *Menopause* 2003;10:45–52
44. Labrie F, El-Alfy M, Berger L, *et al.* The combination of a novel SERM with an estrogen protects the mammary gland and uterus in a rodent model: the future of postmenopausal women's health? *Endocrinology*

# Women's health research: current priorities, future directions

27

*V. W. Pinn*

## INTRODUCTION

Women are raising more questions and demanding more answers about their health and health care than ever before - and the scientific and health-care communities are listening. To effectively address these questions for women and their physicians, needs and strategies must be developed based upon scientifically determined knowledge, and, ultimately, the results of randomized controlled trials.

In the 1980s, public policy and grassroots activists propelled improvement in women's health by calling for dedicated women's health research[1]. In response, the National Institutes of Health (NIH) established the Office of Research on Women's Health (ORWH) in 1990[2,3]. The ORWH sets the national agenda for future directions in women's health research, increases and funds research projects on women's health and related sex/gender factors, ensures that women are appropriately represented in biomedical or behavioral research, and develops opportunities for and supports the involvement and advancement of women in biomedical careers[4].

## WOMEN'S HEALTH RESEARCH IN THE 21ST CENTURY

The last decade brought tangible progress in women's health, along with an explosion of new information fueled by the recognition of several key understandings[5].

(1) *Diseases affect women differently than men.* Women suffer from different diseases, disorders, and conditions than men and, even when they have the same diseases, women often experience different symptoms and responses to treatment than do their male counterparts[6]. Not only may physicians need to make diagnostic and treatment decisions based on the sex of the patient, but they will also need to respond to gender differences in how women and men approach their physicians, their own health, and how they communicate their health concerns[7,8].

(2) *Unacceptable disparities continue to exist among populations of women in health status, health outcomes, and in how women respond to interventions and treatments.* These disparities are the result of an array of interacting variables, including genetics, environment, access to health care, education, behavior, social milieu, and hormonal milieu[9]. Any clinical approach must consider and address these variables when considering treatments.

(3) *Translation of clinical research into practice in women's health is vital.* This becomes particularly significant when research outcomes contradict established clinical practice and the conventional wisdom that dictates standards of care[10]. The historical record in medical research is fraught with episodes where routinely accepted clinical practices were slow to change, despite unassailable evidence in support of marked improvements in patient care. When the outcomes of the estrogen-plus-progestin (E/P) postmenopausal hormone therapy arm of the Women's Health Initiative became available in 2002, definitive evidence advised that - contrary to prevailing scientific and clinical opinion - long-term E/P therapy does not reduce cardiovascular disease in postmenopausal women. Indeed, an increased risk for cardiovascular disease was demonstrated, as well as an

increased risk for breast cancer[11,12]. The Women's Health Initiative underscores a fundamental insight: research leads to workable interventions and measurable benefits to patients, provides data with which to better arm physicians for possible variations in assessment, diagnoses, and therapies, and establishes evidence-based strategies for clinical practice[13-16].

## RESEARCH PRIORITIES AND THE HEALTH OF POSTMENOPAUSAL WOMEN

The term 'women's health' does not imply simply reproductive health, but refers to the comprehensive health of body and mind across a woman's lifespan[17]. Ideally, healthy girls grow into adolescents and mature women, and eventually become healthy, productive postmenopausal and elderly women. In appreciating the connections between early life activities that are antecedents for health or disease in later life – and the role of personal behaviors and lifestyle choices in the health and aging processes of women – we can better understand the nature and import of specific health risks that women might face at every stage in their lives[18]. Studying these risks in the context of other issues and stages in women's development is essential to understanding and improving women's health in the 21st century.

We must also see that the necessary information that allows women to make informed decisions is delivered through a variety of accessible media. Women approaching menopause, in particular, tend to have many complex questions about their health[18]. They want to know the risks versus benefits of hormone therapy. They want information about alternatives to hormone therapy. They ask about early and mid-life behavior modifications that may improve their quality of life. They want to know how to relieve symptoms of menopause such as hot flushes, palpitations, and sexual changes (decreased desire, discomfort with intercourse). They also want information on prevention of cardiovascular disease, the effects on the risks of cancer (of the breast, colon, ovary), and about the role of hormones on cognitive decline and deficit and osteoporosis. With more and better answers to all these concerns, women and their physicians can better decide on optimum ways to facilitate successful aging and excellent quality of life. To answer these questions in comprehensive ways demands an ongoing commitment to basic research – and to translating the results of research into effective clinical strategies.

## FROM HORMONE REPLACEMENT THERAPY TO MENOPAUSAL HORMONE THERAPY

The climacteric is a normal aspect of women's lifespans and, as such, is not a 'disease', biological aberration, or clinical abnormality. The medicalization of menopause is rooted to some degree in the thesis that postmenopausal women are estrogen-deficient and therefore merit 'treatment' with 'replacement' hormones. In fact, reduced circulating estrogen levels reflect the normal climacteric state.

The US Food and Drug Administration (FDA) approved estrogen as a treatment for vasomotor symptoms and vulvar and vaginal atrophy associated with menopause in 1942, and peri- and postmenopausal women have, in the half-century since, turned to menopausal hormone therapy to alleviate the hot flushes and other vasomotor symptoms associated with physiological decline in estrogen production.

Over 65 million prescriptions were written for both estrogen-only and E/P oral agents in 2000. During the 1980s and 1990s, hormone treatment was increasingly prescribed 'off-label', notably for prevention of coronary heart disease on the basis of encouraging data from 1999 that suggested that menopausal hormone therapy was associated with a lowered risk of cardiovascular disease[19]. More recently, menopausal hormone therapy has also been posited as reducing the risk of dementia, stroke, depression, and urinary incontinence as well[11,20]. Almost half of all postmenopausal women in the US report having used hormone replacement therapy, usually in pill form[21].

The growing off-label use of hormone therapy to prevent coronary heart disease was based on observed and assumed sex/gender differences, animal studies, laboratory studies, and, most importantly, on observational studies. The sex difference is real, but it remains unresolved whether estrogen is the sole or even most important factor accounting for it. The animal studies cannot be assumed to apply to humans, and the laboratory studies have revealed mechanisms of harm as well as benefit. The observational studies have flaws, including an inability to capture early coronary events, as well as several biases that tend to overestimate benefit. Hence, the research thrust has moved from basic kinds of research to randomized controlled clinical trials that can provide an unbiased estimate of the true effect of hormone therapy.

Research on menopausal hormone therapy has grown exponentially. The average number of NIH-funded grants and contracts each year for menopausal hormone therapy-related studies was 11 in the fiscal year 1989–1990. Ten years later, in the fiscal year 1999–2000, the average number was 150 per year. And, while progress has been substantial, a need persists for randomized clinical trials to determine benefits and risks of long-term hormone therapy used for disease prevention[22].

## THE WOMEN'S HEALTH INITIATIVE

The Women's Health Initiative is a long-term study sponsored by the National Heart, Lung, and Blood Institute (NHLBI) of the NIH that is testing promising but unproven preventive measures for heart disease, breast and colorectal cancer, and osteoporosis[11].

Clinical consensus regarding MHT saw a fundamental shift in July 2002 when, based on events in one study arm of the WHI, E/P therapy was found to be associated with an increased risk of breast cancer, as well as a possible increased risk for cardiovascular disease, stroke, and thromboemboli[11].

The discontinued arm of the WHI had enrolled 16 608 women with an intact uterus between the ages 50 and 79 years. Study participants were randomly assigned either a daily dose of estrogen plus progestin (0.625 mg of conjugated equine estrogen plus 2.5 mg of medroxyprogesterone acetate) or a placebo. The planned duration of the study was 8.5 years[11,20].

The WHI intended to evaluate the risks and benefits of hormone therapy with regard to several designated outcomes, including breast cancer, coronary heart disease, stroke, venous thrombosis, colon cancer, endometrial cancer, and hip fractures. Limits for adverse findings were set prior to the beginning of the study. In addition, a global index was established to summarize the ongoing balance of risks vs. benefits as the study unfolded[11].

On May 31, 2002, after 5.2 years of follow-up, the Data and Safety Monitoring Board of WHI discontinued the E/P arm of the trial because the predetermined boundary for invasive breast cancer had been exceeded. The global index also supported the investigators' belief that risk outweighed benefit for study indicators, since menopausal hormone therapy also appeared to be associated with increases in the risks of coronary events, stroke, and pulmonary embolism[11]. Participants in the WHI E/P study arm experienced a 26% increase in breast cancer risk, as well as a 41% increased risk of strokes and a 29% increase in heart attacks. (There were also benefits noted, including a 37% reduction in colorectal cancer risk and 34% fewer hip fractures.)

Investigators declared that the risks of menopausal hormone therapy outweigh the benefits when taken to prevent chronic disease in postmenopausal women[23,24].

Based on these results, the US Preventive Services Task Force recommended that E/P not be initiated or continued for the primary prevention of chronic disease. Instead, to prevent coronary heart disease, the recommended focus should be on healthy diet, exercise, smoking cessation, weight control, and control of high blood pressure and high blood cholesterol. Low-dose aspirin may also help[24,25].

The WHI was not designed to address the use of estrogen plus progestin for short-term relief of menopausal symptoms. Indeed, in younger women with moderate to severe menopausal symptoms, the benefits may outweigh the small absolute risks. Nonetheless, the WHI is currently the most reliable source of data on the effects of E/P on younger women (one-third of participants were aged 50–59 years at baseline) and on women with moderate to severe symptoms (more than 2000 women). Subgroup analyses indicate that neither of these subgroups benefited from E/P. The lack of cardiovascular benefit found in WHI is consistent with that found in several other clinical trials. On average, the women in these trials were in their sixties and most trials were conducted in women with clinical disease; however, since postmortem studies show that more than half of women in their fifties already have coronary atherosclerosis, a trial in such women may well yield results similar to those found to date in older women. It may well be that prevention of cardiovascular disease needs to start in early adulthood[11]. (The NIH has also instructed participants in the estrogen-alone arm of the WHI to stop taking their study pills as of March 2004, and to begin the follow-up phase of the study. Letters have been sent to all participants in the estrogen-alone study informing them of a recent NIH study review that concludes that, with an average of nearly 7 years of follow-up completed, estrogen alone does not appear to affect – either increase or decrease – heart disease. At the same time, estrogen *alone* appears to increase the risk of stroke, and this increased risk of stroke in the estrogen-alone study is similar to that found in the WHI study of E/P when that trial was stopped in July 2002. The NIH has determined that the results would not likely change if the estrogen trial were to continue to its planned completion in 2005. Furthermore, enough data have been obtained to assess the overall risks and benefits of the use of estrogen alone in this trial[26].)

After reviewing Women's Health Initiative data, the FDA called for new labels for both estrogen and E/P preparations[27]. These products now note the increased risk for heart disease, heart attacks, strokes, and breast cancer associated with E/P. The risks found for other forms and dosages of E/P are assumed to be similar to those found in WHI unless a drug company can produce evidence to the contrary. The FDA has also modified indications for E/P combination preparations, noting that they should only be used when the benefits clearly outweigh the risks. Estrogen products are now approved for treatment of moderate to severe vasomotor symptoms associated with menopause, such as hot flushes and night sweats. The FDA also recommended its use for moderate to severe symptoms of vulvar and vaginal atrophy associated with menopause (although they advised that topical vaginal products should be considered), as well as for prevention of postmenopausal osteoporosis, but only for women with significant risk of osteoporosis that outweighs the risks of the drug, and only after alternatives have been considered. New labeling advises health-care providers to prescribe estrogen and combined E/P products at the lowest dose and for the shortest possible duration for the individual woman[27].

## LESSONS LEARNED AND FUTURE DIRECTIONS

When do women in the menopausal transition need hormone therapy? What sort of menopausal hormone therapy is best, in what dosages and by what routes of administration? Answering these questions demands an international program in translating research results to clinics and hospitals and physician offices, establishing a new standard of health-care delivery.

Some of the lessons learned from the Women's Health Initiative have major scientific and clinical implications, not the least of which is the reminder that observational or anecdotal data may not be sufficient for reliable clinical decision-making. More than 10 million women use menopausal hormone therapies[22]. To raise awareness about the recent findings on the risks and benefits of menopausal hormone therapy, the FDA has launched a nationwide information campaign[25]. In addition, the results of the Women's Health Initiative will be available for both health-care professionals and consumers in early 2006. A scientific workshop is anticipated to coincide with these announcements, bringing the full results and clinical implications of the WHI to the health-care community – and to celebrate the many women who participated in the WHI.

The Office of Research on Women's Health is co-funding, with the National Heart, Lung, and Blood Institute, and the Health Resources and Services Administration, a 5-year study by the American College of Obstetricians and Gynecologists to evaluate the changes in prescribing and practice patterns of gynecologists in the aftermath of the announcement of the results of the E/P and estrogen-only arms of the WHI. It will be interesting to determine what effect, if any, the results of the WHI and other recent research studies on menopausal hormone therapy have had on prescribing and practice patterns of gynecologists, and other physicians.

Additionally, ORWH has prepared a comprehensive report on NIH-supported research and programs on menopause (see the ORWH web site: *www4.od.nih.gov/orwh*). In September 2003, there were more than 450 current or recent menopause-related research studies funded by the NIH[22]. After the initial WHI E/P results announced 2 years ago, questions were tendered about these studies as well. Has every study using combined E/P provided a plan for review by the Data and Safety Monitoring Board to recommend continuation or discontinuation? Has each study provided a plan for Institutional Review Board review of informed consent and for contacting all study participants to inform them of new findings and implications for their study participants? Was there local compliance with these actions? The answers to these sorts of questions are vital to the ongoing success and strength of women's health research.

## A WOMEN'S HEALTH AGENDA FOR THE 21ST CENTURY

What are the directions for the future of women's health research in the 21st century? One direction is exploring some of the influences contributing to differences in genetic risk manifestations: biology, behavior, environment, and hormonal exposure. Also in the future, research needs to address basic molecular, genetic, biological and physiological properties of hormones and hormone receptors; identification of estrogen-sensitive genetic phenotypes; efficacy and risks and benefits of different formulations (for short- or long-term use), modes of administration, dosages, and when to start or stop; mechanisms and markers for adverse events/risks; and alternatives to hormone therapy in the menopausal woman[8,16].

In the future, the NIH and the ORWH will continue to sponsor research on the natural history of the menopausal transition, as well as fund quality research to understand the menopause transition and aging in women, including proven prevention strategies. A workshop on improving measures of hot flushes was held in January 2004, and in March 2005 a NIH State of the Science Conference will be held on management of menopause-related symptoms. This Conference is a collaboration of the ORWH and the National Center for Complementary and Alternative Medicine, and also enjoys trans-NIH support as well as the support of those interested in women's health from across the Department of Health and Human Services.

Research is helping us to learn about health and to become informed about risks and benefits of preventive interventions. The quest must continue. There is an urgent need for, and appreciation of, the results from current and future research, and further scientific opportunities.

# References


1. Pinn VW. Women's health research: progress and future directions. *Acad Med* 1999;74:1104–5
2. National Institutes of Health Revitalization Act of 1993 (Public Law 103–43), 107, Stat. 22 (codified at 42 U.S.C. 289.a–1), June 10, 1993, at 486 (d)(4)(D)
3. US Department of Health and Human Services, National Institutes of Health, NIH Guidelines on the Inclusion of Women and Minorities as Subjects in Clinical Research; Notice. Federal Register, 59:14508–15413 (March 28, 1994)

4. Pinn VW, Chunko, MT. NIH Office of Research on Women's Health and its DHHS partners: meeting challenges in women's health. *J Am Med Women's Assoc* 1999;54:15–19
5. US Department of Health and Human Services, Public Health Service. Women's Health: report of the Public Health Service Task Force on Women's Health Issues, Volume II. DHHS Pub. No. (PHS) 88-5026. Washington, DC: US Government Printing Office, 1987
6. Wizemann TM, Pardue M-L, eds. Institute of Medicine Committee on Understanding the Biology of Sex and Gender Differences. Exploring the biological contributions to human health: does sex matter? Washington, DC: National Academy Press, 2001
7. Doyal L. Sex, gender, and health: the need for a new approach. *Br Med J* 2001;323:1061–3
8. Gesensway D. Reasons for sex-specific and gender-specific study of health topics. *Ann Intern Med* 2001;135:935–8
9. National Institutes of Health, Office of Research on Women's Health. A report of the Task Force on the NIH Women's Health Research Agenda for the 21st Century. Vol. 1-8. NIH Pub. No. 99-4386. Bethesda, Md: NIH, 1999
10. Grunberg SM, Cefalu WT. The integral role of clinical research in clinical care. *N Engl J Med* 2003;348:1386–8
11. Rossouw JE, Anderson GL, Prentice RL, *et al.* Risks and benefits of estrogen plus progestin in healthy postmenopausal women: principal results from the Women's Health Initiative randomized controlled trial. *J Am Med Assoc* 2002;288:321–33
12. Fletcher SW, Colditz GA. Failure of estrogen plus progestin therapy for prevention. *J Am Med Assoc* 2002;288:366–8
13. Sumaya CV, Pinn, VW, Blumenthal SJ. Women's Health in the Medical School Curriculum: report of a survey and recommendations. HRSA-A-OEA-96-1. Rockville, Md: Health Resources and Services Administration, National Institutes of Health, Department of Health and Human Services, 1996
14. Silverton S, Sinkford J, Inglehart M, *et al.* Women's Health in the Dental School Curriculum. Women's Health: report of a survey and recommendations. NIH Pub. No. 99-4399. Bethesda, Md: National Institutes of Health, 1999
15. Health Resources and Services Administration, National Institutes of Health. Women's Health in the Baccalaureate Nursing School Curriculum: report of a survey and recommendations. BHPR-98-0584 (P). Rockville, Md: Health Resources and Services Administration, National Institutes of Health, 1998
16. Women's health in the next millennium. *Harv Womens Health Watch* 2000;7:4–6
17. Healy B. The Yentl syndrome. *N Engl J Med* 1991;325:274–6
18. DeAngelis DC, Winker MA. Women's health: filling the gaps. *J Am Med Assoc* 2001;285:1508–9
19. Mendelsohn M, Karas R. The protective effects of estrogen on the cardiovascular system. *N Engl J Med* 1999;340:1801–11
20. *Questions and Answers on Hormone Therapy: In Response to the Women's Health Initiative Study Results on Estrogen and Progestin Hormone Therapy.* American College of Obstetricians and Gynecologists (ACOG), available at www.acog.org
21. Brett, KM, Chong Y. *Hormone Replacement Therapy: Knowledge and Use in the United States.* Hyattsville, Maryland: National Center for Health Statistics. 2001
22. Pinn VW, Bates A. *NIH Research and Other Efforts Related to the Menopausal Transition: A Working Document*; Bethesda, MD: Department of Health and Human Services, National Institutes of Health, Office of Research on Women's Health, Nov. 2003: www4.od.nih.gov/orwh/MenopauseWorkingDoc-print.pdf
23. *NHLBI Stops Trial of Estrogen Plus Progestin Due to Increased Breast Cancer Risk, Lack of Overall Benefit.* National Heart, Lung, and Blood Institute press release available at: http://nhlbi.nih.gov/new/press/02-07-09.htm
24. Nelson HD, Humphrey LL, LeBlanc E, Miller J, Takano L, Chan BKS, Nygren P, Allan JD, Teutsch SM. *Postmenopausal Hormone Replacement Therapy for Primary Prevention of Chronic Conditions.* Summary of the Evidence for the US Preventive Services Task Force. Agency for Healthcare Research and Quality, Rockville, MD. Available at: http://www.ahrq.gov/clinic/3rduspstf/hrt/hrtsum1.htm
25. US Preventive Services Task Force. *Hormone Replacement Therapy for Primary Prevention of Chronic Conditions: Recommendations and Rationale.* October 2002. Agency for Healthcare Research and Quality, Rockville, MD. Available at: http://www.ahrq.gov/clinic/3rduspstf/hrt/hrtrr.htm
26. NIH News: *NIH Asks Participants in Women's Health Initiative Estrogen-Alone Study to Stop Study Pills, Begin Follow-up Phase.* March 2, 2004. Available at: www4.nhlbi.nih.gov/new/press/04-03-02.htm
27. *FDA Approves New Labels for Estrogen and Estrogen with Progestin Therapies for Postmenopausal Women Following Review of Women's Health Initiative Data.* US Food and Drug Administration press release available at: www.fda.gov/bbs/topics/NEWS/2003/NEW00863.html

# Natural history and progress of the menopause

28

*H. G. Burger*

## INTRODUCTION

This report summarizes the major presentations made in the first section of the 4th Workshop of The International Menopause Society and includes the contributions of Drs Naftolin, Huber, Sherman, Samsioe and Dennerstein. As each of these contributors has provided a separate manuscript, no references are given in this summary, which concludes with a position statement regarding the natural history and progress of the menopause.

## THE LACK OF DARWINIAN ADAPTATION TO THE MENOPAUSE

As a background to a consideration of the natural history of the menopause, it is noteworthy that the post-reproductive longevity of the human female is unprecedented biologically. Because the end of reproductive capacity signals the end of the possibility of Darwinian adaptation, positive adaptation to the state of estrogen deficiency may become maladaptive. Post-reproductive longevity is the result of our mastery of the environment, with public health measures and the availability of antibiotics leading to a doubling of the average lifespan. Adaptation to falling estrogen levels or estrogen deficiency occurs in several physiological circumstances, with the puerperium being a useful model. At the time when the mother makes a covenant with her newborn offspring, she must stay alive, keep the newborn alive, and develop the means of nurturing it until puberty. Corresponding activity which represents the maladaptive response to menopause includes increased arterial resistance leading to cardiovascular consequences, conservation of energy and mobilization of fat from the femoral area, bone loss as a result of calcium mobilization, and neurological consequences such as flushing and diminished sleep. In the absence of post-reproductive Darwinian adaptation, it is to be expected that some women will show their responses in the reproductive years and that changes will occur in all tissues, which may be harmful in post-reproductive life. These concepts underlie the fundamental significance of reproductive versus chronological age. Women should be treated from the beginning of their post-reproductive phase of life.

## PRIMARY AND PREMATURE OVARIAN FAILURE, POLYMORPHISMS AND CLINICAL MANAGEMENT

Premature menopause is arbitrarily defined as the permanent cessation of menstruation due to loss of ovarian follicular activity before the age of 40 years. It occurs in 1–2% of women. Its biological consequences are variable, but there is evidence for a decrease in bone density and an increase in cardiovascular morbidity and mortality, although the changes are often less than might be predicted and are highly variable between individuals. This is a result both of genetic variation and varying tissue-specific hormone production. It is clear that the ovary is not the sole source of estrogen and that other tissues have steroid synthetic capacity for estrogen production from cholesterol, e.g. adipocytes, muscle cells and endothelial cells.

## STUDIES OF THE NATURAL HISTORY AND PROGRESS OF THE MENOPAUSE

A number of longitudinal studies of the natural history of the menopausal period have been or are being conducted in various parts of the world, including the USA, Australia and Sweden. These include the Massachusetts Women's Health Study, the Study of Women Across the Nation (SWAN), the Penn Ovarian Aging Study, the Women's Health in the Lund Area Study (WHILAS) and the Melbourne Women's Midlife Health Project (MWHP). Each of these is considered in turn.

### Massachusetts Women's Health Study

This study includes approximately 2570 women, aged 45–55 years, of whom 1178 were premenopausal and had experienced menses within the 3 months prior to recruitment. The study involved six telephone interviews at 9-month intervals. From it, the onset of the menopausal transition was calculated as being at age 47.5 years, its duration 3.5 years and the age at natural menopause 51.3 years. Smokers experienced an earlier natural menopause at age 50.2 years. Hot flushes were recorded in 10% of the premenopausal group and peaked 3–9 months before final menses to a prevalence of 50%. Twenty per cent of women were still experiencing flushes 4 years postmenopausally.

### Study of Women Across the Nation

This large multi-ethnic study in the United States aimed to characterize the endocrinology and physiology of the perimenopause, looking at its biological and psychosocial antecedents, its short-term consequences, its effects on later health and on risk factors for age-related disease. It aimed to distinguish the roles of age versus menopause in the development of the chronic diseases of aging.

Approximately 450 women of varying ethnic composition were recruited at each of seven sites in the United States, the baseline age at recruitment being between 42 and 52 years. All subjects were required to have had menses within the preceding 3 months, and at recruitment 54% were premenopausal and 46% had commenced to experience cycle irregularity and were thus early perimenopausal. Blood samples were collected in the early follicular phase between days 2 and 5 of the cycle. It was noted that baseline levels of serum estradiol, testosterone, dehydroepiandrosterone sulfate (DHEAS), follicle stimulating hormone (FSH) and sex hormone binding globulin (SHBG) varied significantly by race/ethnicity. Body size as measured by body mass index was a major confounder of the observed ethnic differences in sex steroids, FSH and SHBG levels. These analytes were also influenced by other important factors such as age, menopausal status, day of cycle and smoking. A substantial fall in circulating estradiol levels commenced approximately 1 year before prospectively identified final menses and reached a nadir 2–3 years later. There was an inverse increase in levels of serum FSH starting about 3 years before final menses and reaching a peak approximately 1 year afterwards. It was concluded that body mass index had a profound influence on hormone levels and that aging during the middle years was associated with declining estradiol levels and increases in FSH. Similar patterns were seen in all five ethnic groups but, at a given age, estradiol and FSH levels varied significantly by ethnicity. Thus, in reference to the stages of the menopausal transition, there were minimal changes except for a small rise in FSH in the transition from pre- to early menopause, the greatest declines in estradiol and increases in FSH, DHEAS and testosterone occurred in moving from early to late perimenopause, and after final menses there was a continued decline in estradiol.

The prevalence of a given symptom varied markedly by ethnicity, the stage of the transition and other factors such as age, body mass index, smoking and socioeconomic status. Between pre- and early perimenopause, there was an increase in vasomotor symptoms, urine leakage and sleep problems and, from early to late perimenopause, further increases in vasomotor symptoms and sleep problems. In passing from late perimenopause to postmenopause, there were no further changes in vasomotor symptoms or sleep problems and there was some improvement in urine leakage.

Ongoing research in this study involves the search for more sensitive and specific early markers of the onset of the early transition, examination of the relationship between hormonal changes and symptoms, cognitive function, sleep and sexuality, an examination of factors influencing the severity and duration of symptoms and the role of complementary or alternative medicines. Further research also involves study of musculoskeletal and body composition changes and cardiovascular risk factors.

## Penn Ovarian Aging Study

This study recruited 218 African-American women and a similar number of Caucasian women, with an average age of 41 years, range 35–47 years. It was noted that estradiol and DHEAS levels were lower in African-American women and that testosterone increased with body mass index. The overall hot flush prevalence was 31%, but was higher in African-American women at 38% than in Caucasians at 25%. Hot flushes were predicted by higher FSH levels, by anxiety levels and by body mass index.

## The Women's Health in the Lund Area (WHILA) Study

This is a population-based cohort study of women aged 50–60 years by December 1, 1995 (*n* = 10 766). Women completed a questionnaire with 104 questions and were invited to undergo a health screen that included mammography, bone mineral density, body mass index, waist/hip ratio, blood pressure, lipid profile, blood glucose and a personal interview which allowed correction of the 19% of questionnaires in which mistakes were initially made. Additional questions were given to women with incontinence or those on hormone therapy. Those with values outside specified ranges were given secondary screening examinations, including serum lipids, glucose, oral glucose tolerance test with insulin, electrocardiogram, thyroid stimulating hormone (TSH) and leptin. The available data include details of demographics, levels of physical exercise, diet, disease, quality of life, all drug use and cardiovascular and bone risk factors. It was noteworthy that, overall, 52% of the subjects had positive screens. The aim of the study design was to correct for the effects of age so as to be able to look more specifically at the influence of menopausal status, with or without hormone therapy, on measured endpoints. It was noted that non-users of hormone therapy were more likely to consume medical resources. There was a high prevalence of impaired glucose tolerance and diabetes, and some younger women with flushes were actually found to have thyrotoxicosis. A similar study design was being followed in other countries, e.g. People's Republic of China.

## Melbourne Women's Midlife Health Project

This project aimed to document the endocrine changes of the menopausal transition, to document the extent of changes in health parameters and sexual function with reproductive aging and to determine the relative roles of hormonal, aging, lifestyle and psychosocial factors. The investigators adopted the definitions of the stages of reproductive aging agreed by a US workshop in 2001. Late reproductive stage was characterized by the absence of change in menstrual cyclicity, the early menopausal transition by a change in menstrual cycle frequency, the late menopausal transition by more than two skipped cycles or 3–11 months' amenorrhea and the postmenopause by 12 months or more of amenorrhea.

The most common symptoms of the menopausal transition included aching and stiff joints, lack of energy, hot flushes, nervous tension, trouble in sleeping and feelings of being sad and down-hearted. The only changes in symptom scores which were specifically related to the occurrence of the menopausal transition included hot flushes, dryness of the vagina, night sweats and trouble in sleeping, and a disappearance of breast soreness specifically related to the transition. The number of total symptoms increased from 6 years prior to final menses, with an initial peak at 4 years and a continuing rise to a maximum at 2 years after final menses, with a gradual decline thereafter. Hot flush prevalence was maximal at 1 and 2 years postmenopause. Even 6 years from final menses, more than 20% of women were experiencing bothersome hot flushes.

An increase in central abdominal fat was noted during the transition and was associated with baseline weight, weight increase, baseline free testosterone and increase in free testosterone.

Estradiol was the only specific predictor of change in bone mineral density. Loss of bone mineral density was dependent on the final value of estradiol and it was noted that an estradiol level of 240 pmol/l was required for preservation of bone mineral density. No other hormones or changes in hormone levels had a significant effect and body mass index, exercise and calcium did not have significant effects on bone loss during the transition.

Using the prospective cardiovascular Munster study which was a 10-year follow-up of middle-aged men, a PROCAM (Prospective Cardiovascular Munster Study) score for coronary heart disease risk was calculated from age, low density lipoprotein (LDL) cholesterol, systolic blood pressure, serum triglycerides, high density lipoprotein (HDL) cholesterol, smoking status, diabetes and a history of myocardial infarction in the family. An increased risk for cardiovascular disease according to this scoring system was associated with a higher than average body mass index, a lower than average estradiol level, a higher free testosterone index, less exercise and increasing body mass index and decreasing estradiol. Calculations did not include women using hormone therapy.

With regard to mood, it was noted that depressed mood declined significantly with age, but that the transition increased symptoms, which tend to increase depressed mood. An indirect effect was noted in that the transition amplifies the mood effects of job loss, poor health and daily hassles, making the menopausal transition a phase of vulnerability.

In terms of changes in sexual function, the change from early to late menopausal transition was associated with significant changes in a number of parameters of sexual function, including decreased feelings for partner, decreased responsivity, decreased libido, increased vaginal dyspareunia, and an increase in partner problems. No further change in partner feelings occurred in the transition from late perimenopause to postmenopause, but there was a further decline in responsivity and sexual frequency, a small further decrease in libido, an increase in dyspareunia, and an increase in partner problems.

Research in progress includes studies on osteoarthritis, bone mineral density, inflammatory markers, cognitive structure and function, and the applicability of the STRAW scoring system.

## POSITION STATEMENT ON THE NATURAL HISTORY AND PROGRESS OF THE MENOPAUSE

A variety of longitudinal studies are illuminating our understanding of the natural history of the menopause. The major hormonal changes of the perimenopausal period (fall in estradiol, rise in FSH) occur in women with 3–11 months' amenorrhea, i.e. in the late perimenopause. Hormonal concentrations vary with ethnicity.

Symptoms occur maximally during this period and in the first 1–2 postmenopausal years. Symptoms may persist for 4–6 years or longer, and include hot flushes, night sweats, urogenital atrophic symptoms and loss of mastalgia. Mood changes positively but there is a vulnerability to stress, especially among women previously experiencing premenstrual mood disorders. There is a marked decline in libido and sexual responsivity, correlated with the decline in estradiol levels.

Body composition changes with increase in visceral fat and decrease in bone mineral density. Glucose intolerance may develop, particularly in women with high body mass index. Increased cardiovascular risk is seen with higher body mass index, lower estradiol and higher free testosterone.

There are therefore several potential targets for medical intervention for prevention and treatment.

# Recommendations for hormone therapy based on the Women's Health Initiative

29

*D. F. Archer*

## INTRODUCTION

The Women's Health Initiative (WHI) results, first published in July 2002, have significantly changed the prescribing practices of many physicians[1]. These changes have principally affected women who were asymptomatic and were placed on hormone therapy with the expectation of a reduction in the risk (incidence) of cardiovascular disease. The WHI final results in 2003 did not find a statistically significant increase in the incidence of coronary heart disease[2]. The incidence of deep vein thrombosis, pulmonary emboli, and stroke was found to be increased with hormone therapy[1,2]. The implications of this study for younger, recently postmenopausal women with hot flushes, night sweats, sleep disturbances, and vaginal atrophy changes such as burning, itching, or dyspareunia, are unknown at the present time. The incidence of cardiovascular disease is low in younger women and the risk-benefit ratio would support the utilization of hormone therapy (estrogen plus progestin therapy) in younger symptomatic women who have a uterus[3].

This article reviews the guidelines proposed by the North American Menopause Society (NAMS) and the American College of Obstetricians and Gynecologists (ACOG). The NAMS position paper for 2003 is available in the journal *Menopause* and on the web site http://www.menopause.org[4]. ACOG has put forward a position paper based on a committee opinion that was accessed on 8 August 2004, at http://www.acog.org.

## THE POSITION PAPER OF THE NORTH AMERICAN MENOPAUSE SOCIETY

The NAMS position paper contains the following statements regarding the indications and use of estrogen (ET) or estrogen plus progestin therapy (EPT)[4]. These recommendations are divided into categories based on whether or not the expert panel was able to reach consensus on the topic.

### Consensus issues

(1) Treatment of moderate to severe menopause symptoms (i.e. vasomotor symptoms, sleep disruption from vasomotor symptoms) remains the primary indication for systemic ET and EPT. Every systemic ET/EPT product is government-approved for this indication.

(2) Every systemic and local ET/EPT product is government-approved for treating moderate to severe symptoms of vulvar and vaginal atrophy, such as vaginal dryness, dyspareunia, and atrophic vaginitis. When hormones are considered solely for this indication, local ET is generally recommended.

(3) The primary menopause-related indication for progestin use is endometrial protection from unopposed ET. For all women with an intact uterus who are using estrogen therapy, clinicians are advised to prescribe adequate progestin, in either a continuous combined (CC) EPT or continuous sequential (CS) EPT regimen. Women without a uterus should not be prescribed a progestin

(4) Some women with an intact uterus who choose EPT may experience undesirable side-effects from the progestin component. However, there is insufficient evidence regarding long-term endometrial safety to recommend use of long-cycle progestin (i.e. progestin every 3–6 months for 12–14 days),

a progestin-containing intrauterine device (IUD), or low-dose estrogen without progestin as an alternative to standard EPT regimens. If utilizing any of these approaches, closer surveillance of the endometrium is recommended, pending more definitive research.

(5) No EPT regimen should be used for primary or secondary prevention of coronary heart disease (CHD) or stroke.

(6) The effect of ET on CHD and stroke is not yet clear. ET does not have a significant effect on stroke risk in postmenopausal women with known ischemic cerebrovascular disease, but, for healthy older women, effects of ET on stroke risk are not clear. However, unless confirming data become available, ET should not be used for primary or secondary prevention of these conditions.

(7) Breast cancer risk is increased with ET and, to a greater extent, EPT use beyond 5 years. Progestin appears to contribute substantially to that adverse effect. EPT and, to a lesser extent, ET increase breast cell proliferation, breast pain, and mammographic density. HT may impede the diagnostic interpretation of mammograms. One recent observational study suggests that the increase in incidence of breast cancer with oral, transdermal, and implanted estrogens varies little between specific estrogens and progestins or their doses, or between continuous and sequential regimens. The observational data also suggest that breast cancer incidence may begin to increase slightly with less than 5 years of HT use. Observational data from one study suggest that HT use may be associated with increased breast cancer mortality, but insufficient data exist to determine whether ET or EPT, or duration of use of ET or EPT, is associated with any increase in mortality.

(8) There is definitive evidence for EPT efficacy in reducing risk for postmenopausal osteoporosis fracture. There is, to date, no comparable evidence for ET. Many EPT and ET products are government-approved for prevention of postmenopausal osteoporosis (i.e. loss of bone mineral density) through long-term treatment. Because of the potential risks associated with HT, for women who require drug therapy for osteoporosis risk reduction (including women at high risk of fracture in the next 5–10 years), alternatives to HT should also be considered, weighing the risks and benefits of each. Recognition should be given to the fact that there are no published data on osteoporosis drug use beyond 7 years.

(9) Initiating EPT after age 65 cannot be recommended for primary prevention of dementia as it increases the risk of dementia during the ensuing 5 years in this population. The evidence is insufficient to either support or refute the efficacy or harm of ET/EPT for primary prevention of dementia when therapy is initiated during the menopause transition or early postmenopause. However, given other adverse events that may be expected to accrue during long-term HT use, it is by no means clear that theoretical dementia benefits would outweigh known risks. HT does not appear to convey direct benefit or harm for secondary prevention (i.e. symptomatic treatment) of dementia due to Alzheimer's disease.

(10) The effects of HT on risk for breast cancer and osteoporotic fracture in symptomatic perimenopausal women have not been established in randomized clinical trials. The findings from trials in different populations (e.g. WHI) should, therefore, be extrapolated with caution. There is, however, no evidence that symptomatic women differ from asymptomatic women in cancer or bone outcomes.

(11) Data from studies such as the WHI and the Heart and Estrogen/progestin Replacement Study (HERS) should be extrapolated only with caution to women younger than 50 years of age who initiate HT. WHI and HERS involved women aged 50 and over (with mean ages of 63 and 67, respectively), and HERS was conducted solely in women with known coronary artery disease. The data should not be extrapolated to women experiencing premature menopause (< 40 years of age) and initiating HT at that time.

(12) Premature menopause and premature ovarian failure are conditions associated with earlier onset of osteoporosis and CHD, but there are no clear data as to whether ET or EPT will reduce morbidity or mortality from these conditions. The benefit-risk ratio may be more favorable for younger women.

(13) Use of ET and EPT should be limited to the shortest duration consistent with treatment goals, benefits, and risks for the individual woman, taking into account symptoms and domains (e.g. sexuality, sleep) that may have an impact on quality of life.

(14) Lower-than-standard doses of ET and EPT should be considered (i.e. daily doses of 0.3 mg conjugated estrogens tablet, 0.25–0.5 mg micronized 17β-estradiol tablet, 0.025 mg 17β-estradiol patch, or the equivalent). Many studies have demonstrated nearly equivalent vasomotor and vulvovaginal symptom relief and preservation of bone mineral density. Lower EPT doses are better tolerated and may or may not have a more positive safety profile than standard doses; however, lower doses have not been tested for outcomes (including endometrial safety) in long-term trials.

(15) Non-oral routes of administration of ET/EPT may offer advantages and disadvantages, but the long-term benefit-risk ratio has not been demonstrated. Differences would be related to the role of the first-pass hepatic effect, the hormone concentrations in the blood achieved by a given route, and the biological activity of component ingredients. There is some evidence that transdermal 17β-estradiol does not increase the level of C-reactive protein, and also that it may be associated with lower risk of deep venous thrombosis than oral estrogen. A large observational study has shown similar increased risks for breast cancer with both oral and transdermal estrogens.

(16) Extended use of ET or EPT is acceptable under the following circumstances, provided the woman is well aware of risks and there is strict clinical supervision:

(a) Extended use is acceptable for the woman for whom, in her opinion, benefits of symptom relief outweigh risks, notably after failing an attempt to withdraw HT: attempts should be made over time to reduce and cease HT. It is also acceptable for women with moderate to severe menopause symptoms who are at high risk for osteoporotic fracture: attempts should be made over time to lower the dose or cease HT and introduce alternate bone sparing therapy.

(b) Extended use of ET or EPT is also acceptable for prevention of osteoporosis in a high-risk woman when alternate therapies are not appropriate for that woman.

(c) Prior to consideration of any therapeutic regimen, including HT, all women should have a complete health evaluation, including a comprehensive history and physical examination. More specific examinations, such as bone densitometry, should be considered on a case-by-case basis.

(d) The Panel acknowledged that the absolute risks published thus far regarding ET/EPT are small (e.g. the EPT arm of the WHI), as are the benefits for bone and reduction in colon cancer risk. For women younger than 50 or those at low risk for CHD, stroke, osteoporosis, breast cancer, or colon cancer, the absolute risk or benefit from EPT is likely to be smaller than demonstrated in WHI, although the relative risk may be similar. An individual risk profile is essential for every woman contemplating any regimen of EPT or ET. Women should be informed of known risks.

## Areas of non-consensus

The panel could not reach consensus on several issues. The reasons were diverse but were principally due to lack of data, and the fact that it is difficult to individualize a patient's need from a broad recommendation.

*What are the currently acceptable definitions of short-term and long-term HT?*

The Panel could not reach a consensus regarding definitions of these terms, agreeing that delineating specific time periods is arbitrary and that no uniform time can be broadly applied to all women. The Panel recognized that this question is an attempt to assign a safe window for HT. The dilemma is that current data suggest that the risk of breast cancer is significantly increased beyond 5 years of use, with a lower elevation in risk before 5 years, whereas there is evidence of potential early CHD and thromboembolism risk within the first 2 years of use and conflicting evidence of early risk of ischemic stroke. Moreover, there are emerging data showing no association of early increase in CHD events in young (i.e. average age 53), healthy postmenopausal women with HT during the first 2 years of treatment. However, deep venous thrombosis is slightly increased from an expected annualized rate of 0.3 per 1000 to 0.9 per 1000. It is therefore difficult to define any safe window, and an individual risk-benefit profile needs to be considered for every woman considering commencement of HT.

*Is HT associated with early risk of CHD?*

Panelists were divided on the issue as to whether there is definitive evidence for early increased risk of CHD with HT. For women similar to participants in the EPT arm of WHI (average age 63 years; range from 50 to 79 years), the WHI data are the best estimate of early harm from EPT. The WHI demonstrated that EPT may increase the risk of CHD among generally healthy postmenopausal women during the first year after initiation of hormone use. There is also evidence that early harm within 2 years of use may not pertain to healthy menopausal women using ET/EPT for menopause symptom management.

*How long should HT be prescribed for symptom relief?*

No consensus could be reached, although a general guiding principle should be for the shortest time at the lowest possible dose. The Panel recognized that symptoms can recur when therapy is discontinued, independent of age and duration of HT use. Useful information regarding the consideration of reinstituting HT is anticipated from the terminated EPT arm of the WHI, as trial participants are being followed for outcomes after termination. The Panel agreed that the decision to reinstitute HT should be individualized based on severity of symptoms, current risk-benefit considerations, and the woman's preference. Reinstituting therapy at a lower dose may facilitate future attempts at discontinuing.

*Is there a best way to discontinue HT?*

Panelists were divided in their recommendations, including both abrupt therapy cessation and tapering the dose. Past history of severe symptoms may favor tapering, but no specific protocols could be recommended. Some gradually decrease the dose, while others lengthen the time between doses. Matrix transdermal HT patches can be trimmed to provide smaller doses. Current data are inadequate to suggest that one method is better than the other.

*Is it possible to make general conclusions about all members of the estrogen and progestin families?*

The majority opinion was that it is not possible to extrapolate conclusions from the study of one compound directly to another. It was acknowledged that estrogen and progesterone agonists share some common features and effects, and the only way to establish definitively the net clinical outcome for any given agent (alone or in combination) is through randomized clinical trials. In the absence of clinical trial data for each estrogen and progestin, the clinical trial results for one agent probably should be generalized to all agents within the same family, especially with regard to adverse effects.

*Does a CCEPT regimen have an effect different from a CSEPT regimen*

There are some indications that continuous progestin in the dosages administered in studies such as WHI and HERS may be related to these trials' adverse cardiovascular and breast outcomes, but conflicting data preclude a consensus.

*Does HT enhance quality of life?*

There is a lack of consensus on the impact of HT on quality of life (QOL). This has largely been due to a lack of agreement in the scientific community regarding how best to obtain an appropriate evaluation of QOL, including the domains to be incorporated into any survey instruments. There is consensus that validated instruments for determining the impact of HT, or indeed any menopause-related therapy, on QOL should be incorporated into future studies.

## THE POSITION OF THE AMERICAN COLLEGE OF OBSTETRICIANS AND GYNECOLOGISTS

The ACOG position is found as *'Response to Women's Health Initiative Study Results by The American College of Obstetricians and Gynecologists'* on their web site at http://www.acog.org, posted as of 3 June 2003.

The WHI studied only one formulation of hormone therapy (0.625 mg/day conjugated equine estrogen and 2.5 mg/day medroxyprogesterone acetate), and results are applicable only to this regimen. The ability to extrapolate results to other formulations is limited. The following recommendations are based on an ACOG expert panel review of the best currently available data. It should be noted that, for estrogen plus progestin therapy, ACOG uses the abbreviation hormone therapy (HT).

(1) The decision about use of HT requires evaluation of the risks and benefits for each individual woman. For women currently using HT, it is important to assess their reasons for use and to evaluate potential risks, benefits and alternatives.

(2) In the past, short-term use has generally been defined as use of HT for 5 years or less, most often prescribed to treat acute menopausal symptoms. There are no data from this study to establish clearly what constitutes safe short-term use. An increase in the diagnosis of invasive breast cancer appears after 4 years of use, but the influence of continuous estrogen and progestin therapy on breast cancer is unclear after even 1 year of use due to the biology of breast cancer.

(3) Women who take HT for the management of vasomotor symptoms should be encouraged to take it for as short a time as needed, and to use the lowest effective dose. Patients interested in HT for long-term use should be counseled about the risks and benefits of use, and about available alternatives. After counseling, women who want to continue taking HT for general improvement in well-being may do so provided they understand the potential risks, and should not be stigmatized for their choice. In addition, for a postmenopausal woman with a uterus, switching from an estrogen and progestin combination to unopposed estrogen is not recommended, due to the increased risk of endometrial cancer[5]. Women who choose to continue HT for quality-of-life benefits should re-evaluate the need for HT periodically. If they decide to continue, they should be encouraged to use the lowest possible dose.

(4) HT has been shown to be the most effective treatment for symptomatic relief of vasomotor symptoms including hot flushes[6].

(5) For patients who decide not to use HT, non-hormonal alternatives, such as selective serotonin reuptake inhibitors, may be helpful for this indication[7]. Other alternative agents have been proposed; however, there are conflicting data on effectiveness, and safety profiles are not established[8].

(6) Based on the WHI data, combined continuous estrogen and progestin therapy is no longer recommended for the prevention of cardiovascular disease, and, if previously prescribed for that purpose, should be discontinued. In fact, the risk of stroke and pulmonary embolism appears to increase within the first 2 years of the study. Alternatives for improved cardiovascular health, including lifestyle modifications such as exercise, smoking cessation, and weight loss, should be encouraged for all women. The use of cholesterol-lowering medications such as statins and the need for treatment of

hypertension should be evaluated for each individual patient.

(7) For patients with osteoporosis, other preventive therapies such as bisphosphonates and selective estrogen receptor modulators are available. For women at risk of osteoporosis who also have vasomotor menopausal symptoms, HT can be of benefit. In addition, a recent randomized trial found that combined HT taken with alendronate resulted in greater bone mineral density than either medication taken alone[9].

(8) For genitourinary symptoms associated with menopause, estrogen and progestin have been shown to be beneficial. Alternatives to oral delivery of estrogen, such as vaginal creams, tablets or rings, are usually effective. Although these delivery methods do not increase systemic estrogen levels appreciably, there are little data to assess the long-term safety of these alternatives.

(9) For women with a family history of colorectal cancer, the risk–benefit ratio for use of combined estrogen and progestin remains unclear. While there appears to be a benefit with hormone use, the study results do not appear sufficiently robust to recommend its use solely for the prevention of colorectal cancer. In addition, routine periodic screening such as by fecal occult blood testing, flexible sigmoidoscopy, or colonoscopy will help to prevent colorectal cancer by identifying polyps that can be removed before they become cancerous.

(10) A determination of appropriate follow-up for patients who choose HT is also important. Periodic reassessment of the need for HT is recommended at least at every annual visit or more frequently if indicated.

(11) Patients should use the lowest dose of HT that provides relief of symptoms. Some limited data suggest that the adverse effects of HT may be dose-related. In addition, patients may find fewer adverse effects with discontinuation of use on a lower dose.

(12) For women planning to discontinue use of hormone therapy, there are no definitive data to guide this process. Whether stopping abruptly or discontinuing use incrementally, some patients will develop vasomotor symptoms and will have to restart medication. Physicians should be aware that, when discontinuing HT, women may also experience vaginal bleeding, which may at times be heavy. If symptoms recur, more gradual withdrawal should be considered.

These two position statements, indicating that estrogen plus progestin should not be used for the primary prevention of coronary heart disease, are supported by the guidelines of the American Heart Association, which states that hormone therapy should not be used for the primary or secondary prevention of coronary heart disease or cardiovascular disease in women (http://www.americanheart.org).

NAMS and ACOG are consistent in their view that hormone therapy does have an indication for the specific treatment of menopausal symptoms, including vulvovaginal atrophy. Hormone therapy does have a role in the prevention of bone loss and is associated with reducing the incidence of osteoporosis and related fractures. Estrogen plus progestin therapy should not be used for primary or secondary prevention of coronary heart disease events.

Further, ACOG is unsure as to the exact relationship between estrogen plus progestin therapy and breast cancer, and for this reason recommends a duration of active hormone therapy of 5 years or less.

Numerous national organizations have developed and presented information regarding the use of HT in postmenopausal women. This information is available on the web site of each national Menopause Society. A compilation of information from national organizations may be found at http://www.gfmer.ch/Guidelines/Menopause_osteoporosis/Menopause_osteoporosis_mt.htm.

# References


1. Rossouw JE, Anderson GL, Prentice RL, *et al.* Risks and benefits of estrogen plus progestin in healthy postmenopausal women: principal results from the Women's Health Initiative randomized controlled trial. *J Am Med Assoc* 2002;288:321–33
2. Manson JE, Hsia J, Johnson KC, *et al.* Estrogen plus progestin and the risk of coronary heart disease. *N Engl J Med* 2003;349:523–34
3. Naftolin F, Taylor HS, Karas R, *et al.* The Women's Health Initiative could not have detected cardioprotective effects of starting hormone therapy during the menopausal transition. *Fertil Steril* 2004;81:1498–501
4. Estrogen and progestogen use in peri- and postmenopausal women: September 2003 position statement of The North American Menopause Society. *Menopause* 2003;10:497–506
5. Effects of hormone replacement therapy on endometrial histology in postmenopausal women. The Postmenopausal Estrogen/Progestin Interventions (PEPI) Trial. The Writing Group for the PEPI Trial. *J Am Med Assoc* 1996;275:370–5
6. Blake JM, Collins JA, Reid RL, *et al.* The SOGC statement on the WHI report on estrogen and progestin use in postmenopausal women. *J Obstet Gynaecol Can* 2002;24:783–90, 793–802
7. Loprinzi CL, Barton DL, Rhodes D. Management of hot flashes in breast-cancer survivors. *Lancet Oncol* 2001;2:199–204
8. ACOG Practice Bulletin. Clinical Management Guidelines for Obstetrician-Gynecologists. Use of botanicals for management of menopausal symptoms. *Obstet Gynecol* 2001;97(Suppl):1–11
9. Greenspan SL, Resnick NM, Parker RA. Combination therapy with hormone replacement and alendronate for prevention of bone loss in elderly women: a randomized controlled trial. *J Am Med Assoc* 2003;289:2525–33

# What hormone preparations will be available?

30

*H. Kuhl*

The results of the Women's Health Initiative (WHI) study gave rise to a requirement to restrict the use of hormone replacement therapy (HRT) or to recommend alternatives to estrogen/ progestin combinations. Recent re-evaluations of the WHI data revealed, however, that the main adverse effects, i.e. the elevated risk of coronary heart disease and breast cancer, were based on selection bias. The overall hazard ratio (HR) of 1.24 for coronary heart disease was no longer significant, and, for the group of women who were within 10 years of menopause, it was not increased (HR 0.89), suggesting that an early initiation of HRT during the perimenopause may be protective.

The increased breast cancer risk which was observed only in women who had already been pretreated with hormones prior to the initiation of the WHI study was not based on a higher rate of diagnoses during HRT, but on an extremely low rate in the placebo group, which was significantly lower than in never-users.

Despite this, it is generally accepted that long-term use of HRT is associated with an increased relative risk of breast cancer. This refers mainly to the use of estrogen/progestin combinations, while the effect of estrogen-only therapy is considerably less. The increase in risk is obviously associated with an enhanced proliferative effect, which is more pronounced with estrogen/progestin combinations than with estrogen-only preparations.

There are no convincing data suggesting a difference between the various types and doses of estrogens with regard to the breast cancer risk. This might be explained by the dose-dependent elevation of the incidence of breast cancer already at very low serum levels of estradiol. There are also no convincing data with regard to a difference between the various progestins.

One of the consequences of the WHI study was the general demand for individualization of hormone replacement therapy. According to the specific needs of the patient, the physician has to choose that preparation which is suitable for the prevention or treatment of individual symptoms or disease on the basis of a careful risk-benefit evaluation. The aim of future efforts should be the development of targeted drugs, particularly for women with specific risks and specific indications.

The available spectrum of preparations is large. They differ in the type and dose of the estrogen and progestin, the regimen and route of administration.

Concerning the estrogens, which are the logical measure for the treatment of symptoms caused by an estrogen deficiency, estradiol is preferred as the natural estrogen for the human, which has a defined chemical structure. In contrast, conjugated estrogens are a mixture of many compounds with different hormonal activities. The role of these compounds, relating to the composite effect of the preparation on various tissues, is not clarified. The oral administration of conjugated estrogens has a stronger impact on the production of hepatic proteins, e.g. serum binding globulins, lipoproteins, hemostasis parameters, than that of estradiol, while the transdermal, intranasal or vaginal application of estradiol has only a weak effect on hepatic metabolism. The transdermal use of estradiol, which has a low impact on hemostasis, probably does not increase the risk of venous thromboembolic disease. Estriol is a weak estrogen which has specific advantages and disadvantages, while ethinylestradiol has a pronounced action on hepatic parameters.

The various progestins differ in their hormonal pattern and may consequently modulate the effects of estrogens in a different manner. They may exert androgenic, antiandrogenic, glucocorticoid or antimineralocorticoid actions. Progestins with androgenic activity have a favorable effect on hemostasis and do not counteract the beneficial effect of estrogens on the arterial wall. Progestins with glucocorticoid activity may upregulate the thrombin receptor and, hence, the thrombin-induced production of tissue factor in the arterial wall. This may contribute to the elevation of the risk of cardiovascular disease in patients with arterial lesions.

The $7\alpha$-methyl-derivative of the progestin prodrug norethynodrel, tibolone, is also a prodrug that, after oral administration, is rapidly converted in the liver to $7\alpha$-methyl-norethisterone ($\Delta$-4-isomer), which is a weak progestin with a strong androgenic activity, to the potent estrogen $7\alpha$-methyl-ethinylestradiol and to two 3-hydroxytibolone metabolites with weak estrogenic activities. Tibolone is an effective alternative to estrogen/progestin preparations for the treatment of climacteric symptoms and the prevention of osteoporosis. In the Million Women Study, treatment with tibolone was associated with an increase in breast cancer risk by 45%, which was in the range of that of estrogen/progestin preparations. Whether this was due to a preferential prescription to women with high-risk factors for breast cancer remains to be proven by appropriate epidemiological studies.

The only indication for the addition of a progestin to an estrogen therapy is the protection against estrogen-induced endometrial hyperplasia. As the use of progestins contributes to the development of various adverse effects and risks, strategies may be developed which reduce or avoid systemic progestogenic effects. The bone is one of the most sensitive estrogen target organs. Therefore, ultra-low-dosed estrogens may be useful in older postmenopausal women without vasomotor symptoms. It remains to be proven whether the long-term use of this estrogen preparation without additional progestin is not associated with an increased rate of endometrial hyperplasia. Transdermal therapy with daily 14 $\mu$g estradiol caused an estradiol serum level of below 10 pg/ml, which prevented bone loss, caused a slight proliferation of the vaginal epithelium, but did not stimulate endometrial proliferation.

Small levonorgestrel-releasing intrauterine systems may be useful for a local protection against estrogen-induced endometrial hyperplasia. Whether the impact on metabolism of low serum levels of levonorgestrel (120 pg/ml) is of clinical relevance remains to be elucidated.

The menopausal transition is a challenge to develop new drugs which enable the individualization of hormone therapy. The best pharmacotherapy is that which addresses individual symptoms, the disposition and risk factors of the woman and her preferences concerning the therapeutic regimen. Further research on the molecular actions of estrogens and progestins is necessary to understand the mechanisms and pathophysiology of climacteric symptoms. This will provide us with the tools to develop the so-called selective estrogen receptor modulators (SERMs) and selective progesterone receptor modulators (SPRMs) that are possibly approaching the idea of an 'ideal drug'.

The available SERMs (e.g. tamoxifen, raloxifene, toremifene) are useful for the prevention of osteoporosis and their use is associated with a reduced breast cancer risk. In contrast to raloxifene, tamoxifen increases the risk of endometrial cancer. The effect of SERMs on coronary heart disease remains to be clarified, while they increase, similar to estrogens, venous thromboembolic disease. SERMs are not useful to treat vasomotor symptoms in postmenopausal women, but can even cause hot flushes in asymptomatic patients. There are no data on the effect of SERMs on cognition and Alzheimer's disease. The development of SERMs with all favorable effects of estradiol but without the risk of adverse events is rather impossible, but may extend the options for special preventive or therapeutic goals. Because of the many estrogenic compounds contained in conjugated estrogens, they may serve as a source for the development of SERMs.

The development of SPRMs that inhibit the estrogen-induced proliferation of the endometrium and breast tissue, but not the desired effects of estrogens, will be the primary aim of future research. Until such therapeutic options are available, those preparations which are now on the market must be used in an optimal manner. As both beneficial and adverse effects of estrogens and progestins are, to a large extent, dose-dependent, preparations containing lower estrogen doses and the minimal effective dose of the progestin must be developed.

# Guidelines for the hormone treatment of women in the menopausal transition and beyond

31

*Position Statement by the Executive Committee of the International Menopause Society*

Recent communications regarding estrogen or estrogen + progestin treatment and clinical cardioprotection, breast cancer risk and cerebral aging have produced considerable confusion and concerns among women, care-givers and the media. The actions of the United States' Food and Drug Administration (FDA) and other National Safety of Medicine Boards, such as the European Medicine Evaluation Agency (EMEA), in response to publication of data from the Women's Health Initiative (WHI)[1–3] and the Million Women Study (MWS)[4], have also raised concerns. The Executive Committee of the International Menopause Society (IMS) has considered position statements presented at the Fourth Workshop of the IMS, December 2003 and reviewed available information from observational studies, randomized controlled trials (RCTs) and pre-clinical research, and wishes to point out the following:

• *Nomenclature* Administration of hormones to symptomatic, estrogen-deficient women such as those in the observational studies is referred to as hormone replacement therapy (HRT). Administration of hormones to asymptomatic women such as those in the recent RCTs is referred to as hormone therapy (HT)[5]. In general, the administration of hormones to menopausal women is referred to as menopausal hormone treatment (MHT).

• The WHI is the most recent of several RCTs undertaken to test the validity of the cardioprotective effects of HRT shown by observational trials. Others include the Heart and Estrogen/progestin Replacement Study (HERS) and the Estrogen Replacement and Atherosclerosis Study (ERAS), which utilized the same hormonal regimen, and which had the common underlying premise that the study of women beginning HT well beyond the menopausal transition is an acceptable design for this purpose. This statement also addresses the ability of these HT RCTs to reveal effects of HRT. Because of the potential for breast cancer induction by HRT, the MWS[4], a recent prospective cohort analysis, was also included in our considerations. Guidelines are suggested for clinical practice regarding HRT for women going forward from the menopausal transition.

• The WHI is an ongoing RCT on the effects of HT in women aged from 50 to 79 years. Few of these women were in the critical first years after menopause. The full results of the trial will not be available for some time. At the end of the 5th year, the independent drug safety monitoring board (DSMB) terminated the estrogen + progestin arm of the study because of an apparent increase in the risk of breast cancer and an apparent adverse global index. The factors included in the index, in addition to an increased risk of breast cancer, were coronary heart disease, stroke and pulmonary embolism. *A subsequent analysis by the WHI of the full 5-year period has already shown that there was not a statistically significant increase in breast cancer and the apparent increase in the cardiovascular hazard, new breast cancer incidence and thromboembolic event frequency risk in year five had occurred because of a transient fall in the rates of these events/diagnoses in the* placebo group, *rather than a rise in the estrogen + progestin group*[1]. In any case, the lack of statistically significant differences between groups after the full duration of the WHI trial makes conclusions regarding the value of HT highly uncertain and devalues or invalidates the conclusions from the initial publication from which so many clinical implications have been drawn.

• The estrogen-only arm in post-hysterectomy women was stopped in the 7th year by the National Institutes of Health (NIH) (not the DSMB). The decision was based upon lack of proven cardioprotection and higher incidence of stroke, as in the estrogen + progestin arm. In contradistinction to the estrogen + progestin arm, the women taking only estrogen had a 23% lower incidence of new invasive breast cancers than did the placebo group ($p < 0.06$)[6].

• The general applicability of the results of RCTs such as the WHI's estrogen + progestin- and estrogen-only arms, the HERS[7] and ERAS[8] trials has been reviewed. *The WHI's publication indicated that, by design, symptomatic women were limited to ~10% of the study population*[9]. *The HERS and ERAS trials, by design, excluded younger women. The average ages of women in the WHI, HERS and ERAS trials were 63, 67 and 65 years, respectively*[1,6,7,9]. *Results in such populations cannot, and should not, be generalized to women who are unlike those tested (i.e. younger women early in menopause).* Women in the estrogen + progestin arm had a mean age of 63.3 years and were, on average, 12 years postmenopausal (13 years since their last period). The women in the estrogen-only arm were the same age on average, but the length of time since hysterectomy (± ovariectomy) is not known. They had somewhat higher indices of heart disease and predisposing factors at the outset, perhaps reflecting the longer period of diminished estrogen[10]. Few (~10%) of these women were in the critical first few years after menopause[11].

• The MWS is an observational study of UK women volunteering for a national breast-screening program. It reported that all types of HT regimens induce an increase in breast cancer risk, *starting from the 1st year of use*. In addition, the risk disappears from 1 to 5 years after the withdrawal of HT. The appearance of significant risk in the 1st year strongly suggests that the surplus of breast cancers arose from observational bias and was not induced by the hormones[4,12].

• In considering apparent differences between the cardioprotective outcomes of the observational studies that inspired the present RCTs and the 'negative' findings of the recent RCTs, the Executive Committee has identified crucial differences between the experimental populations in the two different types of studies, which tend to be neglected during minute consideration of the outcomes. *In the observational studies, the hormones were prescribed for women in the menopausal transition, most of whom were symptomatic, and who were generally 55 years of age or less at the time of starting treatment. On the contrary, in the three RCTs, the HT was started at 55 years or older in 89% of the subjects*[6,9,11]. Overall, the women in the observational trials were mainly patients in the menopausal transition who sought help for symptomatic hormone deficiency, while the women in the RCTs were, by design, recruited subjects who were largely past the point of being symptomatic, *indicating an altered physiological status that could be related to differences in outcomes. All in all, the age and condition of its subjects do not support contentions that the WHI is a primary prevention trial against cardiovascular outcomes or that it is testing HRT, as was the case in the observational studies.* Rather, the WHI is a RCT on the effects of one particular regimen of combined daily, as opposed to cyclic, estrogen + progestin or estrogen-only HT on aging women, many of whom will have had sub-clinical vascular and cardiovascular disease at the time they entered the trial[10,13]. This is a major difference between the observational studies that showed a cardioprotective effect of HRT and the RCTs that failed to show cardioprotection by HT.

• A power analysis of the WHI estrogen + progestin arm showed that it was ten-fold underpowered to detect an early-estrogen cardioprotective effect of the magnitude reported by the observational Nurses Health Study[11,14]. There was therefore no likelihood that this arm of the WHI could be sufficiently powered to reveal a statistically significant difference between treatment and placebo in women starting treatment during the menopausal transition[11]. (Nevertheless, analysis of such women who started estrogen-only between the ages of 50 and 59 years suggested a different effect with three *fewer* cases of CHD and only one extra case of venous thromboembolism and 0.1 of stroke/10 000 women[6].)

• As is standard practice for the application of the outcomes of RCTs, the results of the WHI may not be generalized to populations that it was not designed to study. This exclusion of comparisons extends to the results of observational trials in women in the menopausal transition who were symptomatic at the initiation of HRT. *Therefore, at present, the only valid studies of MHT for cardioprotection of women in the menopausal transition are the epidemiological and observational studies that generally agree with laboratory and animal studies, indicating cardioprotection by estrogen initiated in women during the menopausal transition.*

*The possibility that contemporary MHT causes an increase in breast cancer is not clarified by either the WHI or the MWS and remains to be resolved*[1–3,6].

*In summary: The HT RCTs reported to date cannot indicate whether contemporary estrogen or estrogen + progestin treatment started during the normal or induced menopausal transition (HRT; the great majority of its use) is effective for primary prevention of cardiovascular disease or other long-term consequences of sex steroid withdrawal.*

**With the above in mind, the Committee proposes the following guidelines for addressing these issues for women during the climacteric.**

I. Available **HT** RCTs do not have the statistical power to test the outcomes of MHT starting during the menopausal transition. *In the absence of new, relevant information on **HRT** started in the menopausal transition (the positive data from the younger women in the estrogen-only arm of the WHI notwithstanding), the Executive Committee recommends the continuation of presently accepted global practice, including the use of estrogen + progestin, or estrogen alone in the case of women who have undergone hysterectomy, for the relief of menopausal and urogenital symptoms, avoidance of bone-wasting and fractures, and atrophy of connective tissue and epithelia.* Possible clinical benefits in the prevention of cardiovascular disease and nervous system protection seem likely but have yet to be confirmed.

II. *There are no new reasons to place mandatory limitations on the length of treatment, including arbitrary cessation of **HRT** in women who started replacement during the menopausal transition and remain symptom-free while on hormones.* Judging from the accelerated rate of cardiovascular events after premature menopause[15,16] and the loss of cardioprotection after stopping MHT[14], such cessation may even be harmful. The conflicting data from the WHI on breast cancer incidence do not clarify this area of concern.

III. *Each patient must be counseled about the current data on the risks and perceived benefits of **HRT** so that she can make appropriate, informed, individual decisions about continuing or stopping treatment.* Such discussions could be part of the annual risk–benefit analysis undertaken with each patient and in the context of timely mammographic and other screening protocols.

IV. *The risk of complications of **HT** remains an important clinical issue; there are no general guidelines that apply, except to indicate that **HT**, both estrogen + progestin and estrogen-alone, has been associated with a small absolute increase in deep venous thrombosis with derivative stroke and pulmonary embolism. The WHI continues the trend of conflicting effects on breast cancer (a small absolute increase in the estrogen + progestin arm and decreased risk in the estrogen-only arm) and reduction in the risk of colorectal cancer and bone fractures, including hip fractures*[1,3,6,10]. These issues remain subjects for discussions between individual patients and their care-givers. None of these generalities should preclude regular testing of the involved systems, regardless of the decision whether or not to begin or continue **HT**. *However, cancer, metabolic diseases, vascular disease and brain dystrophy are not only the concerns of women on **HT**, but are of universal concern to women past the age of reproduction.*

V. The use of hormones/hormone substitutes as part of the care of the aging population will be a subject of increasing importance in both sexes. Governing principles for enhancing the length and quality of life are emerging:

(a) *Prevention, not treatment, is the most feasible goal.* Use of hormone/substitutes should be part of an overall strategy including life-style modification and other preventive measures, especially cessation of smoking and alcohol abuse[17].

(b) *There is no evidence that **HT** is beneficial for existing heart disease or dementia, but the initiation of **HRT** during the menopausal transition appears to provide protection against complications of the climacteric such as fractures and potentially heart disease and brain disease*[18-20]. This conclusion remains based on observational studies and pre-clinical research[21], since no RCTs have adequately addressed women starting treatment during the menopausal transition.

(c) *Appropriate and effective doses should be established for each of the systems to be treated/protected.* The dose and regimen of **HRT** need to be individualized. Older menopausal and postmenopausal women generally require lower doses than younger women.

(d) *The effect of the route of administration remains an issue.* Avoidance of the first-pass effects of oral therapy may be advantageous, especially for those with increased risk factors for venous thrombosis. More long-term data are required on the clinical outcomes of non-oral routes of administration.

(e) The different types and regimens of **HRT** do not necessarily have the same tissue and metabolic effects and should not be grouped together as having a class effect. Ideally, good-quality data should have been obtained for each hormonal preparation, but, since this is not feasible, not having such data does not imply that information on other products could be automatically extrapolated.

(f) *Progesterone/progestins are only required for protection of the endometrium.* This benefit has to be balanced against effects on other tissues and metabolic effects. Direct genital delivery systems may have some advantages. The role of progesterone and progestins and the different routes of administration remain issues for study.

(g) Combinations of hormones with other treatment regimens may be of benefit.

(h) *Evidence from population studies cannot be directly generalized to individual patients.* However, such evidence can be used as general guidance in clinical decision-making, in which case the emphasis should be on absolute rather than relative risk.

*There is a great body of important pre-clinical experimental evidence that bears on these matters.* Clinical research, both observational studies and RCTs, should be encouraged to improve clinical practice. *The quality of experimental design is still a key factor in the evaluation and applicability of even the largest RCT*[12]. In this regard, the Executive Committee of the IMS supports the immediate release of the full database from the estrogen + progestin arm of the WHI and the MWS database for independent review.

*The IMS particularly supports the expansion of research into the effects of hormones on the vascular, musculoskeletal and nervous systems, as well as the role of hormones and hormone-like compounds in carcinogenesis and prevention.* We are facing a tide of post-reproductive women and men. *In addition to prevention by changes in life-style and dietary management, HRT remains a principal tool in preventing illness and maintaining quality of life* in this population; therefore, it must be the subject of continuing scientific investigation.

February 13, 2004, revised August 28, 2004

The Writing Group of the IMS Executive Committee – F. Naftolin, H. P. G. Schneider, D. W. Sturdee

With contributions from the other members of the Executive Committee – M. Birkhäuser, M. P. Brincat, M. Gambacciani, A. R. Genazzani *(Ex officio)*, K. K. Limpaphayom, S. O'Neill, S. Palacios, A. Pines, N. Siseles, D. Tan

The original IMS Position Statement is published in *Climacteric* 2004;7:8–11.

# References


1. Rossouw JE, Anderson GL, Prentice RL, *et al.* Risks and benefits of estrogen plus progestin in healthy postmenopausal women: principal results from the Women's Health Initiative randomized controlled trial. *J Am Med Assoc* 2002;288:321–33
2. Manson JE, Hsia J, Johnson KC, *et al.* Estrogen plus progestin and the risk of coronary heart disease. *N Engl J Med* 2003;349:523–34
3. Chlebowski RT, Hendrix SL, Langer RD, *et al.* Influence of estrogen plus progestin on breast cancer and mammography in healthy postmenopausal women. The Women's Health Initiative Randomized Trial. *J Am Med Assoc* 2003;289: 3243–53
4. Million Women Study Collaborators. Breast cancer and hormone replacement therapy in the Million Women Study. *Lancet* 2003;362:419–27
5. Sturdee DW, MacLennan A. HT or HRT, that is the question? *Climacteric* 2003;6:1
6. The Women's Health Initiative Steering Committee. Effects of conjugated equine estrogen in postmenopausal women with hysterectomy: The Women's Health Initiative randomized controlled trial. *J Am Med Assoc* 2004;291:1701–12
7. Hulley S, Grady D, Bush T, *et al.* Randomized trial of estrogen plus progestin for secondary prevention of coronary disease in postmenopausal women. *J Am Med Assoc* 1998;280:605–13
8. Herrington DM, Reboussin DR, Brosnihan KB, *et al.* Effects of estrogen replacement on the progression of coronary artery atherosclerosis. *N Engl J Med* 2000;343:522–9
9. Hays J, Ockene JK, Brunner RL, *et al.* Effects of estrogen plus progestin on health-related quality of life. *N Engl J Med* 2003;348:1839–54
10. Gambacciani M, Genazzani AR. The missing R. *Gynecol Endocrinol* 2003;17:91–4
11. Naftolin F, Taylor HS, Karas R. Early initiation of hormone therapy and clinical cardioprotection: the Women's Health Initiative (WHI) could not have detected cardioprotective effects of starting hormone therapy during the menopausal transition. *Fertil Steril* 2004;81:1498–1501
12. Shapiro S. Effects of HRT on the risks of breast cancer and cardiovascular disease: the validity of the epidemiological evidence. In Schneider HPG, Naftolin F, eds. *Climacteric Medicine - Where Do We Go?* Proceedings of the 4th Workshop of the International Menopause Society. London, New York: Parthenon Publishing, 2004:166–74
13. Karas RH, Clarkson TB. Considerations in interpreting the cardiovascular effects of hormone replacement therapy observed in the WHI: timing is everything. *Menopausal Med* 2003;10:8–12
14. Grodstein F, Manson JE, Colditz GA, Willett WC, Speizer FE, Stampfer MJ. A prospective, observational study of postmenopausal hormone therapy and primary prevention of cardiovascular disease. *Ann Intern Med* 2000;133:933–41
15. Grodstein F, Stampfer MJ, Colditz GA, *et al.* Postmenopausal hormone treatment and mortality. *N Engl J Med* 1997;336:1769–75
16. Joakimsen O, Bønaa KH, Stensland-Bugge E, Jacobsen BK. Population-based study of age at menopause and ultrasound assessed carotid atherosclerosis. *J Clin Epidemiol* 2000;53:525–30
17. Hu FB, Stampfer MJ, Manson JE, *et al.* Trends in the incidence of coronary heart disease and changes in diet and lifestyle in women. *N Engl J Med* 2000;343:530–7
18. Mack WJ, Hameed AB, Xiang M, *et al.* Does elevated body mass modify the influence of postmenopausal estrogen replacement on atherosclerosis progression: results from the estrogen in the prevention of atherosclerosis trial. *Atherosclerosis* 2003;168:91–8
19. Tang MX, Jacobs D, Stern Y, *et al.* Effect of oestrogen during menopause on risk and age at onset of Alzheimer's disease. *Lancet* 1996;348:429–32
20. Zandi PP, Carlson MC, Plassman BL, *et al.* Hormone replacement therapy and incidence of Alzheimer disease in older women: the Cache County Study. *J Am Med Assoc* 2002; 88:2123–9
21. Adams MR, Kaplan JR, Manuck SB, *et al.* Inhibition of coronary atherosclerosis by 17β-estradiol in ovariectomized monkeys: lack of an effect of added progesterone. *Arteriosclerosis* 1990;10;1051–7


Note: Further detailed information and guidelines will be found in *The Health Plan for the Adult Woman: Management Handbook*, to be published on behalf of the IMS by Parthenon Publishing, UK.

# Index